# THE NEUROSCIENCE OF AUTISM

# THE NEUROSCIENCE OF AUTISM

*Edited by*

Rajesh K. Kana

ELSEVIER

ACADEMIC PRESS

An imprint of Elsevier

Academic Press is an imprint of Elsevier
125 London Wall, London EC2Y 5AS, United Kingdom
525 B Street, Suite 1650, San Diego, CA 92101, United States
50 Hampshire Street, 5th Floor, Cambridge, MA 02139, United States
The Boulevard, Langford Lane, Kidlington, Oxford OX5 1GB, United Kingdom



ISBN 978-0-12-816393-1

For information on all Academic Press publications
visit our website at https://www.elsevier.com/books-and-journals

*Publisher:* Nikki P. Levy
*Acquisitions Editor:* Joslyn Chaiprasert-Paguio
*Editorial Project Manager:* Barbara Makinster
*Production Project Manager:* Swapna Srinivasan
*Cover Designer:* Matthew Limbert

Typeset by STRAIVE, India

# Dedication

To my wife Bhumika, my children Advitiya and Naanya, and my parents Karunakaran and Saudamini, for their unconditional love and support.

# Contents

## 4. Social, cognitive, perceptual, and other models of autism spectrum disorder

Meagan E. Beckerson, Kaitlyn E. May, and Rajesh K. Kana



## 5. The neuroanatomy of autism

Charlotte M. Pretzsch and Christine Ecker



## 6. Brain function and brain connectivity in autism

Julie A. Trapani, Haley M. Bednarz, and Rajesh K. Kana



## 7. White matter microstructure in autism

Michael Connaughton, Erik O'Hanlon, and Jane McGrath

# Contributors

**Irene Antony** Department of Developmental Biology, Washington University School of Medicine, Saint Louis, MO, United States

**Meagan E. Beckerson** Department of Psychology, The Center for Innovative Research in Autism, University of Alabama, Tuscaloosa, AL, United States

**Haley M. Bednarz** Department of Neuropsychology, Children's Healthcare of Atlanta & Emory University School of Medicine, Atlanta, GA, United States

**Elizabeth L. Berg** Department of Psychiatry and Behavioral Sciences, MIND Institute, University of California Davis School of Medicine, Sacramento, CA, United States

**Neill Adams Broderick** Departments of Pediatrics and Psychology, Vanderbilt University Medical Center; Vanderbilt Kennedy Center/Treatment and Research Institute for Autism Spectrum Disorders, Nashville, TN, United States

**Gareth Chapman** Department of Developmental Biology, Washington University School of Medicine, Saint Louis, MO, United States

**Michael Connaughton** Psychiatry, Trinity College, Dublin, Ireland

**Christine Ecker** Department of Forensic and Neurodevelopmental Sciences, Institute of Psychiatry, Psychology and Neuroscience, King's College London, London, United Kingdom; Department of Child and Adolescent Psychiatry, University Hospital, Goethe University, Frankfurt am Main, Germany

**Rachel Elman** Department of Developmental Biology, Washington University School of Medicine, Saint Louis, MO, United States

**Nicole R. Friedman** Center for Youth Development and Intervention and Department of Psychology, University of Alabama, Tuscaloosa, AL, United States

**Joshua Golt** Department of Psychology, The Center for Innovative Research in Autism, University of Alabama, Tuscaloosa, AL, United States

**Caitlin M. Hudac** Center for Youth Development and Intervention and Department of Psychology, University of Alabama, Tuscaloosa, AL; Department of Psychology, University of South Carolina, Columbia, SC, United States

**Rachel J. Hundley** Vanderbilt Kennedy Center/Treatment and Research Institute for Autism Spectrum Disorders; Departments of Pediatrics, Psychology, and Psychiatry, Vanderbilt University Medical Center, Nashville, TN, United States

**Rajesh K. Kana** Department of Psychology, The Center for Innovative Research in Autism, University of Alabama, Tuscaloosa, AL, United States

**Erin Kang** Psychology Department, Montclair State University, Montclair, NJ, United States

**Kristen L. Kroll** Department of Developmental Biology, Washington University School of Medicine, Saint Louis, MO, United States

**Kaitlyn E. May** Department of Educational Studies in Psychology, Research Methodologies, and Counseling, University of Alabama, Tuscaloosa, AL, United States

**Rachel G. McDonald** Psychology Department, Montclair State University, Montclair, NJ, United States

**Jane McGrath** Psychiatry, Trinity College; Consultant Child and Adolescent Psychiatrist, ADMiRE, Linn Dara CAMHS, Health Service Executive, Dublin, Ireland

**Mishka Narasimhan** Department of Developmental Biology, Washington University School of Medicine, Saint Louis, MO, United States

**Erik O'Hanlon** Psychiatry, Trinity College, Dublin, Ireland

**Charlotte M. Pretzsch** Department of Forensic and Neurodevelopmental Sciences, Institute of Psychiatry, Psychology and Neuroscience, King's College London, London, United Kingdom

**Renata Shen** Department of Developmental Biology, Washington University School of Medicine, Saint Louis, MO, United States

**Jill L. Silverman** Department of Psychiatry and Behavioral Sciences, MIND Institute, University of California Davis School of Medicine, Sacramento, CA, United States

**Julie A. Trapani** Department of Neuropsychology, Children's Healthcare of Atlanta & Emory University School of Medicine, Atlanta, GA, United States

**Tychele N. Turner** Department of Genetics, Washington University School of Medicine, St. Louis, MO, United States

**Susan W. White** Department of Psychology, The University of Alabama, Tuscaloosa, AL, United States

**Diane L. Williams** The Pennsylvania State University, University Park, PA, United States

# Foreword

This volume on *The Neuroscience of Autism* edited by Rajesh Kana represents the remarkable progress of the past 25 years in understanding the nature of autism, largely in terms of its biological basis. What was once a mysterious and enigmatic condition has now become a particular psychological and biological state with its own known characteristics. This accumulation of knowledge about autism has come about because of a concerted national and international effort to apply the most powerful of contemporary scientific methods to the understanding of autism. The volume describes the new understanding in terms of the various facets of autism, such as developmental and genetic perspectives.

The volume is composed of chapters contributed by some of the leading researchers in their subspecialties within autism. The reason that there are separate chapters on topics such as genetics, white matter, and brain connectivity is that brain function and autism, like any complex system, can be described at different levels of molarity. White matter, the myelin-coated bundles of axons of neurons constituting about 45% of the volume of the human brain, provides the communication infrastructure that enables the multiple regions of the brain to coordinate with each other in the execution of all forms of thinking. At the same time, it is the exquisite programming of the genomic code that enables the axons from one set of neurons to find their path to another set of neurons during fetal development. So both levels of description are necessary to begin to understand why at the age of 6–9 months there are clearly detectable alterations in the white matter of children who will ultimately be diagnosed with autism. So too at the behavioral level is it necessary to understand not only the diagnosis of autism but also the subsequent interventions. The necessity for multiple levels of description explains why there are 12 different chapters in this book written by different authors. The multiplicity of levels of description is just a reflection of the nature of nature: it is inherently multilaminar.

The motivation for this volume arose from the editor's need for a text for the autism course that he regularly teaches. This strongly resonates with my own needs for the autism course that I teach. The chapters would provide an excellent introduction for advanced undergraduates and graduate students to the various scientific approaches to understanding autism. In addition, the collection will serve as resource for anyone with a scientific perspective, including families affected by autism as well as clinicians and educators.

The chapters collectively depict a complex neural systems-level disorder, each chapter contributing a meaningful component of the entire depiction. For example, the chapters on neuroanatomy, brain connectivity, and white matter each present some of the central findings from their research approach to understanding brain structure and function. A thread that winds through several of the chapters and is centrally focused in one of them addresses the lifespan nature of autism development, from fetal stages to adulthood and aging. Other chapters deal with some of the pragmatics of dealing with autism. This state-of-the-art collection presents autism from its many possible scientific perspectives that readers will find interesting and useful, transforming an enigma into a complex but understandable puzzle whose shape is gradually coming into view. It is a view not to be missed.

*Marcel Just*
*D.O. Hebb University Professor of Psychology, Carnegie Mellon University, Pittsburgh, PA, United States*

# Introduction to the neuroscience of autism

Several years ago, when I was a graduate student, I would visit a special education school as part of collecting data for my PhD dissertation. During my very first visit to this autism center, I noticed a young boy, Jay, about 16–17 years old, standing at the other end of the hallway. When he spotted me from distance, he started asking "Can I laugh now?" As I got closer, he would repeat this question several times accompanied by his own answer "yes, you can." In other words, this was an oft-repeated question-answer routine "Can I laugh now? Yes, you can." This was my first visit to the center, and I was completely baffled and struggled to understand the intent of this conversation and to appropriately respond to his question. Later that day, I would learn two important lessons: First, my responses were likely not expected in Jay's question-answer routine. In fact, the purpose of it seemed something completely different. Second, my conversations with his parents later on revealed a story behind this routine. As a child, Jay had a habit of laughing out loudly at everything other people would say. Of course, this led to many uncomfortable situations and awkward conversations. To remedy this, Jay's parents told him that it is not polite to laugh at everything people say. Instead, if you feel like laughing in the middle of a conversation, you may ask others' permission. He captured this advice like a sponge and began using these lines often in his interpersonal interactions, mainly with an intent to initiate conversations. It is likely that his attempt at initiating a conversation would fall short of following the linguistic maxims of interpersonal communication. In addition, perhaps his attempt at conversation with me would have resulted in less successful social interaction more often than not. Nevertheless, this interaction attests the nature of social communication in autism spectrum disorder (ASD) and at the same time highlights the need for understanding it better. This first experience of meeting someone with ASD was interesting, and certainly intriguing. It also taught me about the layers of complexity inherent to autism: what you see at the surface of autism may be very different from what is beneath. And a better understanding of autism may need a closer and deeper look and an active engagement in opening a series of boxes within boxes to discover the precious gift lying inside the tiniest of boxes.

I have been actively engaged in autism research for more than two decades. Why think about writing a book now? The seeds of it were sown when I was teaching an undergraduate course focusing on the cognitive and neurobiological bases of ASD. This course was structured cyclically, from the obvious to the unknown, and back to the obvious. This class began with what we first notice when we see a person with autism, or for that matter anyone: their behavior. We thus started with behavioral characteristics of people with autism, examining the cognitive, neuropsychological, and neurobiological mechanisms underlying behavioral differences. We then turned to the process of changing some of the behaviors, encouraging desired behaviors and mitigating undesired or harmful behaviors. As I was teaching this course, I realized that there is no one book on autism out there, at least in my knowledge, that traverses this path and covers these topic areas exclusively. As the course heavily relied on scientific papers, the need for a book on the neuroscience of autism was also expressed constantly by my students over the years. Although the book is titled *The Neuroscience of Autism*, it tries to follow the above-mentioned structure and tries to cover the A to Z of ASD. Perhaps what makes it even more attractive is that the book is stitched together with contributions from a collection of some of the world's most renowned autism researchers! The primary aim is to provide students, researchers, professionals, and public with fundamental knowledge of the history, definition, diagnosis, and cognitive and neurobiological make-up of autism, as well as training and intervention strategies available for helping autistic individuals in their overall functioning. While a detailed summary of each chapter of the book is not needed at this stage, in the following paragraphs, I provide an overview of what to expect from each chapter.

Conceptualization of autism as a disorder as well as the public perception of autism has gone through massive changes over several decades of research. In Chapter 1, Golt and Kana examine the historical evolution of the definition and diagnosis of autism, starting from the consideration of autism as a symptom of schizophrenia to the current classification of autism according to the fifth edition of *Diagnostic and Statistical Manual of Mental Disorders* (DSM-V). From Leo Kanner's and Hans Asperger's first scientific publications in 1943 and 1944, respectively, this chapter reveals the timeline of the major historical events in the study of ASD. While understanding the historical changes in the definition of a disorder like autism is important for researchers, it is also equally important for families and professionals to learn and appreciate the changes in how autism has been perceived over the past 8–9 decades.

As Chapter 1 outlines the historical timeline of the conceptualization of autism, in Chapter 2, Williams provides an overview of the current definition, prevalence, and behavioral symptoms of autism. The diagnostic criteria for ASD are persistent deficits in social communication and interaction as well as restricted and repetitive behaviors that interfere with daily functioning. In the most recent definition and classification of autism, the severity of ASD is differentiated by the level of support required.

Milder forms of ASD may be regarded as a matter of neurodiversity rather than a disorder. While it is important to define a disorder clearly with measurable criteria, what is also equally important is applying it to the real world and identifying autism as early in life as possible.

In Chapter 3, Hundley and Broderick provide a comprehensive account of the methods and procedures involved in early identification and diagnosis of autism. Although autism can be diagnosed by 2 years of age, in the real world, the diagnosis is usually delayed several years. In this process, families lose a significant amount of valuable time in beginning treatment and intervention. Thus, early identification is absolutely critical not only in easing the stress of families but also in targeting early brain developmental stages through intervention. This chapter also takes a detailed look at the screening tests and procedures available for identifying autism early and also describes the gold standards of autism diagnosis, the autism diagnostic observation schedule (ADOS), and the autism diagnostic interview (ADI).

Chapters 1–3 entail the behavioral and diagnostic features of autism and the historical evolution of the definition of the disorder. Chapter 4 by Beckerson, May, and Kana takes a step back to understand the social, cognitive, and perceptual mechanisms that may underlie the behavioral features. Prominent theoretical models of autism are explored in detail, such as theory-of-mind deficit, executive dysfunction, complex information processing difficulty, weak central coherence, enhanced perceptual functioning, temporal binding, social motivation, extreme male brain, Bayesian priors, and multisensory integration difficulty. The chapter emphasizes the role of these theoretical models in understanding the behavioral characteristics of autism.

From behavior to cognitive and social level explanations, the book takes another step deeper to explore the neurobiological mechanisms underlying cognitive and behavioral features of autism. In Chapter 5, Ecker and Pretzsch focus on neuroanatomical differences in autism that emerge during infancy and persist into adulthood. By examining structural neuroimaging studies and postmortem brain studies, these authors provide a comprehensive overview of brain morphology and its developmental trajectory in autism. The chapter also alludes to the growing recognition of neuroanatomical variability across the autism spectrum and the current research efforts directed at parsing this heterogeneity to help improve our understanding of disease mechanisms.

While neuroanatomical differences are an important index of the organizational differences of the brain in autism, it may also determine functional and connectional differences. Chapter 6, by Trapani, Bednarz, and Kana, examines the insights gained from neuroimaging studies that have illuminated brain activity and functional connectivity differences in individuals with autism. In recent years, neuroimaging research has largely shifted to examining the brain at a *network* level. Functional connectivity research has lent way to the disrupted connectivity hypothesis, which postulates that autism is a distributed disorder marked by inefficiencies in the synchronization of brain activity. This line of research has, of late, led to efforts in identifying reliable and firm neural markers for autism. The pursuit of sensitive and accessible biomarkers remains at the forefront of research efforts, and disruptions in functional connectivity are emerging as a potential future tool for assessing risk, classifying symptom presentation, and determining treatment response and prognostic status. It is likely that functional connectivity differences may be one of the characteristic features of the complex neurobiology of autism. However, such differences may underlie differences or disruptions in anatomical connectivity or the organization of white matter. In Chapter 7, Connaughton, O'Hanlon, and McGrath focus on a relatively new and innovative neuroimaging technique, diffusion-weighted imaging, to understand the white matter connectivity in autism. Diffusion-weighted imaging relies on water diffusion in the brain, the anisotropy of which may indicate insights into the micro- and macrostructural organization of white matter. This chapter also provides a detailed review of some of the sophisticated analytical techniques in diffusion imaging, along with examining the developmental trajectory of white matter in autism and the influence of age and sex in white matter development.

Chapters 5–7 focus on investigating the neurobiology of autism with emphasis on structure, function, and white matter connectivity. Chapters 8–10 take us deeper to unearth cellular, molecular, and genetic mechanisms underlying autism. In Chapter 8, Silverman and colleagues embark on a journey to analyze the valuable insights gained from research using animal models in autism. Since the diagnosis of autism is based solely on behavioral criteria, modeling autism-relevant behaviors in animals is critical for studying the disorder's etiology and evaluating the efficacy of candidate therapeutics. While various animal models have been used in autism research, the most commonly used are rodent models due to their rich social and cognitive behavioral repertoire and to the ease with which targeted genetic mutations can be made. Thus, Chapter 8 is a comprehensive summary of the utility of animal models and that line of research in understanding autism. Despite evidence of a strong biological basis for autism, finding a single gene or a cluster of genes solely responsible for ASD has been challenging. Perhaps, this reflects the distributed and highly complex nature of the disorder. In Chapter 9, Hudac, Friedman, and Turner provide an overview of historical and modern approaches for understanding genetic causes of autism, thought to account for around 10%–30% of ASD. Innovations in modern genome and exome approaches and targeted sequencing within recent decades have implicated more than 100 genes and genomic regions in autism. The chapter showcases recent advances from a genetics-first approach to characterize unique phenotypes of genetic subgroups in autism. The chapter also describes future directions of autism genetics, including the growing consensus of polygenic risk, relevance of noncoding regions, and rare inherited variants.

In Chapter 10, Kroll, Chapman, Narasimhan, Antony, Shen, and Elman examine the cellular and molecular neurobiological mechanisms underlying autism. While many genetic risk factors are currently associated with ASD, no single mutation accounts for more than a minor fraction of cases. Understanding how these mutations contribute to ASD etiology has proven challenging, due both to the inaccessibility of the developing human brain and to limitations of animal models, which diverge from humans both genetically and in multiple aspects of brain development. In recent years, human pluripotent stem cell (hPSC) models have been used to recapitulate aspects of human neurodevelopment and study how these are affected in ASD. In the chapter, the authors describe common genetic liabilities associated with ASD, approaches used to model these in stem cells, and a range of cellular and molecular phenotypes previously observed in stem cell models of ASD. The work highlights the potential for stem cell-derived models of ASD to define contributors to clinical phenotypes and to suggest potential avenues for intervention in affected individuals.

Beginning with behavioral characteristics and historical changes in the definition of autism, this book has attempts to understand the cognitive, neurobiological, and genetic differences that may underlie autism. In the last chapter, Chapter 11, Kang, White, and McDonald take us back to where we started: How can the insights gained from various forms of research be used to improve the behavioral difficulties in individuals with autism? The chapter provides an overview of the literature examining evidence-based interventions for individuals with ASD. The authors examine a wide range of treatment options and intervention approaches with empirical support, including several psychosocial interventions (e.g., early intensive behavioral interventions, cognitive-behavioral and mindfulness-based approaches, and social skills interventions). The chapter also discusses pharmacological and biological interventions as well as emerging approaches that are less supported but promising. The review concludes with challenges the field now faces and implications for future research and clinical practice.

One of the main goals of this book is to provide readers with a comprehensive understanding of ASD at behavioral, cognitive, social, neurobiological, and genetic levels. An additional goal is to provide readers the opportunity to understand and appreciate the massive amount of scientific research that has illuminated the field of autism during the past 80 years or so. As mentioned earlier, the book is designed as a journey from behavior to cognition, to brain, to genetics, and then back to modifying behavior.

The expectation is that the book will appeal to researchers, undergraduate and graduate students, professionals working in the field of autism, parents of children with autism, and the lay public.

The scientific research on ASD that spans the past eight decades has been rich and diverse and has produced significant insights on the behavioral, neuropsychological, and biological aspects of this disorder. As the book attempts to uncover the wealth of knowledge gained from a large body of work, it is important to assess the value of insights gained and also consider future directions. The prevalence estimates reported by the Centers for Disease Control and Prevention (CDC) over the years have been providing indications of a steady increase in the number of cases of autism diagnosis. This may largely be due to the massively increased awareness of the disorder, refinement in the criteria for autism diagnosis, and agencies more actively monitoring potential cases of autism (e.g., pediatricians' offices in the United States nowadays ask families to complete an autism screening form, usually the Checklist for Autism in Toddlers, during their child's first visit. Thus, the chances of a child with some symptoms of autism to be referred for additional screening and/or diagnosis are significantly more now than that perhaps years ago). Many chapters in the book examine the causal factors underlying autism, from genetic, neurobiological, and cognitive perspectives. While a firm answer to such questions is still somewhat elusive, the role of fundamental biological differences cannot be ignored. While there are a large number of genes implicated in autism, perhaps attesting to the complexity of the disorder, it is also worth considering environmental factors, if any, that may be contributing to altered patterns of gene expression and/or brain development. Understanding the etiology of autism more clearly has implications in terms of early identification and diagnosis, and in targeting brain plasticity in the early years through treatment and intervention. Through different chapters of the book, we also discuss various methods of scientific research in autism. It should be noted that there is an added value of integrating multiple layers and levels of inferences gained from these methodological approaches. For example, a specific profile of white matter tract organization or brain activity pattern can be used to predict the efficacy of a given behavioral intervention method on an individual participant; or the machine learning techniques can be used to learn attributes and features of a dataset to classify the participants into groups or subgroups. It is also encouraging to see that more and more studies are addressing neurodiversity, subgroups of autism, sex differences at mechanistic level and in the manifestation of the disorder, and consideration and participation of stakeholders and advocacy groups in the conceptualization, design, and implementation of research studies. Such attempts help reducing the gap between science and society in general, which is vital in studying neurodevelopmental disorders like autism. As future directions, more studies are needed to address the widespread heterogeneity in autism, more longitudinal studies are needed to address the dynamic developmental changes at behavioral and neurobiological levels and to address transition to adulthood, higher education, employment, and aging in autism, and more novel and innovative clinical trial studies are needed to test treatment effectiveness. One of the most promising signs is the significant increase in the number of collaborative and integrative nature of autism research studies, of late. Such efforts have been, and continue to be, influential in beginning reciprocal conversations and collaborations across laboratories, clinic, and community. Indeed, the hope is that these are explicitly and implicitly contributing to reducing the gap between basic research and applied research, the fruits of which can be highly promising for individuals, families, and professionals involved in education and care of people with ASD. With the massive technological revolution and its applications to scientific research, the next few decades will be vital in refining our understanding of autism and in bridging the gaps across laboratory, clinic, and community.

*Rajesh K. Kana*
*Department of Psychology, and The Center for Innovative Research in Autism, The University of Alabama, Tuscaloosa, AL, United States*

CHAPTER

# 1

# History of autism

*Joshua Golt and Rajesh K. Kana*

**Department of Psychology, The Center for Innovative Research in Autism, University of Alabama, Tuscaloosa, AL, United States**

The term "autism" was coined by the German psychiatrist Eugen Bleuler in 1908 to describe some of the symptoms (e.g., being withdrawn or aloof and oblivious to the surroundings) of patients with schizophrenia. The word autism comes from the Greek word "autos" referring to self, which may encapsulate the increased focus on oneself, often observed in children and adults with autism. In 1943, Leo Kanner (a psychiatrist at the Johns Hopkins University), in the first official publication of a collection of case studies on autism, documented the symptoms of autism as "autistic disturbances of affective contact." Since then, the conceptualization of autism as a disorder has gone through many levels of revisions. In this chapter, we attempt to examine the history and evolution of the definition and characterization of autism over last several decades and the impact of it on how the disorder is perceived by families and professionals.

## Early accounts and descriptions of autism

Donald T was a 5-year-old child, in a series of case studies, first seen by Dr. Leo Kanner in 1938, who was then a psychiatrist at the Johns Hopkins Hospital. Donald is also referred to as Case 1.[1] Donald's parents brought him to Dr. Kanner after being hospitalized 2 years prior. He presented different than other children, uniquely different according to Kanner. Donald refused to feed himself, he had behavioral problem, and his parents were told they overstimulated him and he needed to be removed from the home. At the age of 18, Donald would encounter Franz Polgar, a Hungarian hypnotist who was intrigued by Donald. Donald was distant, but he had perfect pitch recognition, naming any tone played on the piano, and he could calculate complicated multiplication problems, instantly, in his head.[2] At the time, someone like Donald was so misunderstood that Polgar asked


https://doi.org/10.1016/B978-0-12-816393-1.00002-6

Donald's parents if he could travel with him as a part of his performances, which his parents declined. As described in many accounts of Kanner's early work, his evaluation of Donald would shortly lead him to describe Donald as autistic. This makes Donald the first to be diagnosed as autistic, initiating an entirely new diagnosis, field of research, and a new way of describing thousands of people around the world.

In a world in which Donald was Case 1, providers did not yet have a grasp on what it meant to have autism, no less how to help. Donald was institutionalized at age 3. His parents were told they overstimulated him, and this caused his behavioral problems. The solution was to remove him from his home to a place that was not made for him, nor understood him. Donald was described as often sitting motionless and disengaged from everything.[2] Later that year, Donald's parents removed him, and the physicians attributed his behavior to a glandular disease. Following his departure from the hospital in which he seemed to receive no help, Donald's parents made him an appointment with one of the top psychiatrists in the United States, Dr. Leo Kanner and the Johns Hopkins Hospital. Interestingly, Donald's father had sent an incredibly detailed 33-page document outlining all of Donald's symptoms to Dr. Kanner prior to their arrival. This document is now considered one of the first listings of autism symptoms.

Kanner's observations of Donald baffled him and his first diagnostic query, schizophrenia. There was no diagnosis to fully capture a child like Donald, but over time, Kanner would make the case for something new. Donald continued to be observed by Kanner for 4 years during which he continued to assess children who had similar behavioral characteristics. Donald and eight other children would soon be known as autistic. Prior to Kanner, autism was considered as a symptom of schizophrenia. Specifically, it was used to describe an individual being withdrawn from social contact, but following his work with those nine children, autism would soon change the field of behavioral sciences and the lives of many like Donald.

Characterization and descriptions of autism spectrum disorder (ASD) have evolved since the 1940s to today. Currently, ASD is described as a pervasive developmental disorder consisting of deficits in social communication and interaction, as well as the presence of restricted, repetitive behaviors and interests.[3] The first descriptions of autism began to emerge in the early 1940s with Kanner's publication titled "Autistic Disturbances of Affective Contact."[1] Kanner described a group of 11 children as lacking the predisposition to be social, and described autism as being a combination of social impairment and a resistance to change, which could be considered today as rigidity.[4] He first described these symptoms as childhood schizophrenia until he coined the term, infantile autism. Additionally, Kanner noted that several of the children he studied did not speak. While that was not a criterion in his work, this foreshadowed what would become a significant factor in modern autism diagnoses. Two things Kanner seems to have emphasized in his account of autism are: (1) the primary difficulty in autistic children is in emotionally relating to others (disturbance in affective contact); and (2) a fundamental biological disturbance may underlie the behavioral symptoms seen in autistic children. It is important to note that these two observations are at the core of autism even in its present characterization.

Unknowingly, but almost simultaneously, Hans Asperger, an Austrian pediatrician, was making observations of his patients in Vienna and developing his theory of autistic individuals.[5] He named many of the same characteristics as that of Kanner, with Asperger's definition of autism including social isolation, lack of social reciprocity, motor clumsiness, abnormal but above average language skills, highly-specific interests, and significantly better performance in certain cognitive domains.[6] This cluster of symptoms would later be named after Hans Asperger himself in a clinical characterization done by Lorna Wing, an English Psychiatrist, in 1981.[7] Asperger's description of autism included many positive aspects of an individual. At the time, Asperger's description of autism focused heavily on the idea that autism could be an extreme variant of male intelligence, and dedicated some of his time to strategizing how these children, with such remarkable intelligence, could be taught.[8] Asperger himself referred to his patients as "little professors." He felt as though the children he was working with had extremely high intelligence and understood the nuances of advanced knowledge at the same time having some pronounced difficulties in social, emotional, and interpersonal domains.

Asperger and Kanner included criteria in their descriptions of the differences in the way individuals with autism thought, not necessarily problems in their ability to think. Both physicians made this distinction with the purpose of distinguishing autistic individuals from individuals with intellectual disabilities, or what would have been considered at the time, mentally retarded.[9] In the 1940s, there was significant stigma surrounding individuals with intellectual disabilities, and it was important to both Kanner and Asperger to not mislead people into believing that autistic individuals inherently had intellectual difficulties. Additionally, as mentioned earlier, Kanner made a note that there were fundamental biological differences (genetic and/or neurobiological differences) in an autistic child, compared to neurotypical peers. This insight into the etiology of autism was incredibly impressive given the knowledge, resources and limited technological advancement at that time.

While it seems, Hans Asperger was potentially focused on what might be considered as more positive traits of autism, Kanner's perspective on the development of autistic traits may have created a divide in their descriptions of autism. So much so, that at the time Kanner and Asperger felt as though they were describing different children. Kanner's description of autism was heavily focused on disturbances in typical social interactions, whereas Asperger put a greater emphasis on autistic traits that would have been described as talents rather than deficits. Asperger himself referenced Kanner's original article describing autism and made sure to distinguish the children he was describing from Kanner's.[10]

Interestingly, while Kanner and Asperger's accounts were written approximately during the same time period, Asperger's writings were not recognized by the rest of the world until much later. In the 1980s, Lorna Wing wrote a description of Asperger's syndrome using his original descriptions written in German[5] which became the first modern account of Asperger's Syndrome. Shortly after, Asperger's work was translated to English and began being used by scientists and clinicians. Asperger's description of autistic individuals was used to describe a set of children who lacked social reciprocity and used precocious language.[7] At this time, Wing was the first person to characterize that the individuals described by Kanner and the individuals described by Asperger were likely both part of the same autism spectrum. While Wing described them on the same spectrum, the idea that these were distinct client presentations persisted until recently.

Later, Kanner wrote about the origins of autism and his hypothesis of refrigerator mothers.[11] Kanner believed that the etiology of autism lied in a lack of warmth and empathy in the child's environment. This lack of warmth could contribute to a child's lack of social reciprocity and a desire to maintain sameness. Kanner's description of an emotionless parenting style contributing to autism became popularized in, "The Empty Fortress," a book written by Bruno Bettelheim in 1967 that set out to explain the origins of autism. Bettelheim gave the term "refrigerator mother" to emotionless parenting and popularized it as a theory. The Refrigerator mother hypothesis created a stigma around an autism diagnosis and would later be refuted by new etiological theories developed by Dr. Bernard Rimland, an American research psychologist.

A much needed departure from psychoanalytic explanations, the neurobiological models of autism were first described in Rimland's book titled "Infantile Autism: the syndrome and its implications for a neural theory of behavior."[12] His book, published in 1964, would influence how researchers, providers, and the public viewed autism.[13] Rimland brought the focus from an environmental perspective (nonemotional parenting) to a focus on individual biology and differences in brain development. Rimland's motivation for changing the way the world saw and interacted with autistic people was close to home as his son was diagnosed with autism, and Rimland was told that it was because his child's mother was too distant. Rimland then used science to refute and disprove this theory entirely. In addition to Rimland's work in dismantling refrigerator mother hypotheses, Rimland created the first diagnostic checklist for autism, the E-2 Checklist,[14] increasing the scientific rigor surrounding autism research and diagnoses. Lastly, Rimland is credited with large advocacy and policy changes in respect to autism. Rimland spent much of his life advocating for individuals with autism and creating foundations to support autism research and intervention. Later in his career there was a shift in Rimland's adherence to scientific evidence and he began advocating for the idea that mercury in vaccines contributed to the development of autism,[15] a hypothesis that has been overwhelmingly disproven. While toward the end of his career, many professionals disagreed with Rimland's assertions, he is still credited with groundbreaking changes in the conceptualization of autism, especially the neurobiological origins of the disorder.

Kanner and Asperger are most popularly credited with identifying and conceptualizing autism and beginning to form hypotheses on the etiology of autism. Over time, many have added to the definition of autism and change its criteria. As research has grown, so has the understanding of autism and the factors that influence autism. As reports of autism related symptoms and difficulties became more apparent, autism began to be included in diagnostic classification of disorders and training manuals. Since the beginning, a key component of autism descriptions has been the idea that while there is heterogeneity among the individuals with Early Infantile Autism, there were key characteristics that formulated that same diagnosis. Kanner writes in 1944, "Among the individual patients, there are great variations in the degree of the disturbance, in the manifestation of specific features, and in the step-by-step development in the course of time. Yet, despite this seeming divergence, they all present essential common characteristics to such an extent that they cannot but be considered as fundamentally alike from the point of view of psychopathology." From the beginning, there was a clear understanding that autism presents differently across individuals and therefore existed in a spectrum, a term that would later be included in the formal diagnosis of autism. Throughout the development of autism as a diagnosis, both Kanner and Asperger have demonstrated valuable insights and understanding into the qualities and characteristics of an autism diagnosis.

## Autism in the DSM

The way autism is described has changed over time and throughout its history, it had had different meanings. While always representing the same core symptoms, autism has changed names, and changed the focus of impairment. In 2013, Verhoeff proposed three phases of the history of autism.[16] **Phase 1,** encompassing the year 1943–65, starts with Kanner's description of autism as aloneness and insistence on sameness. Kanner's descriptions at this time focused on a life-long impairment of any affective engagement with others and the repetitive behaviors that accompanied the social withdrawal. Verhoeff describes **Phase 2** of autism, lasting between the year 1960 and 1980, to be rooted in language and other perceptual and cognitive abnormalities. Research studies that followed Kanner's description of autism provided empirical evidence supporting several claims that Kanner made in his case studies. This first longitudinal study of autism was published and it demonstrated that the desire to withdrawal improved with age, but other autistic symptoms persisted into adulthood[17] giving credibility to the diagnosis. Additionally, Verhoeff describes the emergence of language focused research during this time. Studies demonstrated the difficulty in understanding both verbal and nonverbal language, in addition to deficits in processing different sensory stimuli. During this time, much of what Kanner described persisted, but there was not an empirical base for it. Social deficits were not coupled with language delays, and they would present this way in the first diagnostic criteria of autism. Lastly, Verhoeff's **final phase** is from 1980 to present day and includes a focus on social cognition and instinct. Lorna Wing would conduct the first epidemiological study on autism in London in 1981.[18] Wing would define what went on to be known as the trifecta of autism symptoms. The trifecta included social impairment, communication delay and impairment, and restricted and repetitive behaviors and interests, noting that based on her empirical research, these cluster of symptoms cooccurred with such significance. It is also at this time that Wing would bring Asperger's work into play and create a type of autism that was related yet, at that time, distinct mostly based on impairment and intelligence. This progression in empirical research has led to the inclusion of autism as a diagnosis and its changes as researcher's understanding of autism has developed over time.

The Diagnostic and Statistical Manual of Mental Disorders (DSM) is the taxonomic and diagnostic tool for diagnosing mental disorders used by mental health professionals. Disorders with autism traits have changed names throughout DSM revisions but first appeared in DSM-III, published in 1980. In this context, it should also be noted that in the first edition of DSM in 1952, children with autistic symptoms were labeled as having childhood schizophrenia. Following Kanner's theories on the etiology of autism, a new body of research emerged focusing on potential neurobiological mechanisms for autism.[12] This body of research demonstrated that autism was clearly different from schizophrenia, or any other already characterized mental disorder, and provided evidence for classification as its own mental disorder in the DSM. This research resulted in the inclusion of Infantile Autism in the DSM-III in 1980. Infantile Autism was focused on early development and encompassed the same autistic characteristics discussed by Kanner, but there were several barriers to the utility to autism in the DSM-III.[4,5] For example, to receive a diagnosis of autism using the DSM-III, an individual was required to meet eight of 16 diagnostic criteria (Lack of awareness of feelings in others, no or abnormal seeking of comfort in times of distress, no or impaired imitation, no or abnormal social play, gross impairment in ability to make peer friendships, no mode of communication, markedly abnormal nonverbal communication including eye contact, absence of imaginative activity, abnormalities in speech production, abnormalities in the form or content of speech including stereotyped or repetitive speech, marked impairment in the ability to initiate or sustain a conversation, stereotyped body movements, persistent preoccupation with parts of objects, marked distress over changes in trivial aspects of the environment, unreasonable insistence on following routines in specific detail, markedly restricted or repetitive interests, onset in early childhood). Additionally, the DSM-III discussed residual infantile autism, demonstrating there was an expectation that the symptoms demonstrated by an individual with autism would resolve with age, although it is currently known this is not the case.

There were significant changes made to the description of autism in the DSM when DSM-III was updated to DSM-IV. What stands out most significantly is the change in name from infantile autism to autistic disorder and a separate diagnosis of Asperger Syndrome to demonstrate what was considered a higher functioning form of autistic disorder. There is significance in the name change as it demonstrates an understanding that autism symptoms are pervasive and not likely to resolve. Additionally, by removing the term "infantile" from the name, the DSM-IV reflected the new idea that developmental problems and approaches were not limited to the young children.[4,19,20] The criteria for autism were adjusted to be more flexible and to better capture individuals with autism. The new diagnostic criteria were split in to three different domains: Impairment in reciprocal social interaction, problems in communication, and restricted interests and repetitive behaviors.

To be diagnosed with autism in DSM-III, individuals had to meet all eight criteria of autism, which was problematic given the varied presentation by individuals; this was changed in DSM-IV. In DSM-IV, an individual needed to meet 8 of 16 criteria with the guidelines that two required characteristics needed to be from the impairment in reciprocal social interaction domain, and then at least one criterion from each the problems in communication and restricted interest domains. As discussed before, widening the diagnostic criteria would allow for greater clinical flexibility and potentially more reliable diagnoses. Volkmar and McPartland[4] synthesize the potential impacts resulting from changes made from DSM-III to DSM-IV. The potentially most significant, positive change is the shift in focus to developmental levels of the child being assessed. While moving away from infantile autism allowed for less emphasis on the idea that autism existed only at a young age but removing a need for early onset contributed to an increase in false positive diagnoses. On the other hand, the DSM-IV field trials of DSM-IV criteria demonstrated acceptable interrater reliability and internal consistency among clincians.[21] Lastly, the use of Asperger Syndrome in the DSM-IV was somewhat controversial as it differed from Asperger's original writings and it was synonymous with "high functioning autism." Research has demonstrated that clinical application of autism and Asperger Syndrome did not significantly differ, and this contributed to the removal of Asperger Syndrome as a diagnosis in DSM-V.

Another important aspect of the DSM-IV is the inclusion of diagnoses that captured autism symptoms but were not classified as an autism spectrum disorder. Most predominant is Pervasive Developmental Disorder-Not Otherwise Specified (PDD-NOS). PDD-NOS is often described as synonymous with autism,[22] and providers had a hard time distinguishing between a true autism diagnosis and PDD-NOS. As a result of the lack of differentiation, PDD-NOS became a catch-all diagnosis for neurodevelopmental disorders. The inclusion of PDD-NOS was designed to reflect the idea that autism includes a broader phenotype. Autism is considered a pervasive developmental disorder, meaning that it is a life-long developmental disorder. The not otherwise specified classification indicates that an individual may be experiencing autism-type symptoms but may not fully meet a more specific developmental disorder diagnosis. PDD-NOS is also sometimes referred to as atypical autism. It makes sense that PDD-NOS was later removed during revision to the DSM-V. PDD-NOS became a diagnosis of exclusion and seemed to not outline any specific clinical impairment different from an autism diagnosis.[23] More importantly, when children diagnosed with autism were compared to children diagnosed with PDD-NOS, there were no behavioral or neurophysiological differences between the two groups, when controlling for nonverbal IQ.[24] This led to false heterogeneity in diagnoses, even when diagnosed individuals were experiencing the same type of symptoms, and they were given the profile of different disorders.

In addition to PDD-NOS, the DSM-IV included several other diagnoses in the autism category of Pervasive Developmental Disorders. In total, the Pervasive Developmental Disorders include autistic disorder, Asperger disorder, Childhood Disintegrative Disorder (CDD), Rett Syndrome, PDD-NOS, and atypical autism. At this point, there was consensus that pervasive developmental disorder as an umbrella term did not accurately represent the autism spectrum[25] and in future iterations of the DSM, other diagnoses would not be included with pervasive developmental disorders. In the DSM-IV, autistic disorder is characterized by a qualitative impairment in social interaction and communication, as well as the presence of restricted and repetitive behaviors and delays in functioning. Impairment may include poor eye contact, failure to develop relationships with peers, lack of shared enjoyment with others, delay or lack of spoken language, difficulty in sustaining conversation, stereotyped language, or lack of imaginative play. Additionally, restricted interests and repetitive behaviors may include an interest that is abnormal in intensity, inflexible adherence to routines, stereotyped and repetitive motor mannerisms, and preoccupation with parts of object, such as hyper focus on the wheels of a vehicle.[22] In comparison, Asperger disorder shared many of the same characteristics with autistic disorder but required that an individual had no clinically significant language delay. Additionally, individuals diagnosed with Asperger disorder would demonstrate normal or near-normal intelligence. The idea that autistic disorder and Asperger disorder are distinct would later change in the DSM-V. Also included as a pervasive developmental disorder was Childhood Disintegrative Disorder (CDD). Other names for CDD include Heller's syndrome, dementia infantilis, or disintegrative psychosis. CDD is considered a very rare disorder with only about 1.7 cases per 100,000 children.[26] CDD is characterized by a significant loss in skills and abilities after the age of two. This must occur in a minimum of two developmental domains. Examples of developmental domains include social interaction, language, bowel or bladder control, adaptive skills, play, and motor skills. Regression, or loss of skills, is considered a potential symptom of ASD,[27] but CDD presents differently than autism regression. Studies have found that individuals with CDD and autism share core symptoms, but in the case of CDD, children's symptoms are more severe, and regression happens faster, includes more emotional symptoms, and have a greater overall global skills deficit.[28]

Additionally, the DSM-IV also included Rett syndrome as a pervasive developmental disorder. Rett syndrome, identified by an Austrian physician named Dr. Andreas Rett, is a neurodegenerative disorder which emerges after a period of typical functioning from birth.[29] Additionally, Rett syndrome is limited to females. Children with Rett syndrome usually exhibit autistic-like behaviors in the early stages. Rett syndrome typically presents with regression in skills, changes in hand and finger dexterity, loss of acquired language, gait abnormalities, and stereotypic hand movements. Other symptoms may include changes in sleep, abnormal muscle tone, teeth grinding and difficulty chewing, growth delay, and breathing disruptions. While Rett syndrome can present itself as regression, there are clear physical changes that differentiate it from autism and therefore are not considered part of the description of autism spectrum in DSM-V.

## Current characterization of ASD

The DSM-V[3] further changed the conceptualization of autism and made some changes that have been considered controversial to the definition of autism. An important change from DSM-IV to DSM-V is the nomenclature used for autism. In DSM-V, autism spectrum disorder, or ASD, became the new name for the overarching diagnosis. Additionally, Asperger Syndrome was removed from the DSM-V, and the description of ASD was focused more specifically on the idea that all ASD symptoms exist on a spectrum and are distinguished by how impairing they are, but they are all one diagnosis. These changes have been critiqued for several reasons, one being that the more restrictive and less inclusive criteria would mean that up to 40% of individuals meeting diagnostic criteria on the DSM-IV for autism would not meet criteria for ASD using the DSM-V.[30] The implications of this change in diagnostic criteria could mean that some individuals may not meet the inclusion criteria for services they need. Additionally, research with individuals with ASD could be complicated given that a large portion of the sample could no longer be included.

The three diagnostic categories in the DSM-IV were consolidated into two domains in the DSM-V: Problems with social communication (which was previously deficits in social interaction and language and communication) and restricted and repetitive behaviors and interests. Additionally, a criterion of onset was added to DSM-V after being removed in DSM-IV. In DSM-V, individuals must have had evidence of ASD symptoms at an early age. Furthermore, symptom severity specifiers were added. Specifiers were included to be able to describe the level of care an individual with ASD may need. Given that there is no longer a differentiation between Asperger Syndrome and autism, for example, specifiers allow for a diagnosis to better reflect the needs of an individual diagnosed with ASD. In addition to the level of care needed, DSM-V allows for identification of etiological factors, if known, underlying ASD symptoms (see Table 1 for the timeline of major historical events in the study of autism spectrum disorder).

## Prevalence rates of autism over time

ASD diagnostic criteria have evolved and refined over the years. Consequently, the rate at which individuals have been diagnosed have also changed significantly. Increases in the prevalence of ASD have been attributed largely to awareness of the disorder, changes in diagnostic criteria, and increases in diagnostic competency among community providers such as pediatricians and school counselors.[8] For example, most pediatricians' office these days ask parents to fill out a screening form at their child's first visit, the Checklist for Autism in Toddlers (CHAT), meaning that the likelihood of identifying early symptoms of autism and getting a referral is significantly more than perhaps a decade or two ago. Additionally, the conceptualization of ASD has also changed over the

TABLE 1 Summary of major historical events in the study of autism spectrum disorder.

| Year | Major historical milestones in autism spectrum disorder |
|---|---|
| 1943 | Leo Kanner publishes first paper describing autism in children |
| 1944 | Hans Asperger published his description of highly intelligent children with social deficits |
| 1952 | First edition of DSM labels children with autism symptoms as having childhood schizophrenia |
| 1964 | Bernard Rimland changes public perception by publishing book on neurobiology of autism |
| 1967 | Bruno Bettelheim popularizes the "refrigerator mother" idea through his book "Empty Fortress" |
| 1980 | Diagnostic criteria for Infantile Autism first added to DSM-III |
| 1981 | Lorna Wing characterizes Asperger Syndrome |
| 1987 | Infantile Autism replaced with "autism disorder" in the DSM-IV |
| 1990 | Autism is included as a disability in the Individuals with Disabilities Education Act (IDEA) |
| 1994 | Asperger's syndrome added to the DSM |
| 1996 | Temple Grandin's autobiographical book "Emergence Labeled Autistic" is published |
| 1998 | Paper published suggesting vaccine may be associated with autism (an idea formally debunked later) |
| 2006 | U.S. President signs the Combating Autism Act to support autism research and treatment |
| 2013 | DSM-V combines all subcategories of autism into autism spectrum disorder |

years with more input from parents of children with ASD and individuals with ASD becoming self-advocates for themselves and for the ASD community at large.

It is important to note the once popular public opinion of ASD being caused by vaccines, the measles, mumps, and rubella (MMR) vaccine specifically. This false and misleading information has led to disruptions in parents giving their children vaccines which can lead to its own host of problems. Even though there have been many scientific reports of vaccines not causing ASD,[31] this perception still exists among some. Media sources often cite thimerosal, a vaccine preservative, as the cause of autism in children[32] because the preservative will overload the infant's immune system. Proposal of this entire idea began in 1998 with a study published in the journal, *The Lancet*.[33] This study claimed that in a sample of 12 children, there was a link between the MMR vaccine and autism.

However, it is of utmost importance to note that this study was found to be fraudulent, and the publisher later discovered that the research had been funded by lawyers representing parents who were suing vaccine companies. In the end, this published paper was retracted by the journal in 2010. Unfortunately, the vaccine idea has since outlived the false science it was founded on. Since then, multiple large-scale studies have demonstrated the absence of any association between vaccination and ASD. In a Danish longitudinal study of 657,461 children, it was determined that after 10 years, having received the MMR vaccine did not increase a child's risk for developing ASD when compared to children who did not receive the MMR vaccine.[34] Additionally, the Centers for Disease Control and Prevention (CDC) provides up-to-date information on the safety of vaccines, specifically related to autism.[35] It is the CDC's stance that vaccines are safe and do not have a causal relationship with autism. They support the statement made by the Institute of Medicine in which they assessed vaccine safety and rejected a causal relationship between vaccines and autism. Lastly, the CDC has assessed antigen levels as a potential cause of autism, when compared to unvaccinated children, and it was discovered that there is no difference in level of antigen in vaccinated children with and without ASD. Given the large extent of vaccine research done by health institutions and researchers, it remains clear that the claim of vaccine-autism link is a myth. In this context, it is also worth noting that perhaps the single most influential scientific discovery in human history is the discovery of vaccines as it has eradicated many life-threatening illnesses in humans.

Recent estimated indicate that the current rate of prevalence of autism in the United States is 1 in 54 children.[36] This has risen since 2002 when the CDC reported the rate of autism being 1 in 150 children.[37] Many people have questioned and hypothesized the change in prevalence. First, it is important to understand the difference between rate of prevalence and rate of incidence. The statistics previously presented (and the ones usually seen reported in media and in other sources) are rates of prevalence, the total number of individuals with autism in the population. This is in comparison to rates of incidence, the number of new cases of autism in a population. Incidence statistics may provide a better index on the change in new cases, and prevalence rate may be inflated given their inclusion of new as well as previous diagnoses. One of the most prevailing reasons for increases in autism diagnosis over time is change in understanding and classification of autism.[38] Additionally, introduction of the DSM-V criteria have allowed for increased identification of younger children and less severe children, both of which could contribute to the increase is ASD prevalence.[39] Change in diagnostic criteria, better diagnostic tools, and increased training and competency of providers are likely the major factors contributing to the increased rate of ASD.

## Conclusion

Since the early 1940s, scientists and clinicians have been describing qualities of autism in children, descriptions that have persisted till now, contributing to the modern-day diagnosis of autism spectrum disorder. While ASD diagnostic criteria have not been without critique or problems over time, research continues to demonstrate the validity of ASD diagnoses. Rigorous scientific research backs current diagnostic approaches and assessments, including continually testing validity and reliability of ASD assessment techniques. The history of ASD is rich, broad, and ever-changing to ensure that ASD diagnoses are not only accurate but provide a basis to develop and research effective interventions to help the ASD community. Decades of research, scientific publications, DSM changes, and experiences of clinicians and individuals with autism have all contributed to improve identification and treatment of ASD. As time moves on, more individuals, especially self-advocates, add their voice to the discussion of ASD and will contribute to improving the science and meeting the needs of individuals with ASD.

## References

1. Kanner L. Autistic disturbances of affective contact. *Nerv Child.* 1943;2(3):217–250.
2. Donovan J, Zucker C. *Autism's First Child.* The Atlantic; October 10, 2010:1–19.
3. APA. *Diagnostic and Statistical Manual of Mental Disorders.* 5th ed. Washington D.C.: American Psychiatric Association; 2013.
4. Volkmar FR, McPartland JC. From kanner to DSM-5: autism as an evolving diagnostic concept. *Annu Rev Clin Psychol.* 2014;10:193–212. https://doi.org/10.1146/annurev-clinpsy-032813-153710.
5. Barahona-Corrêa JB, Filipe CN. A concise history of Asperger syndrome: the short reign of a troublesome diagnosis. *Front Psychol.* 2016;6(2024):1–7. https://doi.org/10.3389/fpsyg.2015.02024.
6. Wing L, Gould J, Gillberg C. Autism spectrum disorders in the DSM-V: better or worse than the DSM-IV? *Res Dev Disabil.* 2011;32(2):768–773. https://doi.org/10.1016/j.ridd.2010.11.003.
7. Wing L. Asperger's syndrome: a clinical account. *Psychol Med.* 1981;11(1):115–129.
8. Wolff S. The history of autism. *Eur Child Adolesc Psychiatry.* 2004;13(4):201–208. https://doi.org/10.1007/s00787-004-0363-5.
9. Baker JP, Lang B. Eugenics and the origins of autism. *Pediatrics.* 2017;140(2). https://doi.org/10.1542/peds.2017-1419.
10. Asperger H, Frith UT. *'Autistic Psychopathy' in Childhood.* Cambridge University Press; 1991.
11. Matson JL, Sturmey P. *International Handbook of Autism and Pervasive Developmental Disorders.* Springer Science & Business Media; 2011.
12. Rimland B. *Infantile Autism: The Syndrome and its Implications for a Neural Theory of Behavior.* Appleton-Century-Crofts; 1964.
13. Benedict C. *Bernard Rimland, 78, Scientist Who Revised View of Autism, Dies.* New York Times; 2006.
14. Rimland B. The differentiation of childhood psychoses: an analysis of checklists for 2,218 psychotic children. *J Autism Child Schizophr.* 1971;1:161–174.

15. Rimland B. The autism epidemic, vaccinations, and mercury. *J Nutr Environ Med.* 2000;10(4):261–266. https://doi.org/10.1080/13590840020013248.
16. Verhoeff B. Autism in flux: a history of the concept from Leo Kanner to DSM-5. *Hist Psychiatry.* 2013;24(4):442–458. https://doi.org/10.1177/0957154X13500584.
17. Lockyer L, Rutter M. A five-to fifteen-year follow-up study of infantile psychosis. *Br J Psychiatry.* 1969;115:865–882. https://www.cambridge.org/core. Accessed June 28, 2021.
18. Wing L. Language, social, and cognitive impairments in autism and severe mental retardation. *J Autism Dev Disord.* 1981;vol 11:31–44.
19. Waterhouse L, Wing L, Spitzer RL, Siegel B. Diagnosis by DSM-III-R versus ICD-10 criteria. *J Autism Dev Disord.* 1993;23(3):572–573.
20. Siegel B, Vukicevic J, Elliott GR, Kraemer HC. The use of signal detection theory to assess DSM-III-R criteria for autistic disorder. *J Am Acad Child Adolesc Psychiatry.* 1989;28(4):542–548.
21. Volkmar FR, Klin A, Siegel B, et al. Field trial for autistic disorder in DSM-IV. *Am J Psychiatry.* 1994;151:1361–1367.
22. Filipek PA, Accardo PJ, Baranek GT, et al. The screening and diagnosis of autistic spectrum disorders. *J Autism Dev Disord.* 1999;29:439–484.
23. Towbin KE. Autism and Asperger's syndrome. *Curr Opin Pediatr.* 1997;9(4):361–366.
24. Rapin I, Allen D, Aram D, et al. Classification issues. In: *Preschool Children with Inadequate Communication: Developmental Language Disorder, Autism, Low IQ.* London: MacKeith; 1996:190–213.
25. Wing L. The history of ideas on autism. *Autism.* 1997;1(1):13–23.
26. Fombonne E. Prevalence of childhood disintegrative disorder. *Autism.* 2002;6(2):149–157.
27. Rogers SJ. Developmental regression in autism spectrum disorders. *Ment Retard Dev Disabil Res Rev.* 2004;10(2):139–143. https://doi.org/10.1002/mrdd.20027.
28. Mehra C, Sil A, Hedderly T, et al. Childhood disintegrative disorder and autism spectrum disorder: a systematic review. *Dev Med Child Neurol.* 2019;61(5):523–534. https://doi.org/10.1111/dmcn.14126.
29. Neul JL, Kaufmann WE, Glaze DG, et al. Rett syndrome: revised diagnostic criteria and nomenclature. *Ann Neurol.* 2010;68(6):944–950. https://doi.org/10.1002/ana.22124.
30. Mazefsky CA, Mcpartland JC, Gastgeb HZ, Minshew NJ. Brief report: comparability of DSM-IV and DSM-5 ASD research samples. *J Autism Dev Disord.* 2013;43:1236–1242. https://doi.org/10.1007/s10803-012-1665-y.
31. Hare O, A. Severing the link between MMR and autism. *J R Coll Physicians Edinb.* 2002;32(3):167–169.
32. Hotez P. The physician-scientist: defending vaccines and combating antiscience. *J Clin Invest.* 2019;129(6):2169. https://doi.org/10.1172/JCI129121.
33. Knopf A. Vaccines do not cause autism: pediatricians fight back against anti-science. *Brown Univ Child Adolesc Behav Lett.* 2017;33(S2):1–2. https://doi.org/10.1002/cbl.30195.
34. Hviid A, Hansen JV, Frisch M, Melbye M. Measles, mumps, rubella vaccination and autism: a nationwide cohort study. *Ann Intern Med.* 2019;170(8):513–520.
35. DeStefano F, Shimabukuro TT. The MMR vaccine and autism. *Annu Rev Virol.* 2019;6(1):585–600.
36. Maenner M, Shaw K, Baio J, et al. Prevalence of autism spectrum disorder among children aged 8 years—autism and developmental disabilities monitoring network, 11 sites, United States, 2016. *MMWR Surveill Summ.* 2020;69(4):1–12.
37. Center for Diseases Control (CDC). Prevalence of autism spectrum disorders—Autism and Developmental Disabilities Monitoring Network, six sites, United States, 2000. *MMWR.* 2007;56(SS-1):1–11.
38. Fombonne E. Epidemiology of pervasive developmental disorders. *Pediatr Res.* 2009;65(6):591–598. http://www.dds.ca.gov/Autism/docs/AutismReport2003.pdf. Accessed 27 June 2021.
39. Bent CA, Barbaro J, Dissanayake C. Change in autism diagnoses prior to and following the introduction of DSM-5. *J Autism Dev Disord.* 2017;47:163–171. https://doi.org/10.1007/s10803-016-2942-y.

CHAPTER

# 2

# Definition, prevalence, and behavioral symptoms of autism

*Diane L. Williams*

**The Pennsylvania State University, University Park, PA, United States**

## Definition of autism

Autism is a neurodevelopmental disorder.[1] This means that the development of the brains of children with an autism spectrum disorder (ASD) differs from that of children with more typical development. This developmental difference affects the way the brain of a child with ASD responds to environmental input. The brain response then results in a cascade of differences in learning and social functioning that are the behaviors we call autism.

Although ASD is a neurodevelopmental disorder, the neurofunctional basis of ASD has not as yet been fully determined. Therefore, the definition and diagnosis of ASD continue to be based on characteristic behaviors. These characteristic behaviors are delineated in the fifth edition of the *Diagnostic Statistical Manual of Mental Disorders of the American Psychiatric Association* or the DSM-5.[2] According to the diagnostic criteria for ASD, an individual must have persistent deficits in three areas of social communication and interaction, and two of the four areas of restrictive and repetitive behaviors to be given a diagnosis of ASD. The deficits in social communication/interaction can be in social emotional reciprocity, in nonverbal communicative behaviors that are used for social interaction, or in developing, maintaining, and understanding relationships. The restrictive and repetitive behaviors can be stereotyped or repetitive motor movements, stereotyped or repetitive speech, inflexible insistence on sameness, restricted interests that are unusual in their subject or intensity, or hyper- or hyporeactivity to sensory input. Furthermore, these core behaviors must not be explained by an intellectual disability or a global developmental delay.


https://doi.org/10.1016/B978-0-12-816393-1.00008-7

Deficits in social emotional reciprocity include ineptness with holding a back-and-forth conversation, a reduction in the sharing of interests or emotions with others, or the failure to initiate or respond to social interactions. Deficits in nonverbal communicative behaviors include problems with the integration of verbal and nonverbal communication or abnormalities in eye contact and body language. Other weaknesses in nonverbal communication could include difficulty understanding and using gestural communication, a lack of differentiated facial expressions, or inappropriate nonverbal communication that does not match the emotional content of a spoken message. Deficits in social relationships include struggles with adjusting one's behavior to accommodate different social contexts, difficulty in imaginative play or making friends, or an absence of interest in others.

The restrictive and repetitive behaviors can manifest very differently across individuals and also at different ages. For example, restricted interests may be intense in childhood but may change or become lessened as the individual matures. Some examples of stereotyped or repetitive motor movements are lining up toys, spinning objects, or repeatedly flipping objects such as wads of string. Repetitive speech includes immediate echolalia, that is, repeating what an adult says (Adult: Let's get on the bus. Child: Get on the bus.). Immediate echolalia can also be demonstrated by answering a question with a repetition of the question (Adult: Do you want a cookie? Child: You want a cookie?). In addition, echolalia may be delayed, for example, use of an idiosyncratic phrase ("crispy chicken") with no clear meaning or other formulaic speech ("we'll be back after these messages") that was previously heard by the individual with ASD in another context.

Repetitive, restrictive behaviors may include an insistence on sameness or inflexibility, for example, an expectation that the same schedule will be followed even on weekends or holidays or that the same food will be eaten at every meal. Individuals with ASD may exhibit ritualized patterns of behavior such as touching door knobs and light switches in a certain pattern when entering a room. Small changes in schedules or interruptions that prevent completion of patterns of behavior may cause individuals with ASD extreme distress. Individuals with ASD may have difficulty making transitions from one activity to the next without a verbal warning to help prepare them for the change.

Other forms of restricted behaviors may be fixation on specific interests that are abnormal in intensity or focus such as a strong preoccupation with unusual objects. For example, an individual with ASD may amass a collection of knives because of an intense interest in their reflection in the shiny metal blades. Other intense interests may not be as clearly different from that of other children or adults except when interpreted with respect to other behaviors characteristic of ASD. For example, a fascination with American history, the weather, outer space, or trains may not be unusual in subject but may be unusual in intensity or a failure to understand that others do not share this interest.

Included under the diagnostic criteria for restricted, repetitive behaviors is an unusual response to sensory input. Individuals with ASD may have a hyperactive response to touch, smell, sights, or sounds. For some individuals with ASD, light touch causes great distress and they may prefer deep touch if they tolerate touch at all. Individuals with ASD may be hypersensitive to smells such as perfume or scents from personal care products or foods. They may find bright lights in a room intolerable or the noise from the rheostats of neon lights highly disturbing. Individuals with ASD may react to loud or unfamiliar noises by covering their ears as if in pain and may only be able to remain in noisy environments by wearing noise-canceling headphones.

On the other hand, individuals with ASD may be hyposensitive to sensory input. They may be indifferent to pain and harm themselves by touching hot objects. Children with ASD may walk barefoot on toys scattered across the floor seemingly unaware that the toys are there. They may not react when their name is called, leading parents to be concerned that their child is deaf. Individuals with ASD may repeatedly sniff food or other objects as if they are having difficulty interpreting the smell. They may also have a visual fascination with lights or movements, watching the flickering light through their fingers or fixating on the pattern of movement created by ceiling fans.

### Summary

To meet the diagnostic criteria for ASD, an individual must have a deficit in social communication and interaction and demonstrate restricted, repetitive behaviors that interfere with daily functioning. However, the specific behavior or combination of behaviors that a person exhibits may differ from that of other individuals who are also diagnosed with ASD.

## Must ASD manifest in childhood?

In an earlier version of the DSM, the behavioral characteristics of ASD were required to be manifested before the age of 3 to meet the diagnostic criteria for autism.[3] However, according to the DSM-5, this is no longer the case. The newer diagnostic guidelines allow for cases in which the behavioral characteristics are not fully manifest until demands for social functioning exceed the individual's ability to compensate for these.[2] In cases recognized at older ages, the assumption is that the individual has always had ASD. However, their behaviors were in a mild form and the individuals around them may have ascribed their behaviors to idiosyncratic personality traits or other related diagnoses such as attention deficit/hyperactivity disorder (ADHD) or anxiety. Alternately, individuals may have masked or mitigated the effects of the hallmark ASD behaviors by using compensatory strategies.[4] Diagnosing individuals who are less severely affected with ASD can be quite challenging. As for all individuals with ASD, to meet the diagnostic criteria, the behaviors must cause clinically significant impairment in social life, occupational pursuits, or other areas of current functioning.

## Prevalence of ASD

The prevalence of a condition or disorder is the proportion of a population who have that condition or disorder in a given time period. The prevalence of ASD in a 2016 survey of 8-year-olds diagnosed with ASD from 11 states was 18.5 per 1000 children or 1 in 54 according to estimates from the Center for Disease Control's Autism and Developmental Disabilities Monitoring (ADDM) Network.[5] In that survey, the prevalence by racial/ethnic groups per 1000 children was similar for White (18.5), Black (18.3), and Asian/Pacific Islander children (17.9) with a slightly lower prevalence per 1000 (15.4) for Hispanic children.[5] Black children with ASD with below average cognition were more likely to be diagnosed later than similar White children with a median age at diagnosis of 48 months versus 42 months.[5] In that survey, ASD was 4.3 times more prevalent in boys than in girls. The 4:1 ratio of males to females is generally reported for clinical samples.[6] However, a metaanalysis of prevalence studies that included a total of 53,712 participants with ASD reported a male-to-female ratio that was closer to 3:1.[7]

### Is ASD caused by vaccines?

Social media is filled with blogs and other reports that claim that ASD is caused by vaccines, specifically the measles/mumps/rubella or MMR vaccine. Why is the MMR shot blamed for ASD? The toxin myth began with a report by Dr. Andrew Wakefield of autism onset in association with the MMR immunization at 15 to 18 months and an increase in measles antibodies in the gut; this study had a small sample size ($n = 12$), a poorly controlled design, and conclusions that were not well-supported.[8] This study was subsequently retracted and Wakefield was discovered to have failed to disclose that his work had been funded by lawyers who were representing families who were suing vaccine-producing companies.[9] Other epidemiological studies failed to find a link between the MMR vaccination and autism.[10,11]

## Autism is a spectrum disorder

Autism is a spectrum disorder. This means that individuals who have all been diagnosed with ASD may present very differently. While sharing common primary problems in social communication/interaction and restricted, repetitive behaviors, the overall effect of the difference in neurodevelopment is very heterogenic with different effects on behaviors and the capacity for learning and independent functioning. In its more severe forms, the effect on learning is so significant that an individual may develop little to no functional spoken language and may have a life-long dependency on others for care and mediation with the world. The estimates for the number of individuals with ASD who have intellectual disability varies. The results of a prevalence survey of 11 sites in the United States completed in 2016 indicated 33% of 8-year-old children with ASD had an intellectual disability; 24% had IQs between 71 and 85; and 42% had IQ scores that were average or above.[5] In its less severe forms, ASD may go unrecognized until later childhood or adulthood until the effects begin to interfere with daily living, academic performance, or an ability to develop independence in adulthood.[4] Milder forms of ASD are not universally considered as a "disorder" but rather a variation of neurological development or a neurodiversity that requires understanding and acceptance rather than intervention.[12]

In addition to being very heterogenic in severity and presentation, individuals with ASD can exhibit very different developmental pathways or trajectories. A study of 6975 children with ASD who were born in California from 1992 through 2001 revealed six different developmental profiles.[13] Children who had the least severe symptoms at diagnosis made the most improvement, while children who were the most severely affected continued to have significant challenges. However, at least some of the children who began among the lowest group, showed rapid improvement attaining levels similar to those of the more mildly affected group.

### ASD differentiated by levels of support

According to the DSM-5, once an individual meets the diagnostic criteria for ASD, then the Level of Support needed should be determined for the two core areas of social communication/interaction and restricted, repetitive behaviors.[2] The level of support that an individual requires to meet the challenges of daily living is the basis for determining the severity of the spectrum disorder of ASD. The three levels of support are:

Level 1: Requiring support.
Level 2: Requiring substantial support.
Level 3: Requiring very substantial support.

### *Level 1*

Individuals with ASD who are at Level 1 require minimal support to function in the community. They can generally communicate their thoughts and feelings through sentence-level communication and typically have some social relationships. However, they may be viewed as strange or odd by their peers and may struggle to form and maintain friendships. Others may consider individuals with Level 1 ASD as rude or offensive, although this is usually unintentional on their part. Individuals with ASD at this level may have difficulty interpreting the intentions of others and may be gullible and naïve, putting them at risk for bullying or being taken advantage of by others.[14] Even though individuals with Level 1 ASD can usually communicate using spoken language, they have difficulty with pragmatics or interpreting the implicit social rules of communication. That is, they may say too much, providing overly detailed information about a topic or their intense interest, missing the cues that their listener is not interested in the subject. Alternately, an individual with ASD may say too little and require their conversational partner to continue to prod them to provide more information. Other reported behavioral observations of individuals with ASD at Level 1 who communicate through spoken language are a monotone or odd voice tone or abnormal prosody—the rhythm, intonation, and pitch of speech.[15] They may also use odd or overly precise words, for example addressing individuals by their full names. Other notable language features can include the overuse of idiosyncratic similes or metaphors ("you're as smooth as a jazz trombone") or overuse of words such as "actually" as a sentence starter. At Level 1, the restricted, repetitive domain may present as an obsession with facts, certain topics, details, or collections of specific objects.

The behavioral characteristics of individuals with ASD at Level 1 are consistent with their diagnosis of ASD. However, their capacity for independent functioning is greater than for individuals with ASD at levels 2 and 3. During school-age, children at Level 1 are typically enrolled in classes with children without ASD who are typical learners. In fact, children with ASD at this level may perform very well academically and display advanced skills in areas such as math, science, and reading fluency or decoding of written language. In adulthood, individuals with ASD at Level 1 may attain higher education degrees but, by definition, do not achieve full independence in adulthood and continue to require support such as having a family member manage their finances or their living situation. Individuals at Level 1 are candidates for a wide variety of different types of employment and can be successfully integrated into a work environment, especially if the individuals who manage their work are supportive and appreciative of their talents while accepting their differences.

Some individuals, diagnosed with ASD in childhood, may no longer meet diagnostic criteria in adulthood and do not continue to require support.[16] Interestingly, the behavioral presentation of these individuals may be indistinguishable from comparison individuals with typical development; however, neurofunctional results are more similar to those who continue to meet the criteria for an ASD diagnosis.[17]

### *Level 3*

Individuals who are diagnosed with ASD at Level 3 require very substantial support. They may have minimal use of spoken language or only speak sporadically. Their restrictive and repetitive behaviors typically interfere with independent functioning and the successful completion of many daily activities. At younger ages, individuals with Level 3 ASD have difficulty communicating their wants and needs clearly to others. Repetitive body movements such as hand flapping or rocking may be exhibited. Individuals with ASD at this level may use objects in nonfunctional ways, for example, lining objects up or repeatedly turning an object around in their hands as they visually examine it. They generally have difficulty establishing joint attention through referential looking or pointing and have limited use of gestural communication. Individuals at Level 3 may use the hands of others for requesting, for example, putting an adult's hand on a door knob to request open, rather than using pointing gestures or spoken words. Communication partners may struggle to interpret their communication signals. Individuals with Level 3 ASD frequently use *augmentative/alternative communication* (AAC) to meet their complex communication needs.[18] AAC includes the use of manual signs, pictures, picture symbols, or voice output communication devices to communicate with others. In addition to having difficulty with producing spoken language, individuals at Level 3 may have difficulty with understanding the spoken language of others. Communication partners may need to use simplified language or to support their spoken language with visual supports, a technique that is referred to as *aided modeling*.[18]

Children with Level 3 ASD are generally diagnosed at younger ages because of the severity of presentation.[19] At school-age, they may be enrolled in a special school or in a self-contained classroom for children with significant learning needs. Despite their significant behavioral and communication challenges, children with ASD at this level may also be main-streamed or included in educational activities with children with typical developmental. As adults, individuals with Level 3 ASD continue to require very substantial support and may continue to live with family members or in supported living environments such as group homes. They may work in the community in supported employment, supervised by a job coach. If they are unable to or choose not to participate in competitive employment in the community, individuals at Level 3 may work in sheltered workshop settings, completing routine activities such as sorting nuts and bolts for packaging, assembling papers for mailings, potting plants, or shredding documents.

### *Level 2*

By definition, individuals with ASD functioning at Level 2 require substantial support and are in the mid-range of autism severity between those at Levels 1 and 3. They generally have more communication skills than individuals at Level 3, such as an ability to produce sentence-level spoken language. However, some individuals at Level 2 may be multimodal communicators, relying on a combination of spoken language, gestures, and external communication supports such as AAC. Persons with Level 2 ASD may depend on routines and structures to help them function and may become emotionally upset or highly anxious if these supports are changed or otherwise unavailable.

Individuals with ASD at Level 2 who communicate through spoken language may have difficulty using language flexibly and may not take more than a few conversational turns. Their spoken language may also be characterized with frequent "scripting" or delayed echolalia. That is, they may have some spontaneous language production interwoven with dialogue from their preferred television show or movie or other idiosyncratic phrases. They may have difficulty with maintaining eye contact when communicating with others and using varied facial expressions to convey their emotions. Like individuals with Level 3 ASD, individuals with ASD at Level 2 typically have problems with comprehension of spoken language and may need their communication partners to use simplified language or to support their language with scaffolding with visual supports.

At school-age, children with ASD at Level 2 may be in classrooms with children with typical development, receiving support services either part day in resource rooms or specialized classrooms or by receiving push-in support services whereby the speech-language pathologist or special educator provides services to them in a classroom with children with typical development. As adults, individuals with Level 2 ASD are candidates for competitive employment in the community and can learn a wide variety of jobs such as stocking shelves in a retail store, bagging groceries, working in the laundry department of a hotel, preparing food in a bakery, or busing tables in a restaurant. To learn these positions, they may require the services of a community-based service provider who offers vocational assessment, job placement, job skills training, and continuing support at the job site through job coaches who work with the employer to solve any behavioral or social problems that may arise.

## Additional specifiers

Once it has been determined that an individual meets the criteria for the diagnosis of ASD, additional specifiers are added to the diagnosis.[20] One specifier is the type of onset, particularly whether the individual had regression in language, social skills, motor abilities, or adaptive functioning.

Another specifier is whether the individual also presents with or without an accompanying intellectual impairment. A third specifier is whether ASD occurs with or without an accompanying language impairment (see Spoken language section). Any comorbid symptoms such as ADHD, anxiety or mood disorders are noted as well as cooccurring medical or genetic conditions such as Fragile X, Rett syndrome, or Down syndrome.

### What about Asperger syndrome?

In previous versions of the DSM, autism was included in the diagnostic category of Pervasive Development Disorder (PDD).[3] Subcategories included the diagnoses of Autistic Disorder, Asperger's disorder, or Pervasive Developmental Disorder Not Otherwise Specified (PDD-NOS). These categories are no longer represented in the DSM-5.[2] The primary diagnostic category is Autism Spectrum Disorder as described above. The decision to remove the subcategory of Asperger syndrome was recommended based on research on that had been unable to establish meaningful differences between individuals who had a clinical diagnosis of Asperger syndrome and individuals who were diagnosed with autistic disorder who had conversational level spoken language and cognitive functioning in the average range or above.[21] People who might been diagnosed with Asperger syndrome using the previous DSM criteria may be reclassified as ASD-Level 1 using the DSM-5 criteria for ASD.

## Social (pragmatic) communication disorder

Social (Pragmatic) Communication Disorder is a new category that was presented in the DSM-5 for individuals who have deficits in social communication but did not have the other behavioral manifestations of ASD.[2] To meet the diagnostic criteria for a social communication disorder, the alternative diagnosis of ASD is first ruled out. If an individual does not meet the criteria for ASD but has persistent difficulties in using verbal and nonverbal communication, specifically for social interactions, then a social communication disorder is considered. The diagnostic criteria for this category include problems in using communication for social purposes—greeting others, sharing information as appropriate—and making expected adjustments in communication based on the social context. For example, the individual may talk loudly in a waiting room where the expectation is small, private exchanges or may use informal language during a formal occasion. Individuals with a social communication disorder may also have difficulty adjusting their communication based on the needs of the listener, either providing too much or too little information such that their listener has difficulty understanding what they are trying to communicate. That is, the speaker with a social communication impairment may incorrectly assume that that listener has the same circle of friends and may not provide any identifying details when relating a story about a recent misadventure. These difficulties with social communication must occur without other behaviors characteristic of ASD or other forms of developmental language disorders such as problems with structural language (grammar or syntax) or difficulty expressing their thoughts in spoken words (an expressive language problem).

## Behavioral challenges

Individuals with ASD at all ability levels frequently demonstrate behavioral problems[22] or problems with emotional regulation—modifying one's emotional state to promote adaptive or goal-directed behavior.[23] Very young children or more severely affected individuals with ASD, may exhibit externalizing behaviors such as self-injury (e.g., biting one own's hand or arm or slapping one's head), aggression toward others, temper tantrums or "meltdowns," or other forms of noncompliance.[22] Atypical eating behavior and abnormal sleep patterns are also a common complaint.[22] Problems with emotional regulation may also be exhibited as internalizing behaviors such as anxiety or depression.[23] Externalizing and internalizing behaviors may be difficult for the individual with ASD to self-regulate, requiring structure and support from family and care givers.

## Beyond the diagnostic criteria for ASD

Even individuals with ASD who have overall average or above cognitive functioning may have differences in cognitive, motor, and linguistic processing that make it difficult for them to process information quickly and efficiently, to integrate information, and to think flexibly.[24,25] Some of the areas of intact or enhanced abilities and relatively weaker areas for children and adults with ASD with average or above intelligence are listed in Table 1. In this section, we will review research on the performance of individuals with ASD in these domains.

### Attention

Attention is a general learning mechanism by which an individual's cognitive resources are directed, sometimes volitionally and sometime automatically. Attention has been described by the various ways in which this general mechanism is used. *Selective attention* allows automatic or volitional focus on certain stimuli—such as an overhead ceiling fan—to the

TABLE 1 Intact or enhanced abilities and weaknesses in children and adults with autism with average or above cognitive functioning across the cognitive domains.

| Intact or enhanced | Cognitive weaknesses |
|---|---|
| Attention | Social cognition |
| Elementary motor | Complex motor |
| Simple memory | Complex memory |
| Formal language | Complex language |
| Concept identification | Conceptual reasoning |
| Rule learning | Executive functioning |
| Visuospatial processing | Cognitive flexibility |

exclusion of other stimuli. *Sustained attention* is the maintenance of attention to a stimuli or task for a period of time—such as focusing on the light patterns created by the ceiling fan for several minutes or more. *Attentional shifting* is the process by which we disengage our focus from one stimulus to another stimuli—such as ceasing to look at the ceiling fan when a loud noise suddenly occurs. Given the oft-reported problems that children and adults with ASD have with either failing to attend to a presented stimulus or, alternately, over-focusing on a single stimulus, attention has received much attention in autism research. A subgroup of individuals with ASD have such significant difficulty with attention that they may receive a comorbid diagnosis of ADHD.[26] For individuals with ASD without ADHD, attentional difficulties may still be evident. While basic attentional processes appear to be intact, difficulty with shifting attention from one stimulus to another appears to be problematic.[27] The nature of this difficulty is not yet clear. It has been described by some researchers as a problem with "sticky attention" or a prolonged latency to disengage from the point of focus when a new stimulus appears.[28] However, other researchers have described it as a lack of preferential attention to social stimuli.[29]

## Motor abilities

Although not generally considered a disorder of the motor system, motor difficulties are evident across a broad range of ages and levels of functioning in individuals with ASD. Basic motor abnormalities have been reported in a number of studies.[30–32] Reduced postural stability during standing has been reported for both children and adults with ASD.[33–35] Clumsiness in walking or variations in gait have been frequently documented.[36,37] Challenges in learning skilled motor movements, such as handwriting, tying shoes, or skipping, are indications of motor clumsiness and incoordination.[38] Difficulties in motor planning in gross motor movements, fine motor movements, and speech production have been reported even in more mildly affected individuals with ASD.[36–38]

## Memory

Memory is more than simply a storehouse for what we have experienced and thought. It is a dynamic process involving attention, encoding, storage, and retrieval. A robust memory system is an efficient system, using data reduction mechanisms that allow storage and retrieval of the large amounts and types of information that we encounter on a daily basis. Because of some depictions of autistic individuals in the popular media, for example, Dustin Hoffman's character Raymond in Rain Main,[39] it is commonly assumed that individuals with ASD have phenomenal memories. Individuals with ASD may have a relative strength in rote memory or the recall of facts and details. For example, they may have a prodigious memory for the statistics of baseball players on their favorite team, the schedule of arrivals and departures for municipal bus routes, or all of the dinosaurs from the Jurassic Period. However, this does not mean that they do not have challenges with memory functioning. While an individual with ASD may be able to recall detailed encyclopedia entries that they read in childhood on the political system of China, this does not mean that they would be able to engage in a high level discussion of this topic. While informational details may be easily recalled, this does not mean that they can integrate this information into a novel conversation. Similarly, individuals with ASD may remember information but not know how to use that information. For example, a student may tell the teacher the expected behavior in the classroom—"When we come to class, we sit down, we take out a piece of paper and a pencil, and we copy the lesson from the board"--but then not initiate the expected behaviors.

An efficient memory system requires the use of data reduction mechanisms such as the ones that help us to create a *gist*—a synopsis or shortened version containing the central ideas of the event. We use this gist for ease of retrieval and to communicate this information to others. For example, when telling your friend what you did over the weekend, your friend wants to hear the highlights, not the sequential details that start with when you slept in on Saturday morning. However, individuals with ASD have difficulty in creating and relating the gist of an orally heard story or an observed event.[40] Difficulty with creating a gist leads to story retelling that is a recounting of detailed information with an inability to extract the main idea or point of the story.

During the memory encoding and storage processes, new information should be integrated with already stored information. An organizational structure is created so that like items are grouped together and new information is connected to related, previously learned information. Children and adults with ASD have difficulty with spontaneous generation of these organizational structures that would support retrieval. For example, during word list learning tasks, they attempt to recall the list verbatim rather than grouping similar items together, as is typically observed for learners without ASD.[41] Furthermore, when individuals with ASD are provided support for retrieval in the form of cued recall or the use of recognition tests rather than free recall, the performance differences as compared to individuals with typical development are no longer obtained,[42] indicating that they have an underlying problem with organization to support efficient retrieval of information but not the storage of the information.

## Working memory

Through the process of working memory, information is actively maintained and manipulated so that it can be moved into long term storage.[43] Verbal working memory—usually evidenced by being able to repeat a string of numbers or letters or short sentences—has generally been reported to be intact in individuals with ASD who have spoken language when lower level behavioral tasks are used. For example, in an *n*-back verbal working memory task, respondents see one letter at a time and press a button when they see two letters in a row that are the same (1-back) or when they see a letter that is the same as the one two letters prior (2-back). Children and adults with ASD performed similarly to age- and ability-matched controls on this task.[44] However, when the verbal working memory task becomes more complex, individuals with ASD have relatively more difficulty than individuals with typical development. For example, 5- to 14-year-old children with ASD performed similarly to children with typical development when pointing to pictures in the order they were named; however, the children with ASD had more difficulty during a self-ordered pointing task in which they had to remember which pictured objects they had pointed to in order to point to a different picture in each newly presented set.[45]

Visuospatial working memory tasks, such as a "windows" task, are generally more difficult than verbal working memory tasks for children and adults with ASD.[44] In the "windows" task, the examiner holds up a card with window-like openings in a 3×3 grid and then pokes the end of the pencil through the holes to create a pattern. The respondent is asked to use their finger to reproduce the modeled pattern. The position of the pencil is not easily remembered using words, and the respondent must rely on visuospatial working memory to copy the pattern. However, different results have been obtained when other visuospatial working memory tasks are used. In one such task, 9 blocks are presented in a 3×3 grid. The examiner taps the blocks with a finger in a pattern. Individuals with ASD performed similarly to age and ability matched individuals with typical development on this visuospatial working memory task.[46,47] Visuospatial tasks that include an increased memory load have been reported to be more difficult for individuals with ASD. For example, in a task in which the respondents had to search for blue tokens in "boxes" on a computer screen without returning to an empty box, the children and adolescents with ASD had more difficulty.[48] The demand for maintenance of information during this task is very similar to that of the self-ordered picture task described earlier.

## Spoken language

Language is highly variable in individuals with ASD, ranging from individuals who are minimally verbal to individuals who are very verbose. For all individuals with ASD, which includes problems with social communication/interaction as a primary diagnostic criterion, the functional use of communication or pragmatic language is problematic.[49] Individuals with ASD may also have difficulty with understanding spoken language that is directed to them or what is referred to as auditory processing or language comprehension problems.

Minimally verbal individuals with ASD may use 10 or fewer spoken words or produce echolalic or stereotyped phrases without clear communicative intent. These individuals may use augmentative means of communication such as sign language, picture exchange systems, or speech-generating devices.[50] However, the majority of individuals with ASD have potential for the development of functional spoken language. For example, a follow-up study of children with ASD 17 years after initial testing revealed that two thirds of the cohort had developed spoken language exceeding a 3-year-old age equivalency.[51]

Individuals with ASD who have conversational-level spoken language generally do not have problems with phonology or articulation of speech sounds.[15] However, they may have relatively more difficulty with morphosyntax or grammar, producing sentences that are shorter and less grammatically complex relative to developmental peers.[52] They may also have specific difficulties with the use of markers for verb tense and agreement.[53]

Even very verbal individuals with ASD may have difficulty with higher order language skills. These include difficulty with making inferences, especially about the emotions or mental states of others.[54] Understanding of idioms, such as *eat your words*, and metaphors, such as *She is a shining star*, may be challenging. Individuals with ASD can struggle with organizing their spoken language or discourse. For example, when telling a story or event, they may relate excessive details and not have a clear beginning, middle, and end to their narrative.[55] When having a conversation, they may not change what they are saying in response to what their communication partner says, persisting in talking about their original topic.

Word-learning may be challenging for children with ASD who are more severely affected, with delays in the development of spoken language being a common report.[56] Other children with ASD may learn new vocabulary at a rate similar to children with typical development; however, they may have more difficulty learning the multiple meanings of words (e.g., blue as a color and blue as a feeling) and have a related difficulty with interpreting ambiguous meanings (e.g., I saw her *duck*.). In general, even highly verbal individuals with ASD may interpret language literally and have difficulty using and understanding abstract language. They may also exhibit subtle differences in the flexible use of language with relatively higher levels of formulaic language—phrases that appear to be learned rather than generated that are used as unanalyzed chunks.[57] For example, they may overuse a phrase such as *that's what I'm talking about* within more flexible language.

### *ASD and bilingualism*

Traditionally, an assumption was made that, given the difficulty children with ASD have with learning language, learning a second language would be too difficult and would interfere with language learning.[58] However, children with ASD who have been raised in a bilingual environment show no detrimental effect on their acquisition of expressive and receptive language.[59,60] Furthermore, bilingual children with ASD have been found to perform better than monolingual children with ASD on some aspects of social communication.[60,61]

## Written language/literacy

Written language includes comprehension (reading) and production (writing). Formal written language abilities, that is spelling and reading words and nonwords, have been reported to be equivalent or superior to those of age- and ability-matched peers for children and adults with ASD with overall cognitive abilities in the average range or above; however, this is not a universal finding with some children being "poor readers."[62] Other children with ASD exhibit *hyperlexia*, a condition in which they can easily pronounce written words but have difficulty with reading comprehension.[63] For many older children with ASD, reading comprehension may lag behind their peers.[64] Academically competitive adolescents and young adults with ASD may have difficulty with listening and taking notes in classes due to the need to listen, comprehend, and to determine what are the most important points to record in a written note.

## Conceptual reasoning

Even individuals with ASD with overall cognitive abilities in the average range or above may have difficulty with concept formation.[65] Concept formation is the process of generating new ways of looking at or categorizing information. Experimental work has demonstrated that children and adults with ASD have difficulty identifying unusual examples of a conceptual category, for instance, recognizing that a Manx cat with no tail is a cat.[66] Difficulty with concept formation has been proposed as the cognitive basis for the difficulty that individuals with ASD have with flexibility and generalizing what they have learned to a new situation.[65]

### Executive functions

Executive functions, which arise from the frontal lobe of the brain, particularly the prefrontal cortex, are higher order cognitive processes that manage other cognitive resources. Executive functions include planning, working memory, response inhibition, cognitive flexibility, set shifting, and goal monitoring and allow the spontaneous generation of plans, the formation of hypotheses, problem solving, and navigating changing environmental demands. Problems with various aspects of executive function such as difficulty with development of plans that have to accommodate a number of factors and failure to self-monitor are characteristic of individuals with ASD, independent of level of verbal ability and cognitive functioning.[67] Relative weaknesses in executive functions such as cognitive flexibility have been reported to be related to outcomes in adaptive functioning for adults with ASD.[68] However, other aspects of executive function have not been consistently found to be affected in individuals with ASD.

## Conclusion

ASD is a complex neurodevelopmental disorder with core problems with social communication and interaction and repetitive, restrictive behaviors that interfere with daily functioning. As a spectrum disorder, ASD is highly heterogeneous with a range of needs for the level of support and the ability to communicate with spoken language. Persons with ASD may have additional challenges in attention, motor control, memory, working memory, written language, conceptual reasoning, executive functioning, and cognitive flexibility.

### References

1. Moldin SO, Rubenstein JLR, eds. *Understanding Autism: From Basic Neuroscience to Treatment*. Boca Raton, FL: CRC Press; 2006.
2. American Psychiatric Association. *Diagnostic and Statistical Manual of Mental Disorders*. 5th ed. Washington, DC: American Psychiatric Association; 2013.
3. American Psychiatric Association. *Diagnostic and Statistical Manual of Mental Disorders*. 4th ed. Washington, DC: American Psychiatric Association; 2000. Text Revision.

4. Happé FG, Mansour H, Barrett P, Brown T, Abbott P, Charlton RA. Demographic and cognitive profile of individuals seeking a diagnosis of autism spectrum disorder in adulthood. *J Autism Dev Disord.* 2016;46:3469–3480.
5. Maenner MJ, Shaw KA, Baio J, et al. Prevalence of autism spectrum disorder among children aged 8 years—autism and developmental disabilities monitoring network, 11 sites, United States, 2016. *MMWR Surveill Summ.* 2020;69(SS-4):1–12.
6. Fombonne E. Epidemiology of pervasive developmental disorders. *Pediatr Res.* 2009;65:591–598.
7. Loomes R, Hull L, Mandy WP. What is the male-to-female ratio in autism spectrum disorder? A systematic review and meta-analysis. *J Am Acad Child Adolesc Psychiatry.* 2017;56:466–474.
8. Rao TS, Andrade C. The MMR vaccine and autism: sensation, refutation, retraction, and fraud. *Indian J Psychiatry.* 2011;53:95–96.
9. Horton R. A statement by the editors of the lancet. *Lancet.* 2004;363:820–821.
10. Taylor B, Miller E, Farrington CP, et al. Autism and measles, mumps, and rubella vaccine: no epidemiologic evidence for a causal association. *Lancet.* 1999;353:2026–2029.
11. Dales L, Hammer SJ, Smith NJ. Time trends in autism and in MMR immunization coverage in California. *JAMA.* 2001;285:1183–1185.
12. Kapp SK, Gillespie-Lynch K, Sherman LE, Hutman T. Deficit, difference, or both? Autism and neurodiversity. *Dev Psychol.* 2013;49:59–71.
13. Fountain C, Winter AS, Bearman PS. Six developmental trajectories characterize children with autism. *Pediatrics.* 2012;129:e1112–e1120.
14. Maiano C, Normand CL, Salvas MC, Moullec G, Aimé A. Prevalence of school bullying among youth with autism spectrum disorders: a systematic review and meta-analysis. *Autism Res.* 2016;9:601–615.
15. Shriberg LD, Paul R, McSweeny JL, Klin A, Cohen DJ, Volkmar FR. Speech and prosody characteristics of adolescents and adults with high-functioning autism and Asperger syndrome. *J Speech Lang Hear Res.* 2001;44:1097–1115.
16. Fein D, Barton M, Eigsti IM, et al. Optimal outcome in individuals with a history of autism. *J Child Psychol Psychiatry.* 2013;54:195–205.
17. Eigsti IM, Stevens MC, Schultz RT, et al. Language comprehension and brain function in individuals with an optimal outcome from autism. *Neuroimage Clin.* 2016;10:182–191.
18. Drager KD. Aided modeling interventions for children with autism spectrum disorders who require AAC. *Perspect Augment Altern Commun.* 2009;18:114–120.
19. Mandell DS, Novak MM, Zubritsky CD. Factors associated with age of diagnosis among children with autism spectrum disorders. *Pediatrics.* 2005;116:1480–1486.
20. Grzadzinski R, Huerta M, Lord C. DSM-5 and autism spectrum disorders (ASDs): an opportunity for identifying ASD subtypes. *Mol Autism.* 2013;4:1–6.
21. Witwer AN, Lecavalier L. Examining the validity of autism spectrum disorder subtypes. *J Autism Dev Disord.* 2008;38:1611–1624.
22. Dominick KC, Davis NO, Lainhart J, Tager-Flusberg H, Folstein S. Atypical behaviors in children with autism and children with a history of language impairment. *Res Dev Disabil.* 2007;28:145–162.
23. Mazefsky CA, Herrington J, Siegel M, et al. The role of emotion regulation in autism spectrum disorder. *J Am Acad Child Adolesc Psychiatry.* 2013;52:679–688.
24. Williams DL, Goldstein G, Minshew NJ. Neuropsychologic functioning in children with autism: further evidence for disordered complex information-processing. *Child Neuropsychol.* 2006;12:279–298.
25. Williams DL, Minshew NJ, Goldstein G. Further understanding of complex information processing in verbal adolescents and adults with autism spectrum disorders. *Autism.* 2015;19:859–867.
26. Holtmann M, Bölte S, Poustka F. Attention deficit hyperactivity disorder symptoms in pervasive developmental disorders: association with autistic behavior domains and coexisting psychopathology. *Psychopathology.* 2007;40:172–177.

27. Richard AE, Lajiness-O'Neill R. Visual attention shifting in autism spectrum disorders. *J Clin Exp Neuropsychol.* 2015;37:671–687.
28. Landry R, Bryson SE. Impaired disengagement of attention in young children with autism. *J Child Psychol Psychiatry.* 2004;45:1115–1122.
29. Chita-Tegmark M. Social attention in ASD: a review and meta-analysis of eye-tracking studies. *Res Dev Disabil.* 2016;48:79–93.
30. Jansiewicz EM, Goldberg MC, Newschaffer CJ, Denckla MB, Landa R, Mostofsky SH. Motor signs distinguish children with high functioning autism and Asperger's syndrome from controls. *J Autism Dev Disord.* 2006;36:613–621.
31. Bhat AN, Landa RJ, Galloway JC. Current perspectives on motor functioning in infants, children, and adults with autism spectrum disorders. *Phys Ther.* 2011;91:1116–1129.
32. Downey R, Rapport MJ. Motor activity in children with autism: a review of current literature. *Pediatr Phys Ther.* 2012;24:2–20.
33. Fournier KA, Kimberg CI, Radonovich KJ, et al. Decreased static and dynamic postural control in children with autism spectrum disorders. *Gait Posture.* 2010;2:6–9.
34. Minshew NJ, Sung K, Jones BL, Furman JM. Underdevelopment of the postural control system in autism. *Neurology.* 2004;63:2056–2061.
35. Molloy CA, Dietrich KN, Bhattacharya A. Postural stability in children with autism spectrum disorder. *J Autism Dev Disord.* 2003;33:643–652.
36. Rinehart NJ, Tonge BJ, Bradshaw JL, Iansek R, Enticott PG, McGinley J. Gait function in high-functioning autism and Asperger's disorder: evidence for basal-ganglia and cerebellar involvement? *Eur Child Adolesc Psychiatry.* 2006;15:256–264.
37. Rinehart NJ, Tonge BJ, Iansek R, et al. Gait function in newly diagnosed children with autism: cerebellar and basal ganglia related motor disorder. *Dev Med Child Neurol.* 2006;48:819–824.
38. Fournier KA, Hass CJ, Naik SK, Lodha N, Cauraugh JH. Motor coordination in autism spectrum disorders: a synthesis and meta-analysis. *J Autism Dev Disord.* 2010;40:1227–1240.
39. Levinson B, Johnson M, Morrow B, et al. *Rain Man.* Santa Monica, CA: MGM Home Entertainment; 2004.
40. Diehl JJ, Bennetto L, Young EC. Story recall and narrative coherence of high-functioning children with autism spectrum disorders. *J Abnorm Child Psychol.* 2006;34:83–98.
41. Minshew NJ, Goldstein G. The pattern of intact and impaired memory functions in autism. *J Child Psychol Psychiatry.* 2001;42:1095–1101.
42. Bowler DM, Gaigg SB, Gardiner JM. Effects of related and unrelated context on recall and recognition by adults with high-functioning autism spectrum disorder. *Neuropsychologia.* 2008;46:993–999.
43. Baddeley AD. Is working memory still working? *Eur Psychol.* 2002;7:85.
44. Williams DL, Goldstein G, Carpenter PA, Minshew NJ. Verbal and spatial working memory in autism. *J Autism Dev Disord.* 2005;35:747–756.
45. Joseph RM, Steele SD, Meyer E, Tager-Flusberg H. Self-ordered pointing in children with autism: failure to use verbal mediation in the service of working memory? *Neuropsychologia.* 2005;43:1400–1411.
46. Macizo P, Soriano MF, Paredes N. Phonological and visuospatial working memory in autism spectrum disorders. *J Autism Dev Disord.* 2016;46:2956–2967.
47. Verte S, Geurts HM, Roeyers H, Oosterlaan J, Sergeant JA. Executive functioning in children with an autism spectrum disorder: can we differentiate within the spectrum? *J Autism Dev Disord.* 2006;36:351–372.
48. Landa RJ, Goldberg MC. Language, social, and executive functions in high functioning autism: a continuum of performance. *J Autism Dev Disord.* 2005;35:557–573.
49. Baird G, Norbury CF. Social (pragmatic) communication disorders and autism spectrum disorder. *Arch Dis Child.* 2016;101:745–751.

50. Tager-Flusberg H, Kasari C. Minimally verbal school-aged children with autism spectrum disorder: the neglected end of the spectrum. *Autism Res.* 2013;6:468–478.
51. Pickles A, Anderson DK, Lord C. Heterogeneity and plasticity in the development of language: a 17-year follow-up of children referred early for possible autism. *J Child Psychol Psychiatry.* 2014;55:1354–1362.
52. Eigsti IM, de Marchena AB, Schuh JM, Kelley E. Language acquisition in autism spectrum disorders: a developmental review. *Res Autism Spectr Disord.* 2011;5:681–691.
53. Roberts JA, Rice ML, Tager-Flusberg H. Tense marking in children with autism. *Appl Psycholinguist.* 2004;8:429–448.
54. Bodner KE, Engelhardt CR, Minshew NJ, Williams DL. Making inferences: comprehension of physical causality, intentionality, and emotions in discourse by high-functioning older children, adolescents, and adults with autism. *J Autism Dev Disord.* 2015;45:2721–2733.
55. Barnes JL, Baron-Cohen S. The big picture: storytelling ability in adults with autism spectrum conditions. *J Autism Dev Disord.* 2012;42:1557–1565.
56. Wodka EL, Mathy P, Kalb L. Predictors of phrase and fluent speech in children with autism and severe language delay. *Pediatrics.* 2013;131:e1128–e1134.
57. Boucher J. Language development in autism. *Int Congr Ser.* 2003;1254:247–253.
58. Beauchamp ML, MacLeod AA. Bilingualism in children with autism spectrum disorder: making evidence based recommendations. *Can Psychol.* 2017;58:250–262.
59. Kay-Raining Bird E, Lamond E, Holden J. Survey of bilingualism in autism spectrum disorders. *Int J Lang Commun Disord.* 2012;47:52–64.
60. Hambly C, Fombonne E. The impact of bilingual environments on language development in children with autism spectrum disorders. *J Autism Dev Disord.* 2012;42:1342–1352.
61. Valicenti-McDermott M, Tarshis N, Schouls M, et al. Language differences between monolingual English and bilingual English-Spanish young children with autism spectrum disorders. *J Child Neurol.* 2013;28:945–948.
62. Åsberg Johnels J, Carlsson E, Norbury C, Gillberg C, Miniscalco C. Current profiles and early predictors of reading skills in school-age children with autism spectrum disorders: a longitudinal, retrospective population study. *Autism.* 2019;23:1449–1459.
63. Newman TM, Macomber D, Naples AJ, Babitz T, Volkmar F, Grigorenko EL. Hyperlexia in children with autism spectrum disorders. *J Autism Dev Disord.* 2007;37:760–774.
64. Lucas R, Norbury CF. Levels of text comprehension in children with autism spectrum disorders (ASD): the influence of language phenotype. *J Autism Dev Disord.* 2014;44:2756–2768.
65. Minshew NJ, Meyer J, Goldstein G. Abstract reasoning in autism: a disassociation between concept formation and concept identification. *Neuropsychology.* 2002;16:327.
66. Gastgeb HZ, Strauss MS, Minshew NJ. Do individuals with autism process categories differently? The effect of typicality and development. *Child Dev.* 2006;77:1717–1729.
67. Wallace GL, Kenworthy L, Pugliese CE, et al. Real-world executive functions in adults with autism spectrum disorder: profiles of impairment and associations with adaptive functioning and co-morbid anxiety and depression. *J Autism Dev Disord.* 2016;46:1071–1083.
68. Williams DL, Mazefsky CA, Walker JD, Minshew NJ, Goldstein G. Associations between conceptual reasoning, problem solving, and adaptive ability in high-functioning autism. *J Autism Dev Disord.* 2014;44:2908–2920.

CHAPTER

# 3

# Early identification and diagnosis of autism

*Neill Adams Broderick*[a,b] *and Rachel J. Hundley*[b,c]

[a]Departments of Pediatrics and Psychology, Vanderbilt University Medical Center, Nashville, TN, United States, [b]Vanderbilt Kennedy Center/Treatment and Research Institute for Autism Spectrum Disorders, Nashville, TN, United States, [c]Departments of Pediatrics, Psychology, and Psychiatry, Vanderbilt University Medical Center, Nashville, TN, United States

Significant research and clinical efforts have been directed toward accurately detecting and diagnosing autism spectrum disorder (ASD). This chapter reviews current practice in developmental screening and diagnostic assessment. It ends with a discussion of current issues and future directions.

## Screening for autism spectrum disorder in young children

### Developmental surveillance and screening policies

Surveillance and screening are central to preventive healthcare. They are designed to identify risk for, and early indicators of, a disease or disorder to facilitate, and, even expedite, treatment. Effective screening, and, ultimately, intervention, can improve outcomes for individuals, families, and systems affected by a disease or disorder.

Pediatric healthcare providers are uniquely positioned as the primary point of contact for families regarding surveillance and screening of child development. The American Academy of Pediatrics[1] (AAP) Council on Children with Disabilities defines *surveillance* as the process of recognizing risk for developmental delays in children; it is a critical function, and ongoing effort, for pediatric primary healthcare providers. The AAP[1] recommends that providers embed developmental surveillance into every


https://doi.org/10.1016/B978-0-12-816393-1.00009-9

well-child visit. The same council upholds *screening*, which employs standardized tools to identify and elucidate risk for developmental delays.[1] The AAP[1] recommends that providers administer standardized developmental screening tests at the 9-, 18-, and 30-month well-child visits.

The AAP has released multiple policy statements regarding screening specific to ASD within broader developmental surveillance in the pediatric medical home.[2–4] Children with ASD may not display the full range of diagnostic criteria during developmental surveillance.[5] Therefore, the AAP explicitly recommends that pediatric primary care providers conduct ASD-specific screens with formal tools at 18- and 24-month-old visits, in addition to any other time parents report concerns regarding symptoms of ASD.[3,4]

## Evaluating surveillance and screening tools

The utility of a screening tool can be characterized by its ability to accurately differentiate cases versus noncases of a specific disorder[6,7] Various psychometric indices exist to capture this classification accuracy, including: sensitivity, specificity, Positive Predictive Value (PPV), and Negative Predictive Value (NPV).

Sensitivity refers to the proportion of individuals with a disorder who are correctly identified as at-risk by a screening tool.[6–8] Specificity refers to the proportion of individuals who do not have a disorder and who are correctly classified as such by a screening instrument.[6–8] Sensitivity and specificity are both calculated by comparing the outcome of a screening measure to the outcome of a gold standard instrument or best estimate clinical diagnosis.[6,8] PPV captures the proportion of individuals who screen positive for a disorder and receive a confirmed diagnosis of the disorder, divided by the number of screen-positives.[7,8] NPV refers to the proportion of individuals who screen negative for a disorder for whom the absence of diagnosis is confirmed, divided by the number of screen-negatives.[7,8] Values for all four indices range from 0.0 to 1.0, with higher values reflecting greater accuracy of classification.[8] Values of 0.70 or 0.80 or higher are acceptable for all four indices.[6–9] It is not uncommon, however, to see PPV levels ranging from 0.30 to 0.50.[9]

Screening may be influenced by error or other factors. Someone who is detected by a screener as a positive case but does not have the disorder is considered a false-positive error.[6,7] An individual who is excluded from the screener as a negative case, and, yet, warrants a diagnosis is considered a false-negative, though these may be harder to detect as follow-up for negative screens is less likely.[7] Additionally, the PPV and NPV of a tool are influenced by the base rate or prevalence of a disorder in a population.[6–8] ASD is considered a low base rate disorder with a prevalence between 1% and 2%.[10] Research suggests that a systematic, multistage screening model could offset these psychometric concerns.[6]

## Importance of screening

Extant evidence clearly supports that participation in early intervention optimizes outcomes for young children with ASD.[11–16] In their review, Zwaigenbaum et al.[17] support the integration of developmental and behavioral interventions as best practice for children under 3 years of age with diagnosed or suspected ASD, as it yields improved developmental scores/cognitive performance, adaptive functioning, and language skills. Furthermore, Dawson et al.[18] report that early behavioral intervention may normalize patterns of brain activity, and thus, improve social skills. Furthermore, it is notable that intervention initiated prior to age three may be more effective in improving developmental outcomes than that started after 5 years of age.[17] Early intervention is critical regarding optimal outcomes for children with ASD, and sensitive windows seem to exist regarding the response to early intervention in children with ASD.

Despite substantial evidence regarding the effectiveness of early intervention, some young children may miss the opportunity to participate in such services.[8] Access to early intervention likely requires early identification of risk for, or even diagnosis of, developmental differences, especially ASD.[19] Parents of children with ASD have reported initial concerns regarding ASD symptoms around 14–15 months of age[20]; however, the median age of diagnosis for autism in the United States remains 51 months.[10] Individuals from economically disadvantaged and/or minority groups may be identified even later.[19,21] Lengthy waits may result in children missing months to years of early intervention supports.[8,19] Early screening can facilitate earlier identification of risk, and, thus, earlier referral to evaluation, which expedites access to more targeted early intervention. Screening may also offer access to early intervention, in some capacity, while one waits for a comprehensive diagnostic assessment.[8] Specialized supports can start earlier, operate on brain plasticity sooner, and optimize outcomes.[8,11,13,15,18] The following section examines the types of screening tools available as well as the quality of prominent instruments used to screen for ASD.

## Types of screening

Screening measures were created for different purposes, and, thus, vary in scope and format.[8,22] This section will examine three levels of screening: general developmental screening, Level 1 screening, and Level 2 screening. Across the levels of screening, you will see varying formats, including informant-report (e.g., parent/caregiver), observational, and/or interactive,[8] each of which offers strengths and limitations. Informant-report instruments offer details and insight from daily life, though they may introduce reporter bias.[8] Observational measures provide rater expertise, though they are limited by a single timepoint of measurement.[8] Similarly, interactive measures incorporate administrator knowledge in addition to direct experience with an individual; however, they require more training and time to learn as well as administer and score.[8] Given the advantages and disadvantages of the varying dimensions of screening instruments, a process that entails multiple levels and multiple formats of screening tools may be most effective.[8,23]

## General developmental screening

General Developmental Screening, also known as broad-band screening, refers to efforts to monitor for a wide variety of developmental concerns or delays in the general population.[6] Broad-band measures may assess a range of developmental domains, including: cognition/problem-solving, communication, motor skills, social skills, adaptive skills, and/or behavioral factors.[8] Research suggests that most pediatricians engage in some form of General Developmental Screening, though universal screening has not yet been realized.[24] Pediatricians have reported increasing rates of screening, as indicated by 23% in 2002, 45% in 2009, and 63% in 2016.[25] However, these data suggest that more than one-third of pediatricians are still not using validated procedures. The use of validated measures provides data to support referrals for further evaluation and/or early intervention. Some potential General Developmental Screening tools are discussed in the following section as well as Appendix A.

### Ages and Stages Questionnaire, Third Edition (ASQ-3)

The Ages and Stages Questionnaire, Third Edition (ASQ-3) is a 30-item parent report measure designed to assess developmental functioning across five domains of development in children ages one to 66 months of age.[26,27] The five domains captured include: communication, fine motor, gross motor, personal-social, and problem-solving. Outcomes of the ASQ-3 place children in one of three zones, including at-risk, not-at-risk, or monitoring.[26,27] The measure demonstrates high test-retest reliability (0.92) as well as interrater reliability (0.93).[26,27] Sensitivity (0.83–0.89) and specificity (0.80–0.92) are also good across ages, which suggests that the ASQ-3 screens appropriately for general developmental functioning.[8,26,27] It is not ASD specific.

### Parents' Evaluation of Developmental Status (PEDS)

The Parents' Evaluation of Developmental Status (PEDS) is a 10-item, yes/no parent questionnaire created to assess five domains of development in children one to 95 months of age.[28,29] The five domains assessed include: global/cognitive, expressive language, receptive language, social-emotional, and other. Responses on the PEDS are classified as predictive or nonpredictive of developmental concerns.[28,29] The PEDS demonstrates good sensitivity (i.e., 0.74–0.79) and good specificity (i.e., 0.70–0.80) across ages.[28,29] The psychometric properties of the PEDS suggest that it screens appropriately for general developmental functioning; however, more research is needed for its use as an ASD screening tool.[8,23]

#### Infant Toddler Checklist (ITC)

The Infant Toddler Checklist (ITC) is a portion of the Communication and Symbolic Behavior Scales Developmental Profile (CSBS DP).[30] The CSBS DP assesses language, social communication, and general developmental functioning in children via three measures, including: the ITC, the CSBS DP Caregiver Questionnaire, and the CSBS Behavior Sample.[30,31] The ITC can be used as a broad-band screening instrument whereas the Caregiver Questionnaire and the Behavior Sample can follow concerns detected by the ITC.

The ITC is a standardized instrument that consists of 24 yes/no items and one open-ended question regarding child development in children ages 6 months to 24 months.[30] The ITC generates composite scores for three domains, including social, speech, and symbolic; cut-off scores regarding deficits overall; and standard scores based on a normative sample.[30,31] Initial validation studies indicated good sensitivity (0.94), specificity (0.89), PPV (0.90), and NPV (0.94) for the ITC regarding children diagnosed with ASD,[31] though this sample may have displayed more risk than the general population.[8] Further studies demonstrated good sensitivity (0.77–1.00) for children 9 to 24 months and low sensitivity (0.20) for children 6–8 months.[32] Independent researchers have suggested that the PPV for the ITC is good for children with developmental concerns combined, though the PPV falls below acceptable levels for children with ASD and may lack in sensitivity.[8,33,34] The ITC does not purport to distinguish individuals with ASD versus individuals with developmental delay in screening.

#### Summary of general developmental screening

General developmental screeners are designed to capture developmental concerns in the general population. Despite their utility for this purpose, most of these broad-band measures do not adequately capture all children who may be at risk for ASD.[6] General developmental screeners should continue to be administered in pediatric primary care settings to identify children at risk for varied developmental concerns. ASD-specific instruments should also continue to follow general developmental screening.

### *Level 1 screening*

Level 1 screening refers to tools that assess ASD-specific concerns in the general population. As previously noted, the American Academy of Pediatrics endorses Level 1 screening during well-child checks at 18 and

24 months of age.[3,4] Level 1 screening typically occurs in the primary care setting.[8]

Nearly three-fourths of pediatricians who responded to the 2016 National Survey of Children's Health reported screening for ASD,[33,35] which is an improvement from an independent 2012 survey[36] where 60% of pediatricians reported formal screening for autism at 18 months, and 50% reported it at 24 months. Despite increasing screening efforts, many children with autism may be inadvertently overlooked by their primary care physicians in the absence of formal screening measures. Miller et al.[23] found the use of screening tools to be more effective in detecting ASD than pediatrician's clinical judgment alone. Empirical evidence also suggests that professional training regarding screening instruments can increase provider knowledge of ASD and its early signs as well as foster provider incorporation of screening into practice.[37,38] Moreover, Oosterling et al.[39] demonstrated a significant decrease in the age of ASD diagnosis (i.e., 19.5 months less than baseline) following professional training regarding a formal autism screening tool. Some potential Level 1 screening tools are discussed in the following section as well as Appendix B.

### Checklist for Autism in Toddlers (CHAT)

The Checklist for Autism in Toddlers (CHAT) was the first autism-specific tool created for screening the general population during 18-month-old routine healthcare visit.[40] Using nine items for parents and five items for healthcare providers, the CHAT evaluates several areas of development while emphasizing specific early signs for autism (e.g., differences regarding pretend play, gaze, and pointing).[40] A six-year follow-up study of the CHAT identified low sensitivity and variable PPV, depending on the risk level and score used, despite good specificity.[41] Additional studies have suggested acceptable sensitivity and specificity; however, there are limitations regarding study designs.[8] The CHAT tends to under-identify children who later receive a diagnosis of ASD.[42]

### Modified Checklist for Autism in Toddlers (M-CHAT)

The Modified Checklist for Autism in Toddlers (M-CHAT) adapted the CHAT for use as a Level 1 screening instrument for children 16–30 months of age in primary pediatric care settings in the United States.[43] It is the most commonly used and studied ASD-specific screening instrument for children under 30 months of age in the general population.[4,33,42,44] The M-CHAT entails 23 parent-rated items, nine of which came from the CHAT and 14 that were rigorously studied in development.[8] There are six critical items on the M-CHAT.[43] Results of the M-CHAT are considered positive for ASD risk if two critical items are failed or if three items overall are failed. A follow-up interview is available.[43]

The M-CHAT demonstrates adequate internal consistency reliability overall ($\alpha = 0.85$) as well as for the critical items ($\alpha = 0.84$).[43] Initial validity studies, which examined the checklist and interview combined, yielded good sensitivity (0.95–0.97), specificity (0.95–0.99), and NPV (0.99) despite variable PPV (0.36–0.80) with a sample that may have included participants at high risk for ASD.[43] Additional validity studies have included low- and high-risk samples, and they have demonstrated acceptable PPV levels for children at high-risk when using the M-CHAT with the follow-up interview.[45,46] In the largest sample thus far, Chlebowski et al.[47] screened 18,989 children ages 16–30 months, and the cumulative validity evidence supports that the M-CHAT should be combined with its associated follow-up interview to reduce false positives.

Levy et al.[33] highlighted the variability of the effectiveness of the MCHAT to identify ASD in children across ages, settings, and contexts.[33] Some recent studies have sought clarity regarding the M-CHAT in the general population. Two reviews suggested a PPV of 50%–54% for the MCHAT with its follow-up interview in the general population, though, attrition before follow-up was an issue.[33,42] It is notable, however, that some recent studies have suggested that the M-CHAT may identify some children at risk for ASD prior to documented concerns from parents and/or pediatricians.[23,33,48]

**Summary of level 1 screening**

The AAP upholds the standard that all children should be screened with an ASD-specific screening instrument at 18- and 24-month routine healthcare visits as well as any time caregivers express concerns. Level 1 screening instruments are designed for early identification of ASD symptoms in the general population. Some of the tools demonstrate promising psychometric properties, despite the limitations of low base rate as well as study limitations, including the presence of high-risk participants in samples, lack of validation of cut-off scores, and lack of follow-up for negative screens.[6,8]

Sanchez-Garcia et al.[44] conducted a metaanalysis of studies that emerged from January 1992 through April 2015 to evaluate existing Level 1 screening tools for ASD in children 14–36 months of age in the general population. Overall, the metaanalysis revealed a pooled sensitivity of 0.72 and pooled specificity of 0.98.[44] The Positive Predictive Value (PPV) was 97.78 and the Negative Predictive Value (NPV) was 93.13.[44] Ultimately, Sanchez-Garcia et al.[44] present empirical evidence that Level 1 screening tools for ASD are sufficient to detect autism from 14 to 36 months of age. Please see this review, as well as information in Appendices B and C, for additional insight regarding available Level 1 screening tools.

### *Level 2 screening*

Level 2 screening tools are designed to assess risk for ASD following identification of developmental concerns as well as to discriminate between ASD and other developmental differences, such as speech and/or language disorders or global developmental delay.[8] These instruments are primarily used in community settings, such as early intervention centers or evaluation clinics.[6,8] Level 2 screening may require more training and/or time to administer.[8] Some potential Level 2 screening tools are discussed in the following section as well as Appendix C.

#### Modified Checklist for Autism in Toddlers-Revised/Follow-Up (M-CHAT-R/F)

As previously noted, the M-CHAT is one of the most commonly used Level 1 ASD-specific instruments designed to screen for ASD in the general population.[6,42,44] Ample research suggests that the psychometric properties of the M-CHAT are improved, and false screens may be reduced, when used in conjunction with a follow-up interview.[45,47,49] The Modified Checklist for Autism in Toddlers-Revised/Follow-up (M-CHAT-R/F) formally incorporated a follow-up interview to create a two-step screening process for the detection of ASD symptoms in children ages 16–30 months.[49] In developing the M-CHAT-R step of the M-CHAT-R/F, Robins et al.[49] removed three items from the M-CHAT, adjusted the order of items, simplified language, provided examples to clarify item content, and eliminated critical items.

The M-CHAT-R/F[49] now includes 20 parent-response items, and the results classify risk for autism into low (two points or lower), medium (three to seven points), and high (eight points or higher). Those classified as low risk should continue to participate in surveillance and screening as recommended by the AAP. The follow-up interview, conducted in-person or via telephone, should occur when a score indicates medium risk.[49] If ASD concerns are confirmed via follow-up interview, those individuals should be referred for further evaluation.[49] Individuals classified as high risk by the M-CHAT-R should receive immediate referral for further evaluation and support services.[6]

Robins et al.[50] present evidence demonstrating reliability and validity of the M-CHAT-R/F. Validation studies suggest that the M-CHAT-R/F identifies children with ASD at a higher rate than the M-CHAT.[50] McPheeters et al.[42] suggest a PPV of 48% of the M-CHAT-R/F in the general population. More research is needed regarding the validity of the M-CHAT-R/F, and its utility as a replacement for the M-CHAT. The M-CHAT-R/F administration and scoring materials are available at www.mchatscreen.com.

### Screening Tool for Autism in Toddlers

The Screening Tool for Autism in Toddlers (STAT) is a Level 2 screening instrument designed for children ages 24–36 months.[51] The STAT involves a 20-min play-based interaction with a trained professional designed to capture 12 items across four domains of social communication, including: play (two items), requesting (two items), directing attention (four items), and motor imitation (four items).[51] Each domain generates a score based on the passage or failure of each item within it.[51] The total score, which sums the domain scores, ranges from zero to four.[51] A higher score indicates more ASD symptomatology, with two as the empirically-derived cutoff for "risk for ASD."[51]

Initial validation studies of the STAT demonstrated good sensitivity (0.83), specificity (0.86), PPV (0.77), and NPV (0.90) when comparing 24–36-month-old children with ASD to developmentally-matched children with other developmental disorders.[51] Stone et al.[52] pursued further validation, yielding strong psychometric properties, including: good sensitivity (0.92), specificity (0.85), PPV (0.86), and NPV (0.92); 89% agreement between the STAT risk classification (i.e., at-risk or not-at-risk) and other established measures; and good interrater as well as test-retest reliability. In 2008, Stone et al.[53] pursued validation of the STAT with individuals 12–23 months of age at high risk for ASD. Though this preliminary research is promising, more research is needed regarding the use of the STAT with younger children including the validation of cutoff score.[6,8]

### Summary of level 2 screening

Level 2 screening instruments are designed to discriminate between ASD and other developmental differences. These tools demand clinician involvement—the M-CHAT-R/F through interview and the STAT through interactive observation. While clinician involvement provides a broader perspective on child development, this may prove challenging for some clinical settings. Providers must consider several factors in the screening process, including: clinician training, screening logistics (e.g., physical space, materials, staff support, etc.), family/individual needs (e.g., cultural, linguistic, etc.), professional time for administration and scoring, remuneration, and procedures for follow-up regarding negative and positive screens.[4,6,7] Research suggests that ongoing, multistep screening (i.e., Levels 1 and 2 in the context of general developmental screening) that incorporates family and clinician perspectives may be most effective.[6,7,54] Children who receive a positive screen, or those whose parent or pediatrician has concerns, should be referred for a comprehensive, diagnostic assessment.

## Diagnostic assessment for autism

### Collecting history

The process of diagnostic assessment begins with a careful review of relevant records and any previous evaluations and interventions. Many clinicians have individualized intake questionnaires to capture presenting concerns as well as the referred individual's birth history, attainment of developmental milestones, medical information, and family history. When applicable, it is important to gather information on school functioning through eliciting child-care provider or teacher reports and ratings of classroom behaviors. Teacher observations of behavior and peer interactions from less-structured times of the day, such as recess, lunch, and hallway transitions, may be particularly useful.

Interviews are typically conducted with parents or caregivers and, for adolescents and adults, with the individual themselves. In addition to gathering information, the interview is a valuable tool for building rapport and understanding a family's priorities in seeking an assessment. These priorities may include: confirming an initial diagnosis; determining whether co-occurring disorders or disabilities are present; gaining an understanding of prognosis; identifying service eligibility; and receiving guidance on potential therapeutic, instructional, workplace, community, and financial supports. Parents of younger children may have been notified of a positive screen at their pediatrician's office or they may have more general concerns about their child's rate of development. For example, there may be concerns regarding language and/or motor delays. Individuals first referred for assessment during later childhood or adolescence may not show delays, but typically present with concerns for developmental differences, such as social problems, or with co-occurring emotional and/or behavioral challenges.[55]

Unstructured, semistructured, and structured interviews may all be utilized in collecting a history. In addition to documenting developmental milestones, potential regression, and core features of ASD (i.e., social communication deficits and restricted repetitive behaviors), questions about early history often address specific features regarding a child's emotional regulation and development of social communication skills, including: response to name; initiation and response to bids for joint attention (e.g., pointing to or showing objects); and play. The presence of atypical behaviors, such as: stereotyped or repetitive language; using other's hands as tools or other atypical body movement; rigid and repetitive play routines; and intensive sensory interests or aversions, may also inform case conceptualization. A comprehensive history will also address historical and current behaviors, interests, and skills in the following domains: receptive and expressive language; using and understanding nonverbal communication strategies; social engagement and skills; interest in, and maintenance of, relationships with peers; variety and types of play; psychological or psychiatric history; independence with activities of daily living; and medical and family history. Functional assessment, including questions about the frequency, intensity, and duration of challenging behaviors, as well as their potential antecedents and consequences, may also be embedded in the clinical interview. Please see Hanley[56] and Iwata[57] for more information on functional assessment.

## Assessing core features of autism

### *Structured interviews*

For any psychological assessment, diagnostic instruments must be accurate, reliable, and valid. They must be "fair and appropriate for the evaluation purpose, population, setting, and context at hand" and this is also true in autism.[58,59] Structured tools have been developed for collecting historical and current information relevant to autism diagnosis, and these encompass open-ended questions as well as rigorous, coded, and scored items. Structured interviews often conclude with a diagnostic algorithm indicating whether autism diagnosis is likely. Some of the more commonly used structured interviews are described below.

#### Autism Diagnostic Interview, Revised (ADI-R)

The Autism Diagnostic Interview (ADI) was developed in the 1980s as a tool for research-based assessment of ASD in children age five and above with a mental age of at least 2 years.[60] It was revised to include preschool-aged children.[61] The ADI-R is one of the most used assessment tools in autism research, and it shows good reliability and validity.[62,63] Currently, the Autism Diagnostic Interview-Revised is a comprehensive, examiner-led tool that is administered to parents or caregivers of children aged two through adulthood with suspected autism. It is a 93-item semistructured interview with questions about language/communication; reciprocal social interaction; and restricted, repetitive, and stereotyped behaviors and interests, as well as questions in other domains. Raters complete a diagnostic algorithm based upon specific items at the conclusion of the interview. It requires 2–4h to complete. The ADI-R requires intensive instruction and practice as examiners must demonstrate a high level of interrater reliability to properly utilize the measure. In a review that analyzed results from five studies of preschool aged children being assessed for ASD, summary sensitivity for the ADI-R was 0.52 (results ranging from 0.19 to 0.75) and summary specificity was 0.84 (results ranging from 0.63 to 1.00).[64] Newer algorithms allow the ADI-R to be used with toddlers as young as 12months who have a nonverbal developmental level of at least 10months.[65] As a diagnosis of ASD in a very young child may not be stable, these algorithms result in "ranges of concern" rather than formal classifications. A clinical algorithm, designed to maximize sensitivity and maintain adequate specificity, resulted in sensitivities ranging from 0.80 to 0.94 and specificities ranging from 0.70 to 0.81.[65]

### Diagnostic Instrument for Social Communication Disorders (DISCO)

The Diagnostic Instrument for Social Communication Disorders (DISCO[66] and DISCO-11[67]) is commonly used in Europe. This 300-item measure was designed to provide a holistic description of a person's development and patterns of behavior, including specific skills and vulnerabilities relevant to autism diagnosis. It uses a dimensional approach with a focus on development; current versions provide diagnostic algorithms. The DISCO requires approximately 3h, and it is administered by a trained examiner. Though providing a diagnostic algorithm or classification was not the initial purpose of the DISCO, the DISCO-9 introduced multiple algorithms to align with various international diagnostic criteria of ASD. Assessment of these algorithms indicated a high level of interrater reliability as well as significant relationship to whether individuals were diagnosed with Autistic Disorder or not.[68] The current DISCO-11 has also demonstrated good internal reliability (0.78 for overall score).[69]

### 3di: The Developmental, Diagnostic, and Dimensional Interview

The Developmental, Diagnostic, and Dimensional Interview (3di) was designed as a hybrid of structured and semistructured approaches.[70] Trained examiners read questions from a computer-generated diagnostic interview and code responses. The full autism interview takes approximately 90min, and the abbreviated form may be administered in 45min. The 3di yields a computer-generated report with symptom profiles. Though it requires training to administer this measure, the informal style of questioning and simpler coding structure often yield acceptable (> 0.86) interrater reliability without the need for intensive training. The authors note test-retest and interrater reliability as well as excellent sensitivity (1.0) and specificity (> 0.97).[70]

### MIGDAS-2: Monteiro Interview Guidelines for Diagnosing the Autism Spectrum

The MIGDAS-2 questionnaire is a portion of the MIGDAS-2 assessment system, which involves collecting history and interactive observations (Monteiro Interview Guidelines for Diagnosing the Autism Spectrum).[71] Though no formal scoring is applied, the questionnaire may be utilized to elicit qualitative descriptions in clinical contexts. MIGDAS-2 questionnaires may be administered as an interview or in written form with open fields for parents and/or teachers to complete. Interactive components of the MIGDAS-2 are described below.

### Observational measures

Structured observational measures allow clinicians and researchers to assess and document social communication skills as well as the presence of restricted and repetitive behaviors during face-to-face evaluation. These interactive assessment tools were specifically designed to create opportunities to observe how an individual being assessed for autism initiates and responds to social overtures, maintains reciprocity in interactions, and shows creativity and/or play skills. Across measures, trained examiners may introduce preferred and nonpreferred topics of play/conversation to assess flexibility and reciprocity. They also use specific behavioral techniques, such as briefly holding desired items out of a young child's reach, to assess coordination of verbal and nonverbal communication strategies. In addition, test materials are selected, and in some instances, standardized, to create opportunities to observe sensory seeking and repetitive behaviors. Multiple interactive methods of assessment for core features of autism have been developed for use in research and clinical practice. As previously described, some screening tools also involve interactive assessment. The more commonly used diagnostic measures are described in the following sections.

#### Autism Diagnostic Observation Schedule, Second Edition (ADOS-2)

The Autism Diagnostic Observation Schedule (ADOS) is a widely recognized measure that provides semistructured, standardized assessment of communication and social interaction and also create contexts in which restricted and repetitive behaviors may be observed.[72] It was designed to maximize both sensitivity and specificity. The second edition of the ADOS provided revised algorithms and introduced the calibrated severity score as well as a new module for minimally verbal toddlers (ADOS-2).[73,74] The ADOS-2 consists of five modules based on language and developmental level. It is appropriate for use in clinical and research contexts with individuals aged 12 months through adulthood. After the interactive assessment is completed, trained examiners complete observational codes and an algorithm. Sensitivity (0.72–0.98) and specificity (0.76–0.82) are good across modules.[73,75] The Adaptive ADOS, currently available for use in research, provides two additional modules that allow for the evaluation of minimally verbal adolescents and adults.[76]

#### Childhood Autism Rating Scale, Second Edition (CARS-2)

The Childhood Autism Rating Scale (CARS) is a 15 item rating scale based on direct observation and/or caregiver report that is designed to be completed by a professional who has experience in autism.[77] It includes items on social behavior, communication, emotional regulation, and sensory differences. Across studies, it demonstrated strong agreement with DSM criteria as well as strong sensitivity (0.89–0.94) and specificity (0.85–1.0).[78,79] The CARS-2 includes two separate rating scales based on age and developmental level, as well as a parent questionnaire which is used for gathering information.[80] The examiner is encouraged to consider information gathered from interviews as well as from direct observation.

#### MIGDAS-2: Monteiro Interview Guidelines for Diagnosing the Autism Spectrum

The MIGDAS-2 is a method of gathering and organizing qualitative observations relevant to autism diagnosis in clinical practice.[71] In addition to the caregiver and teacher questionnaires described above, there are three interactive diagnostic interviews based on verbal fluency and age. During the interviews, referred individuals are presented with a range of sensory toys, selected by the clinician, with which they can interact. Individuals with fluent language are given opportunities to talk about their interests and asked questions about their emotional regulation and relationships. As there is no formal scoring, clinicians are encouraged to combine observations generated on this measure with additional evaluation tools.

### *Questionnaires*

Questionnaires may be used to elicit information on the types and intensity of autism related symptoms. Some forms are completed by parents or teachers and others are rated by clinicians after history and observations are gathered. Though not an exhaustive list, some of the more commonly used narrow-band measures are provided in Appendix D. Diagnostic profiles, as well as specific item endorsements, on broad-band screeners of emotional and behavioral adjustment may also be useful.

## Comprehensive assessment

In addition to addressing core features of autism, best practices include assessment across many domains of functioning including cognition, adaptive skills, language, motor skills, and emotional adjustment. For school-aged children and adults, evaluation may also include measures of executive function, attention, and academic skills. Assessment in domains beyond core symptoms of ASD helps to establish the correct diagnosis, determine if co-occurring disability or diagnoses are present, and tailor recommendations to address an individual's current needs. Evaluation results also may serve as a baseline from which to document progress in interventions. As intellectual ability, adaptive skills, facility with language, and autism severity may make differential contributions to outcome, it is important to incorporate multiple measures and multiple sources of information.[81,82]

### *Developmental skills*

Cognitive ability and language skills are two of the strongest predictors of future functioning for autistic individuals and for those who are typically developing.[83,84] Individuals with autism who display an IQ above 70 are more likely to achieve higher levels of education, be employed, be involved in rewarding social relationships, and live independently as adults than those who demonstrate IQ below 70.[85,86] In the most recent report from the Autism and Developmental Disabilities Monitoring Network (ADDM), surveillance data from 11 sites in the United States revealed that, among 8-year-old children with autism, approximately one-third display intellectual disability (IQ ≤ 70 with low adaptive skills), 24% show IQ within the borderline range (IQ 71–85), and 42% exhibit IQ classified in the average range or above (IQ > 85).[10] Multiple studies have indicated that, for most children diagnosed with autism, cognitive ability and language skills increase throughout childhood.[84] There are many standardized tools for assessing developmental, cognitive and language skills that are selected based on an individual's age and range of skills.

Delayed or atypical language is often one of the first indicators that a child may have autism. Though expressive and receptive language deficits do not feature in DSM-5 diagnostic criteria, clinicians should specify the overall level of language for the referred individual and whether language impairment is present.[87] Assessment of receptive, expressive, and pragmatic language skills may be included in the initial evaluation for autism. Clinicians may also refer an individual for further language evaluation and/or therapy as part of the final recommendations.

Adaptive behavior is the expression of conceptual, social, and practical skills needed to function in day to day contexts.[88] Although adaptive behavior is associated with cognition, autistic individuals often score lower on adaptive measures, particularly for social skills, than might be expected from their IQ alone.[89] Adaptive behavior is typically assessed through caregiver or teacher report on standardized interviews and questionnaires. Commonly used measures include the Vineland Adaptive Behavior Scale (Vineland-3) and the Adaptive Behavior Assessment System (ABAS-3).[90,91]

### *Differential diagnosis*

Although ASD exists as a singular diagnosis, it shares characteristics with other clinical concerns and disorders. Clinicians and researchers providing developmental assessments must hold expertise in autism, typical development, other developmental disorders, and psychiatric disorders in order to provide appropriate differential diagnosis.[92] Recent studies have indicated that over 70% of children with autism may meet criteria for a co-occurring emotional or behavioral disorder and up to 40% may have two co-occurring conditions.[93] Common co-occurring diagnoses include social anxiety disorder, attention deficit hyperactivity disorder, language disorders, depression, and oppositional defiant disorder.[94,95] Clinicians may use broad-band emotional and behavioral screening questionnaires as well as more focused interviews and measures to clarify the presence and intensity of a wide range of presenting concerns. As differential diagnosis can be quite complex, it is often helpful to establish whether current behavioral symptoms, such as irritability, increased outbursts, or aggression, represent a new concern or a change from previous functioning.[92] Parent interviews also help to determine whether social communication and behavioral differences characteristic of autism were present in early development. If not, current symptoms may be more easily attributed to other disorders. Many autistic individuals also have co-occurring medical disorders, including gastrointestinal dysfunction, seizures, sleep concerns, and avoidant-restrictive feeding disorder.[96,97] These co-occurring medical issues may be both a cause and, in some cases, an outcome of exacerbated behavioral symptoms.

### *Synthesis and feedback*

Best practices in the diagnostic process require a knowledgeable clinician, who is experienced in autism and related conditions, to synthesize comprehensive information from history, clinical data, and observations. Though current assessment tools are reliable and valid when used by trained professionals, diagnosis should never be based on the results of one test alone.[98] The clinician utilizes all available information to determine whether the referred individual meets diagnostic criteria for ASD as well as to provide a comprehensive impression and recommendations. In addition to clarifying diagnostic status, it is important to address a family's priorities throughout the assessment process, especially when delivering feedback.

Providing both verbal and written feedback in a way that is "honest, clear, and easy to understand" is a critical element in the diagnostic process.[99] Families, and the referred individual themselves, may experience a variety of emotional responses to feedback. It can be difficult to receive or to not receive a diagnosis of autism. If autism is not being diagnosed, it is important to provide information about the individual's current functioning, whether other diagnoses are present, and what interventions may be helpful. It is often appropriate to include the referred individual in some or all of the feedback session.

### *Assessment to intervention*

Receiving a clinical diagnosis gives information about an individual's developmental differences, and their strengths and challenges. Identifying autism may also yield access to interventions or educational placements that would otherwise be unavailable. Most importantly, in addition to a clear diagnostic statement, written reports of evaluations should result in meaningful recommendations and resources for the individual, their family, and other providers. Recommendations may include types of intervention (e.g., ABA therapy, speech therapy, cognitive behavioral therapy, etc.), specific goals for an individual (e.g., improving emotional regulation), and/or guidance on educational supports and placements (e.g., specialized classrooms or tutoring).[55] Evaluation results may also be used as a baseline from which to estimate change and response to intervention.

## Conclusions and future directions

### Current barriers to assessment

The field of autism, and evaluation for autism, has a broad and deep research base; however, it is dynamic and there is still much to learn. At present, most specialty clinics have lengthy waitlists for autism assessment. There are many reasons for this including increased prevalence and awareness of autism as well as the recognition that early intervention can significantly change outcomes.[100] Current demand for autism evaluation significantly exceeds the number of trained, experienced clinicians who can provide a high-quality assessment. Current research and clinical guidelines are beginning to critically consider the following: the length, setting, and types of professionals involved in an assessment; extant and new assessment tools; and novel methods for training a broader range of professionals. These efforts should also examine and address disparities and societal disadvantages that create barriers to timely assessment and intervention.

There have been several recent studies and features regarding health disparities in autism spectrum disorder.[21,101] Bishop-Fitzpatrick's review followed previous work exploring disparities in other aspects of healthcare and indicated that disadvantages may stem from many factors including "race, ethnicity, culture, socioeconomic status, environment, geography, sex, and gender identity."[101,102] Disability status may represent an additional source of societal disadvantage.

Though most clinical and research initiatives have emphasized ways to identify, properly diagnosis, and support children with autism, greater attention is being given to understanding and diagnosing autistic adults than ever before. Please see Mazefsky & White's and Magiati's chapters for more information on adult assessment.[103,104] In addition, as our diagnostic instruments were developed on largely young and male samples, there is still much to learn about the female presentation of autism. Though there are more similarities than differences across gender, it is increasingly clear, that some gender differences are present, and they seem to intensify with age.[105,106]

## Models of assessment

The National Research Council's seminal publication, "Educating Children with Autism,"[107] recommended that evaluations be conducted by a team of experienced professionals, include assessment of multiple domains of functioning, utilize a developmental perspective, and recognize variability of skills across settings. Given the complexity and heterogeneity in the presentation of autism, both across and within individuals, multidisciplinary team assessment has long been recommended as ideal. However, there is little empirical evidence to suggest that this format is more accurate or effective than evaluations involving only one experienced individual clinician who considers multiple areas of functioning.[108] Further, a recent workforce survey regarding developmental-behavioral pediatrics indicated concern that some practice models are "inefficient and unsustainable" in meeting the need for current demands, resulting in lengthy waits, increased patient complexity, and poor reimbursement.[109]

Training a wider range of professionals and developing new types of tools and models of care will likely be needed.[110] For example, telehealth practices involve using videoconference software that allows specialists to provide consultation across geographical distance. The Covid-19 pandemic presented an urgent need for assessment tools that could be reliably and validly administered in socially distanced or remote settings. Though successful models of behavioral intervention and assessment have been described since the onset of available technology, the first systematic evaluation of the accuracy and clinical utility of telehealth assessment for autism was only recently undertaken.[111] Various tools exist for remote assessment of ASD and more are in development.[112–115]

## Summary statement

In summary, autism encompasses a wide variety of symptoms that can vary across and within individuals. Screening and diagnostic evaluation for autism is complex. It is also important to note that ongoing monitoring and reevaluations are valuable for most individuals. Over the last three decades, there has been tremendous progress in the awareness of autism as well empirical evidence regarding assessment and intervention. Notable scientific advances demonstrating the importance of early intervention have recently influenced empirical and clinical efforts serving individuals with autism spectrum disorders. New screening and evaluation tools, and new versions of existing tools, have emerged to facilitate identification of ASD.[8] The current chapter addressed screening for, and evaluation of, ASD as well as some relevant tools and their psychometric properties. Ultimately, the extant knowledge supports the meaningful, sustainable integration of these methods into existing practices and systems. Furthermore, sustainable practices for screening and evaluation must address disparities in healthcare. These developments will contribute to improved outcomes and quality of life for autistic individuals and their families.

# Appendix A

**Commonly used general developmental screening instruments for young children.[a]**

| Measure | Authors | Publication date | Age | Admin time | Completed by |
|---|---|---|---|---|---|
| Ages and Stages Questionnaire (ASQ) | Bricker D, Squires J | 1999 | 1 month of age to 66 months of age for both versions | 10–15 min for administration; 1–3 min for scoring | Parents or caregivers complete; professionals score |
| Ages and Stages Questionnaire (ASQ-3) | Squires J, Bricker D | 2009 | | | |
| Parents' Evaluation of Developmental Status (PEDS) | Glascoe FP | 1998 | Birth to 7 years and 11 months | 2 min or less to administer and score | Parents via questionnaire or interview |
| Communication and Symbolic Behavior Scales Developmental Profile (CSBS-DP) Infant-Toddler Checklist (ITC) | Wetherby A, Prizant B | 2002 | 6 months to 24 months functional communication (6 months to 6 years chronological age) | 5–10 min | Parents or caregivers as well as professionals |

[a] *These are commonly used tools; however, this list is not an endorsement. This table is not designed to be exhaustive.*

# Appendix B

**Commonly used level 1 screening instruments for young children.**[a]

| Measure | Authors | Publication date | Ages | Admin time | Completed by |
|---|---|---|---|---|---|
| Checklist for Autism in Toddlers (CHAT) | Baron-Cohen S, Allen J, Gillberg C | 1992 | 18–24 months of age | 5 min | Parent/caregiver or Physician |
| Modified Checklist for Autism in Toddlers (M-CHAT) | Robins D, Fein D, Barton M | 1999 | 16–30 months of age | 5 min for M-CHAT and M-CHAT-R | Parent/caregiver |
| Modified Checklist for Autism in Toddlers, Revised (M-CHAT-R) | Robins D, Fein D, Barton M | 2001 | | | |
| Pervasive Developmental Disorders Screening Test, Second Edition (PDDST-II) | Siegel B | 2004 | 18–48 months | 15 min to complete; 5 min to score | Parent/caregiver |
| PDDST-I was not published but it was developed in 1993 | | | | | |
| First Year Inventory (FYI) | Reznick JS, Baranek G, Reavis S, Watson LR, Crais ER | 2007 | 12 months of age | Variable (63 items) | Parent/caregiver |
| Early Screening of Autistic Traits (ESAT) | Swinkels SH, Dietz C, van Daalen, E, Kerkhof IH, van Engeland H, Buitelaar JK | 2006 | Designed for birth to 36 months but targets 14 to 15 months of age | 10–15 min | Parent/caregiver with physician |

[a] *These are commonly used tools; however, this list is not an endorsement. This table is not designed to be exhaustive. Please see existing literature, listed in present references and beyond, for additional information regarding available screening tools and their psychometric properties.*[4,7,33,42,44,54]

# Appendix C

**Commonly used level 2 screening instruments for young children.**

| Measure | Authors | Publication date | Ages[a] | Admin time | Completed by |
|---|---|---|---|---|---|
| Modified Checklist for Autism in Toddlers-Revised/ Follow-Up (M-CHAT-R/F) | Robins D, Fein D, Barton M | 2009 | 16–30 months of age | 5 min for M-CHAT-R; 5 min for Follow-up | Parent/ caregiver with medical provider |
| Screening Tool for Autism in Toddlers | Stone WL, Coonrod EE, Ousley OY | 2000 | 24–36 months of age, though research is focusing on 14 months and up | 20 min | Interactive tool for provider and child |
| Systematic Observation of Red Flags (SORF) | Wetherby A, Prizant B | 2002 | 6 months to 24 months functional communication (6 months to 6 years chronological age) | 30–40 min | Observation of interactive tool |
| SCQ (Social Communication Questionnaire) | Rutter M, Bailey A, Lord C | 2003 | Over 4 years with a mental age over 2 years | 10 min | Parents |

[a] *These are commonly used tools; however, this list is not an endorsement. This table is not designed to be exhaustive. Please see existing literature, listed in present references and beyond, for additional information regarding available screening tools and their psychometric properties.*[4,7,33,42,44,54]

# Appendix D

Narrow-band questionnaires used in diagnostic assessment.

| Measure | Authors | Publication date | Ages[a] | Admin time or number of items | Completed by |
|---|---|---|---|---|---|
| Autism Spectrum Ratings Scales (ASRS) | Goldstein S, Naglieri JA | 2009 | 2–18 years | 20 min 4 min for short form | Parents or teachers |
| Autism Spectrum Screening Questionnaire (ASSQ) | Ehlers S, Gillberg C, Wing L | 1999 | 6–17 | 10 min 27 items | Parents or teachers |
| Autism Spectrum Quotient (AQ) | Baron-Cohen S, Wheelwright S, Skinner R et al. | Adult Version: 2001 | Adult form: age 16 + | 50 questions | Self-report |
| | Baron-Cohen S, Hoekstra RA, Knickmeyer R et al. | Adolescent version: 2006 | Adolescent form: ages 9–15 | 50 questions | Self-report |
| Checklist for Autism Spectrum Disorder (CASD) | Mayes S | 2012 | 1–17 years | 15 min | Clinicians |
| Gilliam Autism Rating Scale (GARS) | Gilliam JA | GARS: 1995 GARS-2: 2006 GARS-3: 2013 | 3–22 years | 5–10 min | Parents, teachers, or clinicians |
| PDD Behavior Inventory (PDDBI) | Cohen IL, Sudhalter V | 1999 | 18 months to 18 years 5 months | 20–30 min | Parents or teachers |
| Social Responsiveness Scale (SRS) | Constantino J | SRS: 2005 SRS-2: 2012 | 30 months–Adult | 15–20 min | Parents or teachers Self-report for adults |

[a] *These are commonly used tools; however, this list is not an endorsement. This table is not designed to be exhaustive.*

# References


1. American Academy of Pediatrics, Council on Children With Disabilities, Section on Developmental and Behavioral Pediatrics, Bright Futures Steering Committee, Medical Home Initiatives for Children with Special Needs Project Advisory Committee. Identifying infants and young children with developmental disorders in the medical home: an algorithm for developmental surveillance and screening. *Pediatrics.* 2006;118:405–420. https://doi.org/10.1542/peds.2006-1231.
2. American Academy of Pediatrics, Council on Children With Disabilities. The pediatrician's role in the diagnosis and management of autistic spectrum disorder in children. *Pediatrics.* 2001;107(5):1221–1226. https://doi.org/10.1542/peds.107.5.122.
3. Johnson CP, Myers SM, The Council on Children with Disabilities. Identification and evaluation of children with autism spectrum disorders. *Pediatrics.* 2007;120(5):1183–1215. https://doi.org/10.1542/peds.2007-2361.
4. Hyman SL, Levy SE, Myers SM, The Council on Children with Disabilities. Identification, evaluation, and management of children with autism spectrum disorder. *Pediatrics.* 2020;145(1):e20193447. https://doi.org/10.1542/peds.2019-3447.
5. Gabrielsen TP, Farley M, Speer L, et al. Identifying autism in brief observation. *Pediatrics.* 2015;135(2):e330–e338. https://doi.org/10.1542/peds.2014-1428.
6. Campbell JM, Scheil KA, Hammond RK. Screening methods. In: Matson JL, ed. *Handbook of Assessment and Diagnosis in Autism Spectrum Disorder.* 2016. New York, NY: Springer; 2016:65–86.
7. Zwaigenbaum L, Bauman ML, Fein D, et al. Early screening of autism spectrum disorder: recommendations for practice and research. *Pediatrics.* 2015;136(1):S41–S59. https://doi.org/10.1542/peds.2014-3667D.
8. Ibanez LV, Stone WL, Coonrod EE. Screening for autism in young children. In: Volkmar FR, Paul R, Rogers SJ, Pelphrey K, eds. *Handbook of Autism and Pervasive Developmental Disorders: Assessment, Interventions, and Policy.* vol. 2014. 4th ed. Hoboken, NJ: Wiley; 2014:585–608.
9. Glascoe FP. Screening for developmental and behavioral problems. *Ment Retard Dev Disabil Res Rev.* 2005;11:173–179.
10. Maenner MJ, Shaw KA, Baio J, et al. Prevalence of autism spectrum disorder among children aged 8 years: autism and developmental disabilities monitoring network, 11 sites, United States, 2016. *MMWR Surveill Summ.* 2020;69(SS-4):1–12. https://doi.org/10.15585/mmwr.ss6904a1.
11. Dawson G, Rogers S, Munson J, et al. Randomized controlled trial of an intervention for toddlers with autism: the early Denver start model. *Pediatrics.* 2010;125:e17–e23.
12. Ingersoll B. Brief report: pilot randomized controlled trial of reciprocal imitation training for teaching elicited and spontaneous imitation to children with autism. *J Autism Dev Disord.* 2010;40:1154–1160.
13. Kasari C, Gulsrud AC, Wong C, Kwon S, Locke J. Randomized controlled caregiver mediated joint engagement intervention for toddlers with autism. *J Autism Dev Disord.* 2010;40:1045–1056.
14. Landa R. Efficacy of early interventions for infants and young children with, and at risk for, autism spectrum disorders. *Int Rev Psychiatry.* 2018;30(1):25–39. https://doi.org/10.1080/09540261.2018.1432574.
15. Landa R, Holman KC, O'Neill AH, et al. Intervention targeting development of socially synchronous engagement in toddlers with autism spectrum disorder: a randomized controlled trial. *J Child Psychol Psychiatry.* 2010;52:13–21.
16. Warren Z, McPheeters ML, Sathe N, et al. A systematic review of early intensive intervention for autism spectrum disorders. *Pediatrics.* 2011;127(5):e1303–e1311. https://doi.org/10.1542/peds.2011-0426.

17. Zwaigenbaum L, Bauman ML, Choueiri R, et al. Early intervention for children with autism spectrum disorder under 3 years of age: recommendations for practice and research. *Pediatrics.* 2015;136(1):S60–S81. https://doi.org/10.1542/peds.2014-3667E.
18. Dawson G, Jones EJ, Merkle K, et al. Early behavioral intervention is associated with normalized brain activity in young children with autism. *J Am Acad Child Adolesc Psychiatry.* 2012;51:1150–1159.
19. Barton ML, Dumont-Mathieu T, Fein D. Screening young children for autism spectrum disorders in primary practice. *J Autism Dev Disord.* 2012;42:1165–1175.
20. Chawarska K, Paul R, Klin A, et al. Parental recognition of developmental problems in toddlers with autism spectrum disorders. *J Autism Dev Disord.* 2007;37:62–72. https://doi.org/10.1007/s10803-006-0330-8.
21. Constantino JN, Abbacchi AM, Saulnier C, et al. Timing of diagnosis of autism in african american children. *Pediatrics.* 2020;146(3), e20193629.
22. Zwaigenbaum L, Stone W. Early screening for autism spectrum disorders in clinical practice settings. In: Charman T, Stone W, eds. *Social and Communication Development in Autism Spectrum Disorders: Early Identification, Diagnosis, and Intervention.* New York, NY: Guilford Press; 2006:88–113.
23. Miller JS, Gabrielsen T, Villalobos M, et al. The each child study: systematic screening for autism spectrum disorders in a pediatric setting. *Pediatrics.* 2011;127:866–871.
24. Lipkin PH, Macias MM, Baer B, et al. Trends in pediatricians' developmental screening: 2002-2016. *Pediatrics.* 2020;145(4). https://doi.org/10.1542/peds.2019-0851, e20190851.
25. Lipkin PH, Macias MM, Council on Children with Disabilities. Promoting optimal development: identifying infants and young children with developmental disorders through developmental surveillance and screening. *Pediatrics.* 2020;145(1). https://doi.org/10.1542/peds.2019-3449, e20193449.
26. Bricker D, Squires J. *Ages and Stages Questionnaires.* 2nd ed. Baltimore, MD: Paul H. Brookes; 1999.
27. Squires J, Bricker D. *Ages & Stages Questionnaire: A Parent-Completed Child Monitoring System.* 3rd ed. Baltimore, MD: Paul H. Brookes; 2009.
28. Glascoe FP. *Collaborating with Parents: Using Parents' Evaluation of Developmental Status to Detect and Address Developmental and Behavioral Problems.* Nashville, TN: Ellsworth & Vandermeer; 1998.
29. Glascoe FP. Parents' evaluation of developmental status: how well do parents' concerns identify children with behavioral and emotional problems? *Clin Pediatr.* 2003;42:133–138.
30. Wetherby AM, Prizant B. *Communication and Symbolic Behavior Scales Developmental Profile.* Baltimore, MD: Paul H. Brookes; 2002.
31. Wetherby AM, Woods J, Allen L, et al. Early indicators of autism spectrum disorders in the second year of life. *J Autism Dev Disord.* 2004;34:473–493.
32. Wetherby AM, Brosnan-Maddox S, Peace V, et al. Validation of the infant-toddler checklist as a broad-band screener for autism spectrum disorders from 9 to 24 months of age. *Autism.* 2008;12:487–511.
33. Levy S, Wolfe A, Coury D, et al. Screening tools for autism spectrum disorder in primary care: a systematic evidence review. *Pediatrics.* 2020;145(1):S47. https://doi.org/10.1542/peds.2019-1895H.
34. Pierce K, Carter C, Weinfeld M, et al. Detecting, studying, and treating autism early: the one-year well-baby check-up approach. *Pediatrics.* 2011;159(3):458–465. https://doi.org/10.1016/j.jpeds.2011.02.036.
35. Hirai AH, Kogan MD, Kandasamy V, Reulan C, Bethell C. Prevalence and variation of developmental screening and surveillance in early childhood. *JAMA Pediatr.* 2018;172(9):857–866. https://doi.org/10.1001/jamapediatrics.2018.1524.

36. Arunyanart W, Fenick A, Ukritchon S, et al. Developmental and autism screening: a survey across six states. *Infants Young Child.* 2012;25:175–187.
37. Swanson AR, Warren ZE, Stone WL, et al. The diagnosis of autism in community pediatric settings: does advance training facilitate practice change? *Autism.* 2013;18(5):107. https://doi.org/10.1177/1362361313481507.
38. Warren Z, Stone WL, Humberd Q. A training model for the diagnosis of autism in community pediatric practice. *J Dev Behav Pediatr.* 2009;30:442–446.
39. Oosterling IJ, Wensing M, Swinkels SH, et al. Advancing early detection of autism spectrum disorder by applying an integrated two-stage screening approach. *J Child Psychol Psychiatry.* 2010;51(3):250–258. https://doi.org/10.1111/j.1469-7610.2009.02150.x.
40. Baron-Cohen S, Allen J, Gillberg C. Can autism be detected at 18 months? The need, the haystack, and the CHAT. *Br J Psychiatry.* 1992;161:839–843.
41. Baird G, Charman T, Baron-Cohen S, et al. A screening instrument for autism at 18 months of age. A 6-year follow-up study. *J Am Acad Child Adolesc Psychiatry.* 2000;39:694–702.
42. McPheeters ML, Weitlauf AS, Vehorn A, et al. Screening for autism spectrum disorder in young children: a systematic evidence review for the U.S. Preventive Services Task Force. In: *Evidence Synthesis No. 129. AHRQ Publication No. 13–05185-EF-1.* Rockville, MD: Agency for Healthcare Research and Quality; 2016.
43. Robins DL, Fein D, Barton ML, et al. The modified checklist for autism in toddlers; an initial study investigating the early detection of autism and pervasive developmental disorders. *J Autism Dev Disord.* 2001;31(2):131–144. https://doi.org/10.1023/a:1010738829569.
44. Sanchez-Garcia AB, Galindo-Villardon P, Nieto-Librero AB. Toddler screening for autism spectrum disorder: a meta-analysis of diagnostic accuracy. *J Autism Dev Disord.* 2019;49:1837–1852. https://doi.org/10.1007/s10803-018-03865.
45. Kleinman JM, Robins DL, Ventola PE, et al. The modified checklist for autism in toddlers: a follow-up study investigating the early detection of autism spectrum disorders. *J Autism Dev Disord.* 2008;38:827–839.
46. Pandey J, Verbalis A, Robins DL, et al. Screening for autism in older and younger toddlers with the modified checklist for autism in toddlers. *J Autism Dev Disord.* 2008;35:625–634.
47. Chlebowski C, Robins DL, Barton ML, et al. Large scale use of the modified checklist for autism in low-risk toddlers. *Pediatrics.* 2013;131(4):e1121–e1127. https://doi.org/10.1542/peds.2012-1525.
48. Robins DL. Screening for autism spectrum disorders in primary care settings. *Autism.* 2008;12(5):537–556.
49. Robins DL, Fein D, Barton M. *Modified Checklist for Autism in Toddlers, Revised, with Follow-UP (M-CHAT-R/F) TM;* 2009. Retrieved from https://mchatscreen.com/mchat-rf/.
50. Robins DL, Casagrande K, Barton M, et al. Validation of the modified checklist for Autism in toddlers, revised with follow-up (M-CHAT-R/F). *Pediatrics.* 2014;133(1):37–45. https://doi.org/10.1542/peds.2013-1813.
51. Stone WL, Coonrod EE, Ousley OY. Brief report: screening tool for autism in two-year-olds (STAT): development and preliminary data. *J Autism Dev Disord.* 2000;30(6):607–612. https://doi.org/10.1023/a:1005647629002.
52. Stone WL, Coonrod EE, Turner LM, et al. Psychometric properties of the STAT for early autism screening. *J Autism Dev Disord.* 2004;34(6):691–701. https://doi.org/10.1007/s10803-004-5289-8.
53. Stone WL, McMahon CR, Henderson LM. Use of the screening tool for autism in two-year-olds (STAT) for children under 24 months: an exploratory study. *Autism.* 2008;12(5):557–573. https://doi.org/10.1177/1362361308096403.

54. Brewer N, Young RL, Lucas CA. Autism screening in early childhood: discriminating autism from other developmental concerns. *Front Neurol.* 2020;11. https://doi.org/10.3389/fneur.2020.594381, 594381.
55. Sheridan E, Lord C. Autism spectrum disorders. In: Youngstrom EA, Prinstein MJ, Mash EJ, Barkley RA, eds. *Assessment of Disorders in Childhood and Adolescence.* New York: Guilford Publications; 2020:327–357.
56. Hanley GP. Functional assessment of problem behavior: dispelling myths, overcoming implementation obstacles, and developing new lore. *Behav Anal Pract.* 2012;5:55–72.
57. Iwata BA. Clinical application of functional analysis methodology. *Behav Anal Pract.* 2008;1(1):3–9. https://doi.org/10.1007/BF03391714.
58. American Psychological Association, APA Task Force on Psychological Assessment and Evaluation Guidelines. *APA Guidelines for Psychological Assessment and Evaluation;* 2020. Retrieved from https://www.apa.org/about/policy/guidelines-psychological-assessment-evaluaiton.pdf. Accessed February 10, 2021.
59. Lord C, Corsello C, Grzadzinski R. Diagnostic instruments in autistic spectrum disorders. In: Volkmar FR, Paul R, Rogers SJ, Pelphrey KA, eds. *Handbook of Autism and Pervasive Developmental Disorders.* 4th ed. Hoboken, NJ: Wiley; 2014:610–660. https://doi.org/10.1002/9781118911389.
60. LeCouteur A, Rutter M, Lord C, et al. Autism diagnostic interview: a semistructured interview for parents and caregivers of autistic persons. *J Autism Dev Disord.* 1989;19:363–387.
61. LeCouteur A, Lord C, Rutter M. *Autism Diagnostic Interview-Revised.* Los Angeles, CA: Western Psychological Services; 2003.
62. Tadevosyan-Leyfer O, Dowd M, Mankoski R, et al. A principal components analysis of the autism diagnostic interview-revised. *J Am Acad Child Adolesc Psychiatry.* 2003;42(7):864–872. https://doi.org/10.1097/01.CHI.0000046870.56865.90.
63. De Bildt A, Sytema S, Ketelaars C, et al. Interrelationship between autism diagnostic observation schedule-generic (ADOS-G), autism diagnostic interview revised (ADI-R), and the diagnostic and statistical manual of mental disorders (DSM-IV-TR) classification in children and adolescents with mental retardation. *J Autism Dev Disord.* 2004;34:129–137. https://doi.org/10.1023/B:JADD.0000022604.22374.5f.
64. Randall M, Egberts KJ, Samtani A, et al. Diagnostic tests for autism spectrum disorders (ASD) in preschool children. *Cochrane Database Syst Rev.* 2018;(7). https://doi.org/10.1002/14651858.CD009044.pub2.
65. Kim SH, Lord C. New autism diagnostic interview-revised (ADI-R) algorithms for toddlers and young preschoolers from 12-47 months of age. *J Autism Dev Disord.* 2012;42(1):82–93. https://DOI. https://doi.org/10.1007/s10803-011-1213-1.
66. Wing L, Leekham S, Libby S, et al. Diagnostic interview for social and communication disorders: background, inter-rater reliability and clinical use. *J Child Psychol Psychiatry.* 2002;43:307–325.
67. Wing L. *Diagnostic Interview for Social and Communication Disorders.* 11th ed. Bromly (UK): Centre for Social and Communication Disorders; 2006.
68. Leekam SR, Libby SJ, Wing L, et al. The diagnostic interview for social and communication disorders: algorithms for ICD-10 childhood autism and wing and gould autistic spectrum disorder. *J Child Psychol Psychiatry.* 2002;43(3):327–342. https://doi.org/10.1111/1469-7610.00024.
69. Anglim M, Conway EV, Barry M, et al. An initial examination of the psychometric properties of the diagnostic instrument for social and communication disorders (DISCO-11) in a clinical sample of children with autism spectrum disorder. *Ir J Psychol Med.* 2020;1–10. https://doi.org/10.1017/ipm.2020.100.
70. Skuse D, Warrington R, Bishop D, et al. The developmental, dimensional and diagnostic interview (3di): a novel computerized assessment for autism spectrum

disorders. *J Am Acad Child Adolesc Psychiatry.* 2004;43:48–558. https://doi.org/10.1097/00004583-200405000-00008.
71. Monteiro M, Stegall S. *(MIGDAS-2) Monteiro Interview Guidelines for Diagnosing the Autism Spectrum.* 2nd ed. Los Angeles, CA: Western Psychological Services; 2018.
72. Lord C, Rutter M, Goode S, et al. Autism diagnostic observation schedule: a standardized observation of communicative and social behavior. *J Autism Dev Disord.* 1989;19(2):185–212. https://doi. https://doi.org/10.1007/BF02211841.
73. Gotham K, Risi S, Pickles A, et al. The autism diagnostic observation schedule: revised algorithms for improved diagnostic validity. *J Autism Dev Disord.* 2007;37(4):613–627. https://doi.org/10.1007/s10803-006-0280-1.
74. Lord C, Rutter M, DiLavore PC, et al. *Autism Diagnostic Observation Schedule. 2nd ed. (ADOS-2).* Torrence CA: Western Psychological Services; 2012.
75. Hus V, Lord C. The autism diagnostic observation schedule, module 4: revised algorithm and standardized severity scores. *J Autism Dev Disord.* 2014;44:1996–2012. https://doi.org/10.1007/s10803-014-2080-3.
76. Bal VH, Maye M, Salzman E, et al. The adapted ADOS: a new module set for the assessment of minimally verbal adolescents and adults. *J Autism Dev Disord.* 2020;50(3):719–729.
77. Schopler E, Reichler R, DeVellis R. Toward objective classification of childhood autism: childhood autism rating scale (CARS). *J Autism Dev Disord.* 1980;10:91–103.
78. Perry A, Condillac R, Freeman N, et al. Multi-site study of the childhood autism rating scale (CARS) in five clinical groups of young children. *J Autism Dev Disord.* 2005;35:625–634.
79. Ventola P, Kleinman J, Pandey J, et al. Agreement among four diagnostic instruments for autism spectrum disorders in toddlers. *J Autism Dev Disord.* 2006;36:839–847.
80. Schopler E, Van Bourgondien ME, Wellman GJ, et al. *Childhood Autism Rating Scale.* 2nd ed. Los Angeles, CA: Western Psychological Services; 2010.
81. Risi S, Lord C, Gotham K, et al. Combining information from multiple sources in the diagnosis of autism spectrum disorders. *J Am Acad Child Adolesc Psychiatry.* 2006;45:1094–1103.
82. Kim SH, Lord C. Combining information from multiple sources for the diagnosis of autism spectrum disorders for toddlers and young preschoolers from 12 to 47 months of age. *J Child Psychol Psychiatry.* 2012;53:143–151.
83. Charman T, Pickles A, Simonoff E, et al. IQ in children with autism spectrum disorders: data form the special needs and autism project (SNAP). *Psychol Med.* 2011;41:619–627.
84. Solomon M, Iosif A-M, Reinhardt VP, et al. What will my child's future hold? Phenotypes of intellectual development in 2-8 years olds with autism spectrum disorder. *Autism Res.* 2018;11(1):121–132.
85. Howlin P, Goode S, Hutton J, et al. Adult outcome for children with autism. *J Child Psychol Psychiatry.* 2004;45:212–229.
86. Howlin P, Savage S, Moss P, et al. Cognitive and language skills in adults with autism: a 40-year follow-up. *J Child Psychol Psychiatry.* 2014;55:49–58.
87. American Psychiatric Association. *Diagnostic and Statistical Manual of Mental Disorders.* 5th ed. Arlington VA: American Psychiatric Association; 2013.
88. *Frequently Asked Questions on Intellectual Disability and the AAIDD Definition.* American Association on Intellectual and Developmental Disabilities (AAIDD) Website; 2008. https://www.aaidd.org/docs/default-source/sis-docs/aaiddfaqonid_template.pdf?sfvrsn=9a63a874_2. Published. Accessed January 20, 2021.
89. Mouga S, Almeida J, Café C, et al. Adaptive profiles in autism and other neurodevelopmental disorders. *J Autism Dev Disord.* 2015;45:1001–1012.
90. Sparrow SS, Cicchetti DV, Saulnier CA. *The Vineland Adaptive Behavior Scales.* 3rd ed. Minneapolis, MN: Pearson Assessments; 2016.

91. Harrison P, Oakland T. *Adaptive Behavior Assessment System.* 3rd ed. Torrance, CA: Western Psychological Services; 2015.
92. Deprey L, Ozonoff S. Assessment of comorbid psychiatric conditions in autism spectrum disorder. In: Goldstein S, Ozonoff S, eds. *Assessment of Autism Spectrum Disorder.* New York: Guilford Press; 2018:308–337.
93. Gjevik E, Eldevik S, Fjaeran-Granum T, et al. Kiddie-SADS reveals high rates of DSM-IV disorders in children and adolescents with autism spectrum disorders. *J Autism Dev Disord.* 2011;41:761–769.
94. Simonoff E, Pickles A, Charman T, et al. Psychiatric disorders in children with autism spectrum disorders: prevalence, comorbidity, and associated factors in a population-derived sample. *J Am Acad Child Adolesc Psychiatry.* 2008;47:921–929.
95. Abdallah MW, Greaves-Lord K, Grove J, et al. Psychiatric comorbidities in autism spectrum disorders: findings from a Danish historic birth cohort. *Eur Child Adolesc Psychiatry.* 2011;20:599–601.
96. Coury D, Jones NE, Klatka K, et al. Healthcare for children with autism: the autism treatment network. *Curr Opin Pediatr.* 2009;21:828–832.
97. Field D, Garland M, Williams K. Correlates of specific childhood feeding problems. *J Paediatr Child Health.* 2003;39:299–304.
98. Huerta M, Lord C. Diagnostic evaluation of autism spectrum disorders. *Pediatr Clin N Am.* 2012;59(1):103–111. https://doi.org/10.1016/j.pcl.2011.10.018.
99. Holliday EL, Stanley HC, Fodstad JC, et al. Stress and satisfaction in the diagnostic process. In: Matson JL, ed. *Handbook of Assessment and Diagnosis of Autism Spectrum Disorder.* New York: Springer; 2016:137–155.
100. Kanne SM, Bishop SL. Editorial perspective: the autism waitlist crisis and remembering what families need. *J Child Psychol Psychiatry.* 2021;62(2):140–142. https://doi.org/10.1111/jcpp.13254.
101. Bishop-Fitzpatrick L, Kind AJH. A scoping review of health disparities in autism spectrum disorder. *J Autism Dev Disord.* 2017;47(11):3380–3391. https://doi.org/10.1007/s10803-017-3251-9.
102. Hill CV, Perez-Stable EJ, Anderson NA, et al. The national institute on aging health disparities research framework. *Ethn Dis.* 2015;25(3):245–254. https://doi.org/10.18865/ed.25.3.245.
103. Mazefsky CA, White SW. Adults with autism. In: Volkmar FR, Paul R, Rogers SJ, Pelphrey K, eds. *Handbook of Autism and Pervasive Developmental Disorders.* 4th ed. Hoboken, NJ: Wiley; 2014:191–211.
104. Magiati I. Assessment in adulthood. In: Matson JL, ed. *Handbook of Assessment and Diagnosis of Autism Spectrum Disorder.* New York: Springer; 2016:191–207.
105. Kaat AJ, Shui AM, Ghods SS, et al. Sex differences in scores on standardized measures of autism symptoms: a multisite integrative data analysis. *J Child Psychol Psychiatry.* 2021;62:97–106.
106. Van Wijngaarden-Cremers PJM, van Eeten E, Groen WB, et al. Gender and age differences in the core triad of impairments in autism spectrum disorders: a systemic review and meta-analysis. *J Autism Dev Disord.* 2014;44:627–635.
107. National Research Council. Educating children with autism. Committee on educational interventions for children with autism. In: Lord C, McGee JP, eds. *Division of Behavioral and Social Sciences and Education.* Washington, DC: National Academy Press; 2001.
108. Penner M, Anagnostou E, Andoni LY, et al. Systematic review of clinical guidance documents for autism spectrum disorder diagnostic assessment in select regions. *Autism.* 2018;22:517–527.
109. Bridgemohan C, Bauer NS, Nielsen BA, et al. A workforce survey on developmental-behavioral pediatrics. *Pediatrics.* 2018;141(3). https://doi.org/10.1542/peds.2017-2164, e20172164.

110. Zwaigenbaum L, Warren Z. Commentary: embracing innovation is necessary to improve assessment and care for individuals with ASD: a reflection on kanne and bishop (2020). *J Child Psychol Psychiatry.* 2021;62(2):143–145. doi. https://doi.org/10.1111/jcpp.13291.
111. Juarez AP, Weitlauf AS, Nicholson A, et al. Early identification of ASD through telemedicine: potential value for underserved populations. *J Autism Dev Disord.* 2018;48:2601.
112. Corona L, Weitlauf AS, Hine J, et al. Parent perceptions of caregiver-mediated telemedicine tools for assessing autism risk in toddlers. *J Autism Dev Disord.* 2021;51:476–486.
113. Smith C, Rozga A, Matthews N, et al. Investigating the accuracy of a novel telehealth diagnostic approach for autism spectrum disorder. *Psychol Assess.* 2017;29(3):245–252.
114. *Brief Observation of Symptoms of Autism (BOSA) Training by Dr. Catherine Lord's Lab. [Video].* UCLA CART Website; 2020. https://www.semel.ucla.edu/autism/bosa-training. Published June 29. Accessed January 28, 2021.
115. Talbott MR, Dufek S, Zwaigenbaum L, et al. Brief report: preliminary feasibility of the TEDI: a novel parent-administered telehealth assessment for autism spectrum disorder symptoms in the first year of life. *J Autism Dev Disord.* 2020;50(9):3432–3439. https://doi.org/10.1007/s10803-019-04314-4.

CHAPTER

# 4

# Social, cognitive, perceptual, and other models of autism spectrum disorder

*Meagan E. Beckerson*[a], *Kaitlyn E. May*[b], *and Rajesh K. Kana*[a]

[a]**Department of Psychology, The Center for Innovative Research in Autism, University of Alabama, Tuscaloosa, AL, United States,** [b]**Department of Educational Studies in Psychology, Research Methodologies, and Counseling, University of Alabama, Tuscaloosa, AL, United States**

## Introduction

The phenotype of a complex disorder like autism spectrum disorder (ASD) is diverse and multidimensional, with substantial heterogeneity in its symptomatology. This makes it challenging to generate an overarching theoretical model that can explain the core and extended symptoms of ASD. Unpacking the defining features of ASD (deficits in social communication; repetitive/restricted patterns of behaviors and interests) will open up an array of functions and skills people with ASD usually struggle with. However, the past few decades of behavioral, neuropsychological, and neurobiological research have provided many compelling hypotheses to explain the etiology of ASD and its diverse set of cognitive, social, and behavioral symptoms. While any of these models may not be enough in itself to explain the breadth of symptoms in ASD, this chapter attempts to bring these models together, to identify their relative strengths and weaknesses, and to understand the emerging consensus across them. We discuss the following 10 theoretical models that have illuminated socio-cognitive and behavioral research in autism: (1) theory-of-mind deficit hypothesis; (2) executive dysfunction hypothesis; (3) complex information


https://doi.org/10.1016/B978-0-12-816393-1.00005-1

processing deficit hypothesis; (4) weak central coherence hypothesis; (5) enhanced perceptual functioning hypothesis; (6) temporal binding deficit hypothesis; (7) social motivation hypothesis; (8) extreme male brain hypothesis; (9) Bayesian priors hypothesis; and (10) audio multisensory integration deficit hypothesis.

## Theory-of-mind deficit hypothesis

One of the major building blocks of human social cognition is our ability to read other people's minds. Social cognition entails a set of processes that allow us to communicate and build relationships with others, which is often difficult for people with ASD. A critical aspect of social cognition is theory-of-mind (ToM) or "mentalizing,"[1] which involves recognizing that other people may have beliefs, intentions, desires, or emotions that differ from our own.[1] Basic ToM is typically acquired between 3 and 5 years of age, but continues to develop through adulthood.[2] Children with ASD are often reported to have an impaired ToM.[2] The ToM deficit hypothesis suggests that ToM deficits, or "mindblindness," may explain the array of social symptoms of ASD, such as poor social judgment, paucity of social interaction, and emotional indifference. Signs of impaired ToM can be observed early in development through basic child-caregiver interactions. For example, *joint attention*, identified as early as 3 months of age, describes two or more people orienting to the same object or event.[3] Children who later develop ASD engage in joint attention behaviors less frequently than typically-developing (TD) children, including fewer instances of orienting to their name, initiating joint-attention, and responding to joint attention cues.[4,5] As responding to and initiating joint attention require a basic understanding of intentionality and perspectives, these deficits are considered a sign of poor ToM. Joint interactions also help infants make word-object associations[6] and is predictive of later language development.[3,7] Proper language development, which is commonly delayed or impaired in many children with ASD,[8] is therefore necessary for achieving ToM. Pretend play is also thought to facilitate ToM development through imagination and role-playing.[2] Children with ASD engage in pretend play less often than TD children, and tend to engage in stereotyped or realistic play rather than symbolic play.[9] In addition, skills such as autobiographical memory, working memory, and generating event schemas are employed in ToM.

ToM is commonly assessed with the canonical Sally-Anne Test,[10] in which a child must demonstrate their understanding that other people have beliefs that contrast with reality (false beliefs), or have different perspectives than their own. In this task, children observe a social scenario in which a character (Sally) puts a marble in a red box and leaves the room.

Another character, Anne, moves the marble from the red box to a blue box while Sally is away. The child is asked where Sally would search for the item upon her return. To pass this task, the child must understand that Sally would not know that Anne moved the item, and should thus choose the red box, rather than the blue box. Children with ASD are often unable to demonstrate ToM skills at the appropriate age. For example, TD children tend to pass the Sally-Anne test by age 4 or 5,[11] while most children with ASD fail this task or pass at a later age.[1,12] Impaired ToM is also seen in more advanced versions of this task. Second-order false belief tasks, which require an understanding of two people's perspectives, is typically mastered by 6 years of age, but not achieved until the teenage years for those with ASD.[2] Children are typically able to recognize faux pas, which are embarrassing or awkward moments in a social situation, between ages 9 and 11, whereas children with ASD cannot do so at this age.[13] Poor performance on ToM tasks is also accompanied by lower activation and functional connectivity among relevant brain regions.[14] Collectively, these data provide converging evidence for a core deficit in ToM that may underlie social difficulties in individuals with ASD.

Although the ToM deficit hypothesis is well-replicated and explains social deficits in ASD relatively well, it does not address other defining symptoms of ASD, nor does it explain skill assets in ASD.[15,16] Additionally, ToM deficits are not always seen in ASD,[16] and occur in other conditions such as Down syndrome, Prader-Willi syndrome, cerebral palsy, Fragile X, and epilepsy.[17] Language and executive function (EF) impairments in ASD may also underlie poor performance on ToM tasks since they involve complex language and integration of information across multiple levels.

## EF dysfunction hypothesis

EFs are a set of higher-order skills that regulate cognition to achieve goals. These functions include planning, working memory, inhibitory control, and mental flexibility. Deficits in EF are extensively documented in the ASD literature.[18,19] The EF Dysfunction Model of ASD suggests that impairments in EF are responsible for many of the core characteristics of ASD, such as rigidity and perseveration, repetitive actions, and social impairments.[19,20] Recent work also suggests a broader influence of EF affecting social cognition, mental health, disability, and quality of life. However, there is substantial interindividual variability in EF performance in ASD, reflective of the diverse cognitive and neurological profiles of the disorder. While there seems to be general EF dysfunction in ASD, the nature and magnitude of such differences is dependent on several factors such as tasks, level of functioning, age at assessment, specific executive skill measured, and even task instructions (explicit vs implicit).

We discuss the primary EF domains that are relatively well-studied in ASD. (1) *Planning and Problem Solving*: Planning requires the individual to monitor, reevaluate, and update a sequence of actions. Individuals with ASD demonstrate impairments in traditional tests of planning (e.g., Tower of Hanoi, Tower of London)[21,22]; however, performance on more novel tasks (e.g., reach-to-grasp tasks, Maze subtests of the Wechsler Intelligence Scale for Children, parent/teacher reports) suggests a lack of universality in planning deficits.[20,23] Thus, it is possible that there may not be a global impairment in planning in ASD, but that deficits occur when the task complexity increases. Alternatively, it may be that deficits in planning are indicative of general intellectual functioning and maturation, rather than ASD symptomatology. Planning or problem solving impairments may manifest as difficulty starting, organizing, monitoring, or completing tasks; difficulty solving problems; inability to balance tasks; problems managing time; or difficulty managing social situations. (2) *Cognitive Flexibility*: Cognitive flexibility (CF) is the ability to shift between tasks or thoughts in accordance with task demands. Both children[24,25] and adults[26] with ASD show impairments in performance on the Wisconsin Card Sort Task (WCST), a traditional test of CF,[27] but no impairments on other measures of CF.[28,29] This may be because of the complex cognitive demands of the WCST, as it fails to provide explicit task instructions and requires multiple additional cognitive processes and a higher degree of disengagement. Impairments in CF may result in difficulty transitioning between tasks; trouble controlling impulses; or rigidity in thoughts and behaviors. (3) *Inhibitory Control*: Deficits in IC vary based on the type of IC assessed. Individuals with ASD show impairments in prepotent response inhibition[30,31]; however, tasks assessing interference control typically show no deficits.[32,33] Likewise, ASD children and adolescents succeed at tasks assessing interference inhibition, such as the Stroop task.[32,33] Individuals with ASD may fail to demonstrate an IC deficit so long as task rules are strictly defined and the developmental age of the participant is 6 years or older.[24] Deficits, if any, in IC may appear as an inability to control emotions or impulses; trouble listening or paying attention, socially inappropriate behavior, emotional outbursts or meltdowns, or hand flapping/stimming. Another line of evidence for the EF dysfunction hypothesis of ASD comes from alterations in the prefrontal cortex (PFC) responses and its connectivity with the rest of the executive control network.[34–36] Cortical and subcortical differences,[37,38] as well as delayed maturation of the frontal lobes,[39] structural abnormalities, and abnormalities in total brain volume[40] have been cited. In addition, abnormalities of the frontoparietal network are suggested to underlie autism symptomatology, particularly EF impairments.[41] Still, there is a large amount of variability in this body of work, perhaps reflecting the heterogeneity of ASD and the comorbidity of EF impairments in other neurodevelopmental disorders. While this variability may partially explain the vast heterogeneity in the manifestation of ASD, it also limits the universality of the EF dysfunction hypothesis as an explanatory model of ASD.[42]

## Complex information processing difficulty hypothesis

During the mid-1990s, the emerging consensus was that multiple cognitive deficits characterized ASD, and subsequent research sought to identify a common underlying pattern in diverse impairments that would better inform understanding of ASD. The largest and most comprehensive of these studies purported that ASD is the result of an impairment in processing complex tasks, deemed the complex information processing difficulty hypothesis of ASD.

This model was initially developed through a neuropsychological profile study of 33 high-functioning adolescents and adults with ASD and matched TD controls.[43] This study examined whether a wide range of impairments (e.g., sensory perceptual, attention, memory, language) presented individually, as single primary deficits, or as comorbid features in ASD. Assessments included simple attention (3 tests), complex attention (2 tests) immediate memory (9 tests), delayed memory (7 tests), formal language (3 tests), pragmatic language (4 tests), and abstract (7 tests). Results suggested reliable differences between tests of complex memory and problem-solving that required language, and tests of simple or complex attention, associative memory, attribute identification, or rule-learning aspects of abstract reasoning. The authors suggested that the commonality of these deficits was higher processing demands, as all intact abilities were low-level cognitive or neurological processes that did not place a large demand on cognition. Thus, the study suggested that ASD is not the result of a single, primary deficit but a wide range of deficits in multiple domains.

The complex information processing difficulty hypothesis proposes that ASD is the result of a selective impairment in cognitive and neural processing of complex information.[44,45] Here, *complex* refers to the level or type of demand inherent to task processing, not the information itself. Specifically, this model suggests that individuals with ASD show deficits in cognitive processing of complex information across domains and sensory modalities, such that cognitive functions are compromised when processing demands exceed neural capacity. Support for this model comes from a multitude of studies indicating poorer performance in individuals with ASD on complex or higher order tasks that are within the range of their general ability, exhibiting selective impairments that are not explained by general ability. In addition, research showing that individuals with ASD are successful in performing simpler skills in the same domain provides further support for this model. Thus, cognitive impairments in

ASD are indicative of weakness in neural processing mechanisms, not with a particular type of information.

In sum, the complex information processing difficulty hypothesis of ASD unifies the syndrome at a clinical level. This suggests that the neural basis of ASD is the underdevelopment of connectivity (coordinated/synchronized brain activity) within and between systems that underlie complex information processing demands. Several neuroimaging studies provided support for this model finding functional underconnectivity across brain regions involved in handling higher computational demands, such as sentence comprehension,[46] problem-solving,[47] social cognition,[48] response inhibition,[36] and narrative comprehension.[49] Collectively, these studies indicate that individuals with ASD increasingly struggle as information-processing demands increase due to less coordinated and less efficient allocation of neural resources.

## Weak central coherence (WCC) hypothesis

The weak central coherence (WCC) hypothesis[50] suggests that individuals with ASD are better at processing local information, such as component details of stimuli, and struggle to combine information into a unified meaning—an aspect of typical information-processing called central coherence.[50] For example, individuals with ASD may perform better and faster, than their TD peers, in spotting Waldo in the *Where's Waldo* illustrations (a series of children's puzzle books created by English illustrator Martin Handford). Increased focus on the visual perception of details along with weak central coherence in ASD individuals may be an advantage in doing such tasks.

Supporting evidence for the WCC hypothesis includes a *strength model* and a *deficit model*. According to the strength model, individuals with ASD are better at processing component details, or local information, translating to superior performance on low-level visual tasks. For example, children with ASD tend to outperform TD children on the Embedded Figures Task (EFT) which requires identifying smaller, simple shapes that are embedded in an image of a larger object, and the Block Design subtest of Wechsler Intelligence Tests, which involves constructing a complex design with individual blocks.[51] The deficit model posits that weak coherence is detrimental to tasks requiring higher-level, holistic perception, explaining impaired global processing in ASD. For example, children with ASD tend to encode faces feature-by-feature rather than using a holistic, configural approach.[52] Additionally, when shown an image of a larger letter constructed from a series of smaller letters (for example, capital letter H made out of a set of small letter s), individuals with ASD have difficulty reporting the larger letter.[53] This cognitive pattern may also play a role in restricted, repetitive behaviors such as being routine-oriented or preoccupied with specific toy parts. People with ASD have been found to show lower prefrontal cortex involvement during EF tasks[54,55] as well as greater activity in relatively posterior brain regions during the block design task,[54] which may represent either a greater role of perceptual processes or atypical frontal processing, or weaker frontal-posterior connectivity that results in the increased/compensatory recruitment of posterior resources. Too many brain areas responding in an isolated fashion, but not in cohesion, may be a neural analog to WCC.

The WCC hypothesis[50] was adapted after contradictory findings such as instances of intact global processing in ASD, global biases, and the ability to overcome local biases when global processing is explicitly instructed.[53] O'Riordan and Plaisted[56] alternatively proposed that those with ASD have a detail-focused cognitive processing approach rather than a deficit in processing global information. Reduced central coherence, or generalization, may then occur as a secondary outcome of enhanced local processing.

Whether WCC sufficiently explains the array of social symptoms of ASD, or if it is an independent deficit, are topics of debate. The linked deficit hypothesis[57,58] suggests that WCC mediates ToM deficits; thus, people with ASD fail false-belief tasks because they focus on where the item's current location is, failing to grasp the "big picture."[50,57] Alternatively, the independent cognitive deficit hypothesis suggests that WCC and ToM deficits coexist separately.[51,58] In other words, WCC is a cognitive abnormality that does not necessarily explain social aspects of ASD, but is present nonetheless. WCC has also been considered a consequence, or aspect, of poor EF. For example, it is possible that WCC occurs due to an inability to flexibly switch between local and global processing.[53] WCC model is limited because it is not a comprehensive account of the social and communicative deficits in ASD, despite associations with ToM.[59] Additionally, this hypothesis is more descriptive than explanatory, as it does not provide a mechanistic or neurological explanation for why these biases may occur.

## Enhanced perceptual functioning hypothesis

In response to the WCC model,[60] Mottron and Burack (2001) proposed the enhanced perceptual functioning (EPF) hypothesis to provide a framework to understand the perceptual abilities of individuals on the spectrum.[61] EPF proposes that the unique symptomatology of ASD is in consequence to superior function and increased independence of auditory and visual perceptual processes. Specifically, EPF argues that individuals with ASD have superior perceptual abilities, including feature detection, pattern recognition, one-dimensional discrimination, and recognition of visual patterns, above social and higher order cognitive processes in ASD. This superior attention to perceptual information impedes higher-order cognitive operations, making perceptual processes difficult to control and possibly disruptive of other behaviors. Still, the superior perceptual abilities can also be adaptive, for example, providing a compensatory role in sensory deprivation.[62]

The EPF hypothesis proposes eight principles that guide the perception in ASD. They are: (1) The default setting of autistic perception is more locally oriented than that of nonautistics; (2) Increased gradient of neural complexity is inversely related to the level of performance in low-level perceptual tasks. According to this principle, the superior performance in ASD may not be universal. While superior performance may be seen in static, simple discrimination tasks, that is not the case in dynamic and complex tasks in both visual and auditory modalities; (3) Early atypical behaviors have a regulatory function toward perceptual input. Early perceptual behaviors like lateral glances in ASD children may be attempts to limit otherwise excessive amounts of information; (4) Perceptual primary and associative brain regions are atypically activated during social and nonsocial tasks, specifically in relatively posterior areas of the brain and in more anterior association cortex in ASD; (5) Higher-order processing is optional in autism and mandatory in nonautistics; (6) Perceptual expertise underlies savant syndrome; (7) Savant syndrome is an autistic model for subtyping pervasive developmental disorders (PDD); and (8) Enhanced functioning of primary perceptual brain regions may account for autistic perceptual atypicalities. The EPF model is supported by research documenting enhanced visual functioning across multiple tasks[63] as well as increased brain activity in areas of the brain used in pattern processing.[64] Moreover, research indicating increased gray matter in perceptual areas, and increased cortical thickness in the visual and primary auditory cortices[65,66] lend further support to the model.[66]

## Temporal binding deficit hypothesis

The temporal binding deficit hypothesis[52] was proposed as a mechanistic explanation of the WCC hypothesis. The brain is composed of specialized regions that coactivate when performing a task. As central coherence involves assimilating information to derive a unified meaning,[50] the temporal binding deficit hypothesis suggests that poorly integrating activity from different neural networks underlies WCC. Thus, the local advantages in visual perception tasks typically observed in ASD may be a result of poorly integrating local features.

It is important to note that this refers to binding *between* networks, not *within*.[52] Neural networks arise from **segregation** (decreases in long-range connections) and **integration** (increases in short-range connections) in the brain.[67] As the human neonatal brain becomes more specialized (segregated) over time, the integration of activity across networks becomes increasingly important. Alternatively, brain regions in ASD are thought to become more isolated over time, with insufficient long-range connections and excessive short-range connections.[52,67] Such a profile may lead to decreased functional efficiency, especially in handling higher computational demand.

The *binding problem* is the question of *how* exactly different brain regions interact and assimilate information from one another.[52] One solution to this problem is **temporal binding**, which suggests that object feature combinations are represented in the brain by different neurons that fire simultaneously. For example, a neuron would fire for "shape" at the same time as another neuron fires for "orientation" during visual processing. Deficits in temporal binding would force the individual to rely on combination coding (particular neurons exist for each combination of object features, such as a single neuron firing for each "shape" and "orientation" pair), considered another "solution" to the binding problem.

Impaired temporal binding is considered responsible for deficits in multisensory processing seen in ASD.[52,68] The *multisensory temporal binding window*, the span of time in which sensory information is combined into single perceptual experience, is considered to be prolonged in ASD,[69] which may explain superior perceptual discrimination.[61] For example, individuals with ASD are less-susceptible to the "flash-beep" illusion, where increasing the number of beeps elicited with a single visual flash stimulus tends to lead to the illusion of multiple flashes.[69] Temporal binding deficits may also explain other symptoms of ASD such as cognitive inflexibility and social impairment, as these tasks require assimilating several pieces of information. While prefrontal brain regions play a role in completing these types of tasks, integration with the parietal cortex is critical. Therefore, poor integration across these regions could result in cognitive and behavioral inflexibility.

## Social-motivation hypothesis

Social motivation involves social orienting (expressed preference for the social world), social reward (finding social experience and social interaction rewarding), and social maintaining (working to develop and maintain social bonds). The social motivation hypothesis posits that disinterest in social experiences early in life impairs the development of the social brain network.[70,71] Specifically, it suggests that because individuals with ASD are less interested in social information from a young age (e.g., gaze, faces), they often have less opportunities for social learning (e.g., decreased engagement in joint attention, collaborative play, friendships), which impairs their social development. It is argued that this altered development of the social brain network (i.e., the amygdala, striatum, orbital-frontal cortex, fusiform face area, inferior frontal gyrus, posterior superior temporal sulcus, and superior frontal gyrus) plays a key role in the social and emotional difficulties in ASD.[72] These impairments result in a lack of attention toward the social environment, resulting in a failure to develop socioemotional cognitive skills.[73,74]

Behavioral evidence supporting the social motivation hypothesis demonstrates that infants and adults with ASD attend less to people and more to background objects,[75] show preference for nonsocial over social sounds,[76] demonstrate poorer friendship quality, develop ToM skills later, and show social cognition impairments into adulthood.[77] In addition, individuals with ASD often hyper-focus on nonsocial stimuli that are disregarded by TD individuals.[78,79] However, neural evidence assessing the social motivation hypothesis is mixed. Whereas some studies indicate hyperactivation of brain areas associated with reward processing while viewing faces,[80] others show hypoactivation.[81,82] Still, a recent meta-analysis of these studies found that across existing studies, individuals with ASD showed aberrant processing of both social and nonsocial rewards.[83] Despite the findings supporting the social motivation hypothesis, social disinterest is not limited to individuals with ASD.[84,85] Moreover, within ASD these behaviors may often be used as compensatory mechanisms (e.g., a lack of eye contact aids concentration) and therefore may not reflect social disinterest, but a need to offload the processing demands of social interaction.

## Extreme male brain hypothesis

Recent estimates of the prevalence rate of ASD indicate that the sex ratio of diagnoses is around 3:1 (male:female).[86] This male-biased prevalence may provide insights into the etiology of ASD. The extreme male brain (EMB) hypothesis suggests that ASD is a case of exaggerated male sex differences in brain and behavior.[87] In the last two decades, factors that tend to show sex differences in the general population have been examined in the context of ASD and provide support for the EMB theory.

For example, the empathizing/systemizing (E-S) hypothesis of typical sex differences posits that females have a tendency to identify, understand, and share others' feelings (empathize), while males are driven to analyze and understand the underlying rules that direct behavior (systemize).[87] When the ability to empathize exceeds the ability to systemize, one is considered to have a "female" brain, while one with a more well-developed ability to systemize is considered to have a "male" brain.[87] People with

ASD tend to score higher on the Systemizing Quotient (SQ) and lower on the Empathizing Quotient (EQ) than TD individuals.[87] Additionally, superior performance on Embedded Figures Tasks in ASD requires systemizing components such as attention to detail and show male performance biases in the general population.[87] Collectively, these data suggest that people with ASD have intensified male-patterns of behavior regarding empathy and analytical thinking.

Neuroimaging studies have revealed unique neuroanatomical patterns in typical males and females that apply to the EMB model as well, including larger total brain volumes and smaller volumes of the posterior region of the corpus callosum.[88] Typical males also tend to show greater growth of the amygdala during childhood, which is pronounced in ASD.[89] Both males and females with ASD also show the typical male developmental trajectory of interhemispheric functional connectivity.[90] Additionally, fetal testosterone (fT), the hormone that influences the development of the male phenotype, is found to be negatively associated with eye contact, vocabulary, and empathy in early childhood.[88] fT is also positively correlated with systemizing and performance on EFT tasks, more autistic traits, left-handedness, and heavier brain weight.[88] As these factors are common characteristics of ASD, increased exposure to fT in-utero may have a role in the development of ASD.

Although supported by different sources of correlational evidence (not causation), many females with ASD are un-diagnosed, calling the current diagnostic sex-ratio into question.[91] In addition, the "extreme" male patterns seen in ASD are not a great deal different than the patterns seen in typical males. Whether this hypothesis merely reflects more males being diagnosed with ASD is a question of debate.

## Bayesian priors hypothesis: Perception as inference

While many theoretical models discussed above are trying to explain specific symptoms of ASD, a more recently-developed model, the *Bayesian brain* perspective,[92] offers a unified explanation of ASD. *Bayesian* describes a method of statistical inference in which causes of events are given probabilities based on prior and current evidence. This framework has been used to describe the processes of perception and cognition, as the brain must constantly extract meaning from various sensory signals, or "noise." The brain continually hypothesizes the causes of events or sensory inputs based on both previous knowledge (*top-down processing*) and current sensory information (*bottom-up processing*) in order to predict, make sense of, and regulate its environment.[93] Deviations in this process may underlie the perceptual, social, and repetitive behavior symptoms of ASD.[92]

The Bayesian Brain hypothesis describes perception as an automatic, computational process in which the causes of sensory input, or events in the environment, are first assigned probabilities based on prior experiences—a *prior probability*.[92] In terms of cognition, this is conceptualized as an expectation. Prior probabilities are then changed to *posterior probabilities* in response to data (i.e., experience). Given prior knowledge, posterior probabilities (i.e., beliefs) reflect inferences of the most likely cause of the experience. This process occurs at many timescales and across several modes such as visual patterns and facial expressions.[94] An example of a perceptual prior is the effect of visual illusions, such that our a priori perceptual experiences and understanding of the physical environment guide our current perceptions.[95] Individuals with ASD are believed to generate *hypo-priors*, in which the top-down influence of prior expectations on perception is reduced, causing greater reliance on bottom-up processing.[96]

Hypo-priors are considered to underlie both social and nonsocial symptoms of ASD.[92] For example, those with ASD are thought to struggle with using previous experience to guide social interactions and understand others' intentions.[96] Additionally, as weak priors cause more weight to be placed on bottom-up processing, the intensity of sensory stimuli is enhanced, which may explain hyper-sensitivity to stimuli such as loud noises in ASD.[92] This may also explain why those with ASD have difficulty adapting to certain stimuli or environments, as they struggle to predict incoming sensory input.[92] Repetitive behaviors and insistence on sameness could therefore serve as a protective mechanism against weak priors that provide a sense of control over their sensory experiences. This hypothesis, however, was developed post hoc to explain years of cognitive research, and a priori empirical tests of this model yield mixed results.

## Multisensory integration deficit hypothesis

Research has identified a variety of impairments in sensory processing in ASD, including abnormalities in sensory modulation,[97] preferential reliance on proximal senses,[98] a dominance of somatosensory stimuli,[98] overselectivity in response to a single aspect of an object,[99,100] and less benefit from visual cues than TD peers.[98] During the 1980s to 1990s, focus shifted toward deficits in higher-order cognitive functions, which reduced the attention toward deficits in sensory processing, diminishing research in this area. Recent years have generated renewed interest in sensory processing[101,102] and unisensory detection and discrimination in ASD.[65,103,104] One aspect of sensory processing that appears to be impaired in ASD is multisensory integration (MSI), or the ability to integrate sensory information from multiple modalities. Difficulty integrating sensory information may underlie many symptoms of ASD, such as sensory hyper- and hypo-sensitivities. A lack of MSI may affect development in a variety of ways, potentially including the vast social, communication, and various other symptoms of ASD.[105]

Multiple studies document impairments in audiovisual MSI in ASD. Support for this hypothesis stems from research demonstrating impaired temporal asynchrony judgments for linguistic stimuli,[106] differential responses to incongruent speech compared to TD controls,[107] diminished multisensory facilitation in reaction time,[108] and less influence of visual speech on auditory speech processing.[109] Collectively, these findings suggest that individuals with ASD may have selective deficits in integrating information across multiple sensory modalities.[110]

Still, there is a lack of agreement in this literature. For example, group differences are often inconsistent, with some research reporting superior performance in ASD participants relative to TD peers in a variety of MSI tasks.[111,112] Likewise, there is disagreement regarding the correlation of MSI with other impairments in ASD. MSI has been shown to be correlated with language,[113] communication skill,[113,114] and broader ASD symptom severity,[115,116] suggesting that audiovisual MSI may be inherently linked to ASD and related symptomatology. Other studies fail to document significant correlations.[117–120]

Few studies have examined MSI networks and MSI integration in ASD. Existing studies suggest that whereas TD individuals show enhanced neural response to multisensory information, individuals with ASD do not. This suggests a lack of neural integration of MSI stimuli could underlie some of the social and cognitive deficits observed in ASD.[121] Moreover, it may be that individuals with ASD activate different processing networks despite similar performance.[122] Future work systematically examining differences in activation during MSI compared to unisensory processing is needed.

## Conclusion

Finding overarching causal explanations for the vast array of behavioral symptoms in a disorder like ASD is a difficult task. Moreover, this becomes more challenging considering the multidimensional profile of ASD and its widespread heterogeneity. This chapter outlined many prevailing etiological hypotheses of autism, some of which address symptoms independently, while others theorize a unified explanation for a collection of symptoms. Finding a global and unifying explanation for a complex disorder like ASD may be arguably impossible. Rather, considering multiple explanatory models at cognitive, social, perceptual, and neural levels allows us to acknowledge the variability of the biological causes, severity, and presentation of symptoms in ASD. The hypotheses discussed in this chapter are called hypotheses for a reason. They are not well-established theories and hence they provide promising directions in explaining the complex profile of ASD. They have ultimately guided research in the field and have improved understanding of the cognitive and behavioral mechanisms that characterize this disorder (Table 1).

**TABLE 1** Table showing the summary of common tests used for measuring various functions in different theoretical models discussed and the general trend in ASD participants' performance on those tests.

| Model | Tests/tools | Function measured | Age group | Main finding in ASD |
|---|---|---|---|---|
| ToM | Sally Anne Test | False belief | 4–5 years | Delayed relative to TD |
| | Faux pas | ToM | 9–11 years | Pass during teenage years (TD around age 6) |
| | Strange stories | ToM | 9–11 years | Poor context-appropriate mental state explanations |
| | RMIE | Emotion from eyes | 6–Adult | Poor relative to TD |
| | RMIV | Emotion from voice | | Impaired |
| EF dysfunction | TOH | Planning | 3–12 years | Impaired |
| | TOL | Planning | 6–89 years | Impaired |
| | Reach-to-grasp | Planning | 6–12 years | Unimpaired. Can plan when task is not overly complex. |
| | Maze subtests of WISC | Planning | 6–16 years | Unimpaired. Can plan when task is not overly complex. |
| | WCST | Cognitive flexibility | 6.5–89 years | Impaired |
| | Go/No-Go | Response inhibition | 5–Adult | Impaired performance |
| | Stop task | Response inhibition | | Impaired performance |
| | Stroop task | Interference | 4–Adult | Unimpaired |

**TABLE 1** Table showing the summary of common tests used for measuring various functions in different theoretical models discussed and the general trend in ASD participants' performance on those tests.—cont'd

| Model | Tests/tools | Function measured | Age group | Main finding in ASD |
|---|---|---|---|---|
| Complex information processing | | Skilled motor; complex memory/language; reasoning | | Impaired |
| | | Attention | | Intact |
| | | Simple memory; simple language; visual-spatial | | Intact or superior |
| WCC/EPF | Embedded figures task | Field dependence/independence | 10 and up | Faster RT and greater accuracy than TD peers |
| | Block design subtest of WASI | Visual-spatial and organizational processing | 16–90 | Faster RT and greater accuracy than TD peers |
| Temporal binding | Audiovisual illusion test | Audio-visual integration | 20 and up | Impaired multisensory temporal function |
| Social motivation hypothesis | SMI | Social desire, interest, and behaviors | 8–17 | Impaired |
| | Eye-tracking with social stimuli | Gaze to socially relevant stimuli | | Reduced gaze to the eyes, less pupillary response to human images, slower to fixate on social elements. |
| EMB hypothesis | EQ and SQ questionnaire | Systemizing and empathizing | 16–84 | Poor at empathizing, normal or superior at systemizing. |

# References


1. Baron-Cohen S, Leslie AM, Frith U. Does the autistic child have a "theory of mind"? *Cognition.* 1985;21(1):37–46. https://doi.org/10.1016/0010-0277(85)90022-8.
2. Korkmaz B. Theory of mind and neurodevelopmental disorders of childhood. *Pediatr Res.* 2011;69(5 Pt 2):101R–108R.

3. Mundy P, Robertson M, Robertson J, Greenblatt M. The prevalence of psychotic symptoms in homeless adolescents. *J Am Acad Child Adolesc Psychiatry.* 1990;29(5):724–731.
4. Mundy P. A review of joint attention and social-cognitive brain systems in typical development and autism spectrum disorder. *Eur J Neurosci.* 2018;47(6):497–514.
5. Werner E, Dawson G, Osterling J, Dinno N. Brief report: recognition of Autism spectrum disorder before one year of age: a retrospective study based on home videotapes. *J Autism Dev Disord.* 2000;30(2):157–162. https://doi.org/10.1023/a:1005463707029.
6. Baldwin DA. Understanding the link between joint attention and language. In: *Joint Attention: Its Origins and Role in Development*; 1995:131–158. Published online.
7. Charman T. Why is joint attention a pivotal skill in autism? *Philos Trans R Soc Lond B Biol Sci.* 2003;358(1430):315–324.
8. American Psychiatric Association. *Diagnostic and Statistical Manual of Mental Disorders (DSM-5®).* American Psychiatric Pub; 2013.
9. Wing L, Gould J, Yeates SR, Brierley LM. Symbolic play in severely mentally retarded and in autistic children. *J Child Psychol Psychiatry.* 1977;18(2):167–178.
10. Baron-Cohen S, Leslie AM, Frith U. Mechanical, behavioural and intentional understanding of picture stories in autistic children. *Br J Dev Psychol.* 1986;4(2):113–125. https://doi.org/10.1111/j.2044-835x.1986.tb01003.x.
11. Wellman HM, Cross D, Watson J. Meta-analysis of theory-of-mind development: the truth about false belief. *Child Dev.* 2001;72(3):655–684. https://doi.org/10.1111/1467-8624.00304.
12. Happe FGE. The role of age and verbal ability in the theory of mind task performance of subjects with autism. *Child Dev.* 1995;66(3):843. https://doi.org/10.2307/1131954.
13. Baron-Cohen S, Ring HA, Wheelwright S, et al. Social intelligence in the normal and autistic brain: an fMRI study. *Eur J Neurosci.* 1999;11(6):1891–1898.
14. Kana RK, Maximo JO, Williams DL, et al. Aberrant functioning of the theory-of-mind network in children and adolescents with autism. *Mol Autism.* 2015;6:59.
15. Tager-Flusberg H. Evaluating the theory-of-mind hypothesis of autism. *Curr Dir Psychol Sci.* 2007;16(6):311–315.
16. Frith U, Happé F. Language and communication in autistic disorders. *Philos Trans R Soc Lond B Biol Sci.* 1994;346(1315):97–104.
17. Gernsbacher MA, Yergeau M. Empirical failures of the claim that autistic people lack a theory of mind. *Arch Sci Psychol.* 2019;7(1):102–118.
18. Demetriou EA, Lampit A, Quintana DS, et al. Autism spectrum disorders: a meta-analysis of executive function. *Mol Psychiatry.* 2018;23(5):1198–1204.
19. Hill EL. Executive dysfunction in autism☆. *Trends Cogn Sci.* 2004;8(1):26–32. https://doi.org/10.1016/j.tics.2003.11.003.
20. Hughes C, Russell J, Robbins TW. Evidence for executive dysfunction in autism. *Neuropsychologia.* 1994;32(4):477–492. https://doi.org/10.1016/0028-3932(94)90092-2.
21. Geurts HM, Verte S, Oosterlaan J, Roeyers H, Sergeant JA. How specific are executive functioning deficits in attention deficit hyperactivity disorder and autism? *J Child Psychol Psychiatry.* 2004;45(4):836–854. https://doi.org/10.1111/j.1469-7610.2004.00276.x.
22. Lopez BR, Lincoln AJ, Ozonoff S, Lai Z. Examining the relationship between executive functions and restricted, repetitive symptoms of autistic disorder. *J Autism Dev Disord.* 2005;35(4):445–460.
23. Bishop DVM, Norbury CF. Exploring the borderlands of autistic disorder and specific language impairment: a study using standardised diagnostic instruments. *J Child Psychol Psychiatry.* 2002;43(7):917–929.
24. Russo N, Flanagan T, Iarocci G, Berringer D, Zelazo PD, Burack JA. Deconstructing executive deficits among persons with autism: implications for cognitive neuroscience. *Brain Cogn.* 2007;65(1):77–86.

25. Yerys BE, Wallace GL, Harrison B, Celano MJ, Giedd JN, Kenworthy LE. Set-shifting in children with autism spectrum disorders. *Autism.* 2009;13(5):523–538. https://doi.org/10.1177/1362361309335716.
26. García-Villamisar D, Della SS. Dual-task performance in adults with autism. *Cogn Neuropsychiatry.* 2002;7(1):63–74.
27. Heaton RK, Chelune GJ, Talley JL, Kay GG, Curtiss G. *Wisconsin Card Sorting Test Manual Revised and Expanded.* 2nd. Psychological Assessment Resources, Inc.; 1993:1–230.
28. Corbett BA, Constantine LJ, Hendren R, Rocke D, Ozonoff S. Examining executive functioning in children with autism spectrum disorder, attention deficit hyperactivity disorder and typical development. *Psychiatry Res.* 2009;166(2–3):210–222.
29. Hill EL, Bird CM. Executive processes in Asperger syndrome: patterns of performance in a multiple case series. *Neuropsychologia.* 2006;44(14):2822–2835. https://doi.org/10.1016/j.neuropsychologia.2006.06.007.
30. Bíró S, Russell J. The execution of arbitrary procedures by children with autism. *Dev Psychopathol.* 2001;13(1):97–110.
31. Geurts HM, van den Bergh SFWM, Ruzzano L. Prepotent response inhibition and interference control in autism spectrum disorders: two meta-analyses. *Autism Res.* 2014;7(4):407–420.
32. Christ SE, Holt DD, White DA, Green L. Inhibitory control in children with autism spectrum disorder. *J Autism Dev Disord.* 2007;37(6):1155–1165.
33. Goldberg MC, Mostofsky SH, Cutting LE, et al. Subtle executive impairment in children with autism and children with ADHD. *J Autism Dev Disord.* 2005;35(3):279–293.
34. Braden BB, Blair Braden B, Smith CJ, et al. Executive function and functional and structural brain differences in middle-age adults with autism spectrum disorder. *Autism Res.* 2017;10(12):1945–1959. https://doi.org/10.1002/aur.1842.
35. May KE, Kana RK. Frontoparietal network in executive functioning in autism Spectrum disorder. *Autism Res.* 2020;13(10):1762–1777.
36. Kana RK, Keller TA, Minshew NJ, Just MA. Inhibitory control in high-functioning autism: decreased activation and underconnectivity in inhibition networks. *Biol Psychiatry.* 2007;62(3):198–206. https://doi.org/10.1016/j.biopsych.2006.08.004.
37. Romero-Garcia R, Warrier V, Bullmore ET, Baron-Cohen S, Bethlehem RAI. Synaptic and transcriptionally downregulated genes are associated with cortical thickness differences in autism. *Mol Psychiatry.* 2019;24(7):1053–1064.
38. van Rooij D, Anagnostou E, Arango C, et al. Cortical and subcortical brain morphometry differences between patients with autism spectrum disorder and healthy individuals across the lifespan: results from the ENIGMA ASD working group. *Am J Psychiatry.* 2018;175(4):359–369.
39. Zilbovicius M, Garreau B, Samson Y, et al. Delayed maturation of the frontal cortex in childhood autism. *Am J Psychiatry.* 1995;152(2):248–252.
40. Freitag CM, Luders E, Hulst HE, et al. Total brain volume and corpus callosum size in medication-naïve adolescents and young adults with autism spectrum disorder. *Biol Psychiatry.* 2009;66(4):316–319.
41. Lin H-Y, Perry A, Cocchi L, et al. Development of frontoparietal connectivity predicts longitudinal symptom changes in young people with autism spectrum disorder. *Transl Psychiatry.* 2019;9(1). https://doi.org/10.1038/s41398-019-0418-5.
42. Pellicano E. The development of executive function in autism. *Autism Res Treat.* 2012;2012:1–8. https://doi.org/10.1155/2012/146132.
43. Minshew NJ, Goldstein G, Siegel DJ. Neuropsychologic functioning in autism: profile of a complex information processing disorder. *J Int Neuropsychol Soc.* 1997;3(4):303–316.
44. Minshew NJ, Goldstein G. Autism as a disorder of complex information processing. *Ment Retard Dev Disabil Res Rev.* 1998;4(2):129–136. 3.0.co;2-x">10.1002/(sici)1098-2779(1998)4:2<129::aid-mrdd10>3.0.co;2-x.

45. Minshew NJ, Johnson C, Luna B. The cognitive and neural basis of autism: A disorder of complex information processing and dysfunction of neocortical systems. *Autism.* 2000;111–138. https://doi.org/10.1016/s0074-7750(00)80008-7.
46. Just MA, Cherkassky VL, Keller TA, Minshew NJ. Cortical activation and synchronization during sentence comprehension in high-functioning autism: evidence of underconnectivity. *Brain.* 2004;127(Pt 8):1811–1821.
47. Just MA, Cherkassky VL, Keller TA, Kana RK, Minshew NJ. Functional and anatomical cortical underconnectivity in autism: evidence from an FMRI study of an executive function task and corpus callosum morphometry. *Cereb Cortex.* 2007;17(4):951–961.
48. Kana RK, Keller TA, Cherkassky VL, Minshew NJ, Just MA. Atypical frontal-posterior synchronization of theory of mind regions in autism during mental state attribution. *Soc Neurosci.* 2009;4(2):135–152.
49. Mason RA, Williams DL, Kana RK, Minshew N, Just MA. Theory of mind disruption and recruitment of the right hemisphere during narrative comprehension in autism. *Neuropsychologia.* 2008;46(1):269–280.
50. Frith U. *Autism: Explaining the Enigma.* Wiley-Blackwell; 2003.
51. Frith U, Happé F. Autism: beyond "theory of mind". *Cognition.* 1994;50(1–3):115–132.
52. Brock J, Brown CC, Boucher J, Rippon G. The temporal binding deficit hypothesis of autism. *Dev Psychopathol.* 2002;14(2):209–224.
53. Happé F, Frith U. The weak coherence account: detail-focused cognitive style in autism spectrum disorders. *J Autism Dev Disord.* 2006;36(1):5–25.
54. Kana RK, Liu Y, Williams DL, et al. The local, global, and neural aspects of visuospatial processing in autism spectrum disorders. *Neuropsychologia.* 2013;51(14):2995–3003.
55. Liu Y, Cherkassky VL, Minshew NJ, Just MA. Autonomy of lower-level perception from global processing in autism: evidence from brain activation and functional connectivity. *Neuropsychologia.* 2011;49(7):2105–2111.
56. O'Riordan M, Plaisted K. Enhanced discrimination in autism. *Q J Exp Psychol A.* 2001;54(4):961–979.
57. Jarrold C, Butler DW, Cottington EM, Jimenez F. Linking theory of mind and central coherence bias in autism and in the general population. *Dev Psychol.* 2000;36(1):126–138.
58. Morgan B, Maybery M, Durkin K. Weak central coherence, poor joint attention, and low verbal ability: independent deficits in early autism. *Dev Psychol.* 2003;39(4):646–656.
59. Scher Lisa J, Shyman E. *Annals of Behavioral Neuroscience Challenging Weak Central Coherence: A Brief Exploration of Neurological Evidence from Visual Processing and Linguistic Studies in Autism Spectrum Disorder*; 2019. Published online https://pdfs.semanticscholar.org/289d/eb5b32e7f6d818fee41f2e456c8fc95478e3.pdf.
60. Frith U. A new look at language and communication in autism. *Int J Lang Commun Disord.* 1989;24(2):123–150.
61. Mottron L, Burack JA. Enhanced perceptual functioning in the development of autism. *The development of autism: Perspectives from theory and research.* Lawrence Erlbaum Associates Publishers; 2001:131–148.
62. Kapur N. Paradoxical functional facilitation in brain-behaviour research. A critical review. *Brain.* 1996;119(Pt 5):1775–1790.
63. Caron M-J, Mottron L, Berthiaume C, Dawson M. Cognitive mechanisms, specificity and neural underpinnings of visuospatial peaks in autism. *Brain.* 2006;129(Pt 7):1789–1802.
64. Samson F, Mottron L, Soulières I, Zeffiro TA. Enhanced visual functioning in autism: an ALE meta-analysis. *Hum Brain Mapp.* 2012;33(7):1553–1581.
65. Bertone A, Mottron L, Jelenic P, Faubert J. Enhanced and diminished visuo-spatial information processing in autism depends on stimulus complexity. *Brain.* 2005;128(10):2430–2441. https://doi.org/10.1093/brain/awh561.
66. Hyde KL, Samson F, Evans AC, Mottron L. Neuroanatomical differences in brain areas implicated in perceptual and other core features of autism revealed by cortical thickness analysis and voxel-based morphometry. *Hum Brain Mapp.* 2010;31(4):556–566.

67. Fair DA, Dosenbach NUF, Church JA, et al. Development of distinct control networks through segregation and integration. *Proc Natl Acad Sci U S A.* 2007;104(33):13507–13512.
68. Stevenson RA, Segers M, Ferber S, Barense MD, Wallace MT. The impact of multisensory integration deficits on speech perception in children with autism spectrum disorders. *Front Psychol.* 2014;5:379.
69. Foss-Feig JH, Kwakye LD, Cascio CJ, et al. An extended multisensory temporal binding window in autism spectrum disorders. *Exp Brain Res.* 2010;203(2):381–389.
70. Chevallier C, Kohls G, Troiani V, Brodkin ES, Schultz RT. The social motivation theory of autism. *Trends Cogn Sci.* 2012;16(4):231–239.
71. Bernier R, Dawson G, Lunde S. EEG imaging of the Mirror neuron system in autism. *PsycEXTRA Dataset.* 2007. https://doi.org/10.1037/e711792007-001.
72. Johnson MH, Griffin R, Csibra G, et al. The emergence of the social brain network: evidence from typical and atypical development. *Dev Psychopathol.* 2005;17(3):599–619.
73. Gaigg SB. The interplay between emotion and cognition in autism spectrum disorder: implications for developmental theory. *Front Integr Neurosci.* 2012;6:113.
74. Misra V. The social brain network and autism. *Ann Neurosci.* 2014;21(2):69–73.
75. Chawarska K, Macari S, Shic F. Decreased spontaneous attention to social scenes in 6-month-old infants later diagnosed with autism spectrum disorders. *Biol Psychiatry.* 2013;74(3):195–203.
76. Klin A. Young autistic children's listening preferences in regard to speech: a possible characterization of the symptom of social withdrawal. *J Autism Dev Disord.* 1991;21(1):29–42. https://doi.org/10.1007/bf02206995.
77. Baron-Cohen S. Theory of mind and autism: A review. *Autism.* 2000;169–184. https://doi.org/10.1016/s0074-7750(00)80010-5.
78. Baranek GT, Little LM, Diane Parham L, Ausderau KK, Sabatos-DeVito MG. Sensory features in autism spectrum disorders. In: *Handbook of Autism and Pervasive Developmental Disorders.* 4th ed; 2014. https://doi.org/10.1002/9781118911389.hautc16. Published online April 1.
79. Gale CM, Eikeseth S, Klintwall L. Children with autism show atypical preference for non-social stimuli. *Sci Rep.* 2019;9(1):10355.
80. Dichter GS, Richey JA, Rittenberg AM, Sabatino A, Bodfish JW. Reward circuitry function in autism during face anticipation and outcomes. *J Autism Dev Disord.* 2012;42(2):147–160.
81. Kohls G, Schulte-Rüther M, Nehrkorn B, et al. Reward system dysfunction in autism spectrum disorders. *Soc Cogn Affect Neurosci.* 2013;8(5):565–572.
82. Scott-Van Zeeland AA, Dapretto M, Ghahremani DG, Poldrack RA, Bookheimer SY. Reward processing in autism. *Autism Res.* 2010;3(2):53–67.
83. Clements CC, Zoltowski AR, Yankowitz LD, Yerys BE, Schultz RT, Herrington JD. Evaluation of the social motivation hypothesis of autism: a systematic review and meta-analysis. *JAMA Psychiatry.* 2018;75(8):797–808.
84. Jaswal V, Akhtar N, Burack JA. *Building Bridges: Cognitive Development in Typical and Atypical Development.* Routledge; 2019.
85. Bishop DVM. Autism, Asperger's syndrome and semantic-pragmatic disorder: where are the boundaries? *Int J Lang Commun Disord.* 1989;24(2):107–121. https://doi.org/10.3109/13682828909011951.
86. Loomes R, Hull L, Mandy WPL. What is the male-to-female ratio in autism spectrum disorder? A systematic review and meta-analysis. *J Am Acad Child Adolesc Psychiatry.* 2017;56(6):466–474.
87. Baron-Cohen S. The extreme male brain theory of autism. *Trends Cogn Sci.* 2002;6(6):248–254.
88. Baron-Cohen S, Lombardo MV, Auyeung B, Ashwin E, Chakrabarti B, Knickmeyer R. Why are autism spectrum conditions more prevalent in males? *PLoS Biol.* 2011;9(6), e1001081.

89. Sparks BF, Friedman SD, Shaw DW, et al. Brain structural abnormalities in young children with autism spectrum disorder. *Neurology.* 2002;59(2):184–192.
90. Kozhemiako N, Vakorin V, Nunes AS, Iarocci G, Ribary U, Doesburg SM. Extreme male developmental trajectories of homotopic brain connectivity in autism. *Hum Brain Mapp.* 2019;40(3):987–1000.
91. Ratto AB, Kenworthy L, Yerys BE, et al. What about the girls? Sex-based differences in autistic traits and adaptive skills. *J Autism Dev Disord.* 2018;48(5):1698–1711.
92. Pellicano E, Burr D. When the world becomes "too real": a Bayesian explanation of autistic perception. *Trends Cogn Sci.* 2012;16(10):504–510.
93. Palmer CJ, Lawson RP, Hohwy J. Bayesian approaches to autism: towards volatility, action, and behavior. *Psychol Bull.* 2017;143(5):521–542.
94. Lawson RP, Rees G, Friston KJ. An aberrant precision account of autism. *Front Hum Neurosci.* 2014;8:302.
95. Geisler WS, Kersten D. Illusions, perception and Bayes. *Nat Neurosci.* 2002;5(6):508–510.
96. Chambon V, Farrer C, Pacherie E, Jacquet PO, Leboyer M, Zalla T. Reduced sensitivity to social priors during action prediction in adults with autism spectrum disorders. *Cognition.* 2017;160:17–26.
97. Stroh G, Buick D. Perceptual development and childhood psychosis. *Br J Med Psychol.* 1964;37:291–299.
98. Hermelin B, O'Connor N. *Psychological Experiments with Autistic Children.* Pergamon; 1970.
99. Lovaas OI, Schreibman L. Stimulus overselectivity of autistic children in a two stimulus situation. *Behav Res Ther.* 1971;9(4):305–310.
100. Lovaas OI, Schreibman L, Koegel R, Rehm R. Selective responding by autistic children to multiple sensory input. *J Abnorm Psychol.* 1971;77(3):211–222.
101. Lane AE, Young RL, Baker AEZ, Angley MT. Sensory processing subtypes in autism: association with adaptive behavior. *J Autism Dev Disord.* 2010;40(1):112–122.
102. Schoen SA, Miller LJ, Brett-Green BA, Nielsen DM. Physiological and behavioral differences in sensory processing: a comparison of children with autism spectrum disorder and sensory modulation disorder. *Front Integr Neurosci.* 2009;3:29.
103. Bertone A, Mottron L, Jelenic P, Faubert J. Motion perception in autism: a "complex" issue. *J Cogn Neurosci.* 2003;15(2):218–225.
104. Bonnel A, Mottron L, Peretz I, Trudel M, Gallun E, Bonnel A-M. Enhanced pitch sensitivity in individuals with autism: a signal detection analysis. *J Cogn Neurosci.* 2003;15(2):226–235.
105. Cascio CJ, Woynaroski T, Baranek GT, Wallace MT. Toward an interdisciplinary approach to understanding sensory function in autism spectrum disorder. *Autism Res.* 2016;9(9):920–925.
106. Bebko JM, Weiss JA, Demark JL, Gomez P. Discrimination of temporal synchrony in intermodal events by children with autism and children with developmental disabilities without autism. *J Child Psychol Psychiatry.* 2006;47(1):88–98.
107. Smith EG, Bennetto L. Audiovisual speech integration and lipreading in autism. *J Child Psychol Psychiatry.* 2007;48(8):813–821.
108. Brandwein AB, Foxe JJ, Butler JS, et al. The development of multisensory integration in high-functioning autism: high-density electrical mapping and psychophysical measures reveal impairments in the processing of audiovisual inputs. *Cereb Cortex.* 2013;23(6):1329–1341.
109. de Gelder B, de Gelder B, Vroomen J, van der Heide L. Face recognition and lip-reading in autism. *Eur J Cogn Psychol.* 1991;3(1):69–86. https://doi.org/10.1080/09541449108406220.
110. Iarocci G, McDonald J. Sensory integration and the perceptual experience of persons with autism. *J Autism Dev Disord.* 2006;36(1):77–90.

111. Bebko JM, Schroeder JH, Weiss JA. The McGurk effect in children with autism and Asperger syndrome. *Autism Res.* 2014;7(1):50–59.
112. Noel J-P, De Niear MA, Stevenson R, Alais D, Wallace MT. Atypical rapid audio-visual temporal recalibration in autism spectrum disorders. *Autism Res.* 2017;10(1):121–129.
113. Patten E, Watson LR, Baranek GT. Temporal synchrony detection and associations with language in young children with ASD. *Autism Res Treat.* 2014;2014, 678346.
114. Woynaroski TG, Kwakye LD, Foss-Feig JH, Stevenson RA, Stone WL, Wallace MT. Multisensory speech perception in children with autism spectrum disorders. *J Autism Dev Disord.* 2013;43(12):2891–2902.
115. Smith E, Zhang S, Bennetto L. Temporal synchrony and audiovisual integration of speech and object stimuli in autism. *Res Autism Spectr Disord.* 2017;39:11–19.
116. Turi M, Karaminis T, Pellicano E, Burr D. No rapid audiovisual recalibration in adults on the autism spectrum. *Sci Rep.* 2016;6:21756.
117. Falck-Ytter T, Rehnberg E, Bölte S. Lack of visual orienting to biological motion and audiovisual synchrony in 3-year-olds with autism. *PLoS One.* 2013;8(7), e68816.
118. Foxe JJ, Molholm S, Del Bene VA, et al. Severe multisensory speech integration deficits in high-functioning school-aged children with autism Spectrum disorder (ASD) and their resolution during early adolescence. *Cereb Cortex.* 2015;25(2):298–312.
119. Grossman RB, Schneps MH, Tager-Flusberg H. Slipped lips: onset asynchrony detection of auditory-visual language in autism. *J Child Psychol Psychiatry.* 2009;50(4):491–497.
120. Walker-Andrews AS, Haviland JM, Huffman L, Toci L. Brief report: preferential looking in intermodal perception by children with autism. *J Autism Dev Disord.* 1994;24(1):99–107.
121. Russo N, Foxe JJ, Brandwein AB, Altschuler T, Gomes H, Molholm S. Multisensory processing in children with autism: high-density electrical mapping of auditory-somatosensory integration. *Autism Res.* 2010;3(5):253–267.
122. Doyle-Thomas KAR, Goldberg J, Szatmari P, Hall GBC. Neurofunctional underpinnings of audiovisual emotion processing in teens with autism spectrum disorders. *Front Psychiatry.* 2013;4:48.

CHAPTER

# 5

# The neuroanatomy of autism

*Charlotte M. Pretzsch*[a] *and Christine Ecker*[a,b]

**[a]Department of Forensic and Neurodevelopmental Sciences, Institute of Psychiatry, Psychology and Neuroscience, King's College London, London, United Kingdom, [b]Department of Child and Adolescent Psychiatry, University Hospital, Goethe University, Frankfurt am Main, Germany**

## Introduction

Autism spectrum disorder (ASD) is a life-long neurodevelopmental condition characterized by (i) impairments in social communication abilities, (ii) the presence of rigid, repetitive, and stereotyped behaviors, and (iii) atypical sensory responses (DSM-5). These symptoms typically manifest during early childhood (i.e., between 1 and 2 years), although most individuals are diagnosed after the age of 4–5 years.[1] There is significant clinical heterogeneity both between individuals who fulfill diagnostic criteria, and within individuals across development.[2] This phenotypic heterogeneity is most likely due to the multifactorial etiology of the condition, which includes genetic and nongenetic risk factors. On the genetic level alone, more than 500 genetic and genomic loci have been implicated in ASD,[3] many of which interact with environmental risk factors (pre)natally (e.g., advanced parental age, maternal physical/mental health, premature birth), or during early development (e.g., exposure to toxins/chemicals).[4] The etiology of ASD is therefore complex and not attributable to a single underlying factor or mechanism. However, despite the large heterogeneity associated with this condition, research converges on the fact that ASD is accompanied by atypical development of brain structure. In the present chapter, we aim to outline the progress that has been made in understanding the neuroanatomy underpinning


https://doi.org/10.1016/B978-0-12-816393-1.00013-0

ASD. In particular, we will provide a brief overview over (i) experimental techniques to assess neuroanatomy postmortem and in vivo, (ii) large-scale brain structure across development, (iii) volume- and surface-based measures of neuroanatomy, (iv) regional neuroanatomy, (v) neuropathology, and (vi) neuroanatomical heterogeneity.

## Assessing neuroanatomy postmortem and in vivo

There are multiple approaches to examining neuroanatomy in autism. Traditionally, researchers have relied on histological analyses of postmortem brain tissue to study ASD. Situated at the junction between neurobiological pathways and macroscopic brain anomalies, such analyses have provided invaluable information, e.g., about microscopic anatomy and cellular characteristics.[5] However, postmortem studies are commonly hampered by limited tissue availability and quality, scarce documentation of life events, and other confounds (e.g., the cause of death). Hence, they are poorly equipped to deal with the phenotypic heterogeneity characteristic of ASD. Nonetheless, the development of novel techniques, such as the stereological estimation of cell numbers and in situ hybridization to evaluate gene expression levels, may significantly enhance the information potential of postmortem analyses.[5] Currently, the gold standard approach to examining neuroanatomy in ASD in vivo is via structural magnetic resonance imaging (sMRI). In brief, MRI harnesses the varying magnetic properties of different tissue types, e.g., gray matter and white matter, to produce high-resolution images of the brain. Commonly used types of MRI include, e.g., T1-weighted images, which provide a high level of structural detail; and diffusion tensor imaging (DTI), which assesses white matter organization by examining water motion along fiber tracts.[5] MRI studies have provided important insights into neuroanatomy both cross-sectionally and longitudinally (i.e., across development). Their advantages include their safety in vivo (including in utero), and their ability to provide noninvasive three-dimensional data at a spatial resolution of approximately one cubic millimeter.[5] In contrast, some of the limitations of MRI are their cost, susceptibility to methodological artifacts (e.g., motion and site effects), acquisition time, and the requirement to exclude subjects with metal objects in their body. Nonetheless, existing MRI methods, and the current development of novel techniques (e.g., new pulse sequences, the integration and combination of multiple imaging modalities, virtual histology, the automation of processing and analysis pipelines, etc.) represent an invaluable tool in the research of ASD pathology and the development of novel treatment approaches.[6]

## Large-scale brain structure across development

The notion that cortical development may be altered in ASD initially arose from early clinical observations that the head circumference of autistic children may be larger than that of neurotypical children. For example, reports by Bailey et al. suggest that more than a third of children with ASD may have a head circumference above the 97th normative percentile,[7] which indicates macrocephaly (i.e., an atypical enlargement of the head). These initial findings linking ASD to macrocephaly were confirmed by a number of subsequent studies, even though the reported prevalence in those studies was significantly lower,[8] with estimates averaging around 21%.[9] Also, at birth, head circumference appeared typical, with a significantly increased rate of growth appearing at around 12 months of age.[10] This is important because it suggests that the maturational trajectory of the brain in ASD deviates from that in neurotypicals, and particular during early development.

Subsequently, sMRI studies confirmed that the increase in head circumference in ASD is accompanied by a commensurate increase in total brain volume.[11] This increase is typically observed in ~ 15% of boys with the condition and appears less commonly in autistic girls.[12] Similar to studies examining head circumference, sMRI studies examining total brain volume indicate that the brain of children with ASD may be enlarged between the ages of 2–4 years, and that this enlargement may persist until the age of 5–6 years,[10,13] after which no significant increase in total brain volume is observed. These early cross-sectional neuroimaging findings have now been confirmed by large, longitudinal studies of brain development in ASD (e.g., Refs. 14,15). Combined, they suggest that the trajectory of atypical brain development in ASD may be subdivided into three stages, namely (1) a period of early brain overgrowth until the age of 4 to 5 years, (2) a period of decelerated or arrested growth during early and late childhood, and (3) a period of accelerated decline in total brain volume across the remaining life span; as shown schematically in Fig. 1. However, neuroimaging studies examining the brain during later adulthood and aging in ASD remain rare.

The altered developmental trajectory of brain maturation in ASD may further vary between lobes and regions of the brain. Across studies, it has been demonstrated that frontal and temporal lobe regions are more affected by atypical neurodevelopment than parietal and occipital brain regions.[16] This is of interest because typical brain development occurs in a highly synchronized and hierarchically organized fashion, where phylogenetically younger brain areas (e.g., in the frontal lobe) typically mature after the maturation of older areas (e.g., in occipital and parietal lobes) is completed.[17] Hence, the above findings suggest that the temporal and

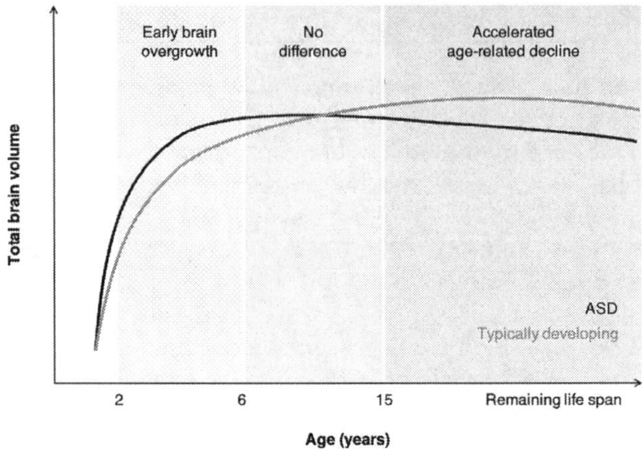


**FIG. 1** Atypical brain development in ASD. Stages are thought to include (1) a period of early brain overgrowth until the age of 4–5 years, (2) a period of decelerated or arrested growth during early and late childhood, and (3) a period of accelerated decline in total brain volume across the remaining life span.

regional sequence of typical early brain development (i.e., from back to front) is perturbed in ASD; which may lead to differences in brain anatomy and connectivity within a wider cortical system. The time point at which differences in the neuroanatomy of ASD first become visible remains unclear. Traditional neuroimaging studies have mostly examined infants with a diagnosis of ASD, which can be made reliably after 1 to 2 years of life.[18] In contrast, to examine brain structure in ASD during the first year of life, studies typically resort to a high-risk family design. Here, infants with a high familial risk of ASD (e.g., siblings of individuals with a confirmed diagnosis of ASD) are compared to low-risk infants (e.g., individuals with no affected family member) prior to obtaining a diagnosis and are typically followed up when a reliable diagnosis can be made. Using such a "prospective" neuroimaging study, Hazlett et al. demonstrated in seminal work that total brain volume first becomes enlarged after the first year of life.[19] This enlargement was only seen in high-risk infants who later obtained a diagnosis of ASD, relative to high-risk infants without a diagnosis of ASD or neurotypical individuals. Moreover, the increase in total brain volume between 12 and 24 months was preceded by an accelerated expansion of the cortical surface between 6 and 12 months, particularly in the middle occipital gyrus, the lingual gyrus, and—to a lesser extent—in the inferior temporal gyrus and middle frontal lobe. This study was important as the findings not only suggest that (i) neuroanatomical differences in ASD appear alongside behavioral symptoms in the first year of life, but also that (ii) neuroanatomical differences in ASD are not restricted to higher-order association areas of the cortex, but also include lower-order sensorimotor areas. Furthermore, the study demonstrated that the regional pattern, magnitude, and direction of neuroanatomical differences observed in ASD depend on various factors, including the age range of the examined sample and the selected neuroanatomical measures (or "features").

## Volume- and surface-based measures of neuroanatomy

Traditional neuroimaging studies have predominantly explored measures of cortical volume (CV). Evidence for atypical regional brain volume in ASD first originated from hand tracing studies, where a brain region of interest is chosen a priori and subsequently manually "segmented" (i.e., outlined). For example, Langen et al. segmented the basal ganglia in ASD, and demonstrated that the head of the caudate nucleus was significantly enlarged in the ASD group compared to neurotypicals.[20] Similarly, using manual tracing, Nordahl et al. demonstrated that the volume of the amygdala, a key component of the social brain, is significantly increased in ASD, with an increased rate of growth in children between 2 and 4 years of age.[21] Hence, hand tracing studies represented important first steps in establishing the regional neuroanatomy of ASD; and provide reliable volumetric measures, particularly for smaller brain structures. However, their disadvantages include that they are very time consuming and labor-intensive, and hence suited only for the examination of few a priori specified regions of interest. Thus, the exploratory analysis of volumetric differences requires advanced computational techniques that allow screening of the whole brain without the need for manual interventions.

One of these techniques is voxel-based morphometry (VBM), which centers on the between-group comparison of local concentrations of gray matter at each location (i.e., voxel) in the brain. Hence, VBM permits the examination of cortical and subcortical brain structures at the same time. Overall, VBM studies indicate that ASD is accompanied by volumetric atypicalities in multiple cortical regions that are spatially distributed across the brain. For instance, a VBM study in children with ASD reported localized gray matter reductions within frontostriatal and parietal networks, as well as in temporal brain regions.[22] Using VBM, Ecker et al. (2012) have also shown increased gray matter volume in anterior temporal and dorsolateral prefrontal brain regions, and reductions in occipital and medial parietal regions, in male adults with ASD compared to neurotypicals.[23] Combined, these VBM studies suggest that the neuroanatomy of ASD is complex and involves multiple brain areas across the cortex, rather than isolated brain regions. However, while volume-based examinations of the brain have been invaluable for characterizing the regional neuroanatomy of ASD, measures of brain volume are—by definition—a product of cortical thickness (CT) and surface area (SA), i.e., CV is not an independent neuroanatomical feature but depends on both CT and SA. CT is typically defined as the closest distance from the gray/white matter boundary, to the gray matter/cerebrospinal fluid boundary (i.e., the outer gray matter surface of the brain), and is measured in millimeters.[24] SA, on the other hand, represents the area of the cortex/a cortical region at a point on the cortical surface (i.e., vertex) expressed in square millimeters.

Increasing evidence suggests that CT and SA not only represent separate aspects of the cortical architecture, but also possess distinct genetic determinants,[25] phylogeny,[26] and developmental trajectories.[27] Therefore, it is crucial to examine these cortical measures separately in order to understand what drives CV differences in ASD. This became possible with the introduction of so-called surface-based morphometry (SBM), which relies on the accurate 3D reconstruction of the cortical gray and white matter surfaces.[28] These reconstructions can subsequently be used to explore a variety of cortical features, including SA and CT, but also curvature and local gyrification.[29] Consequently, SBM has been applied extensively to study the specific neuroanatomical (and associated neurobiological) underpinnings of ASD using multiple aspect of cortical architecture.

For instance, CT anomalies have been reported in a number of studies in both children and adults with ASD. However, findings of studies with samples below $N<200$ vary significantly regarding the direction and pattern of the observed CT differences. For example, in children with ASD, some studies report increases in CT of frontotemporal regions,[30,31] while others note the opposite trend in similar regions.[32] In adults, most studies report thickening of the frontal cortex,[33,34] while the temporal lobe has been reported to be thicker[34] and/or thinner in ASD.[35] Nonetheless, a more consistent picture is now emerging across an increasing number of large-scale investigations ($N>500$), which consistently report increased CT in the temporal lobes in ASD (e.g., Refs. 36,37). Furthermore, the thickness of the cortical sheet is highly age-dependent in ASD (as in the neurotypical brain). Specifically, the developmental trajectory of CT is thought to follow an inverted U-shape, peaking at around 7–10 years of age, and steadily declining across the remaining life span.[38] Longitudinal studies show that cortical thinning is accelerated in ASD compared to neurotypicals, especially in the frontal, parietal and occipital lobe, with relative sparing of the temporal lobes.[39,40] This may explain the observed increase in temporal lobe CT during later childhood and adolescence (see Refs. 36,37). Thus, ASD-associated differences in CT, as well as their spatial pattern, should be interpreted while taking into account the participants' age.

Fewer studies have examined measures of SA in ASD. This may be because areal measures can be derived at various spatial resolutions (i.e., cortical, regional and vertex-level), and are therefore more difficult to interpret than measures of CT. Moreover, areal measures heavily depend on the shape and folding of the cortex. Hence, it is difficult to compare measures across cortical regions that possess different intrinsic organizations (e.g., some regions are more folded than others). Nonetheless, early neuroimaging studies show that early brain overgrowth (in terms of total brain volume) is likely driven by an accelerated expansion of the cortical surface rather than a thickening of the cortical mantle. For example, Hazlett et al. demonstrated that, in all examined cortical regions (frontal, temporal, and parieto-occipital lobes), early brain overgrowth in ASD was associated with an increase in cortical SA before the age of 2 years.[41] This was later confirmed in infants at high-risk for ASD, who displayed a significantly increased SA growth rate from 6 to 12 months compared to infants without ASD (see Refs. 19).

Measures of CT and SA thus contribute differentially to volumetric atypicalities in ASD, with early differences (< 2 years) most likely being caused by the mechanisms underpinning atypical cortical expansion, and later differences across childhood and adolescence being more closely related to atypical cortical thinning and/or a combination of both. Further, while both measures can contribute to volumetric differences in ASD, their spatial patterns may vary. Ecker et al. examined differences in SA and CT between male adults with ASD and neurotypicals and found that patterns of differences in CT and SA were large nonoverlapping and only shared ~ 3% of all significantly different locations on the cerebral surface.[42] Also, CT and SA have distinct neurodevelopmental trajectories in ASD,[43] and particularly during late childhood/adolescence.[40] Combined, these findings show that individuals with ASD display significant differences in regional brain volume, which may be underpinned by (separable) variations in CT and SA.

Last, SBM studies have shown that the brain in ASD differs from the neurotypical brain in terms of its pattern of cortical folding. As the cortex expands during development, it eventually needs to fold to fit an increasing SA into the restricted (i.e., finite) space of the skull. Based on the studies described above, which report an accelerated expansion of the cerebral cortex in ASD (e.g., Refs. 19), one would expect the brain in ASD to be more heavily folded. In line with this, visual neuroradiological studies have reported a significantly higher incidence of cortical malformations in ASD compared to neurotypicals. These malformations include (i) polymicrogyria (too many small folds, thought to arise from atypical prenatal brain maturation); (ii) schizencephaly (clefts linked within the cortical gray matter); and (iii) microgyria (increased size of gyri).[44] Early neuroimaging studies also suggest significantly increased gyrification of the frontal lobe in both children and adolescents with ASD,[45] and that some sulci (e.g., the Sylvian fissure) appear displaced along the principal axes of the brain in children with ASD.[46] Using various surface-based shape characteristics, subsequent computational neuroimaging studies confirmed that the central, intraparietal and frontal medial sulci show abnormalities across different geometrical indices including the length and depth of sulci, which are closely related to the amount of SA buried within the cortical folds.[47] Also, using SBM, it is possible to measure cortical gyrification. For instance, the local gyrification index (LGI) reflects the amount of cortex buried within the sulcal folds at any given point on the cortical surface. It is computed as the ratio between the surface of a circular patch on the smooth outer surface of the brain, and the surface of the corresponding patch on the actual cortical gray-matter surface.[29] While the LGI is a powerful technique to examine cortical folding in vivo, findings remain inconsistent across studies. In males with ASD, the LGI has been reported to be increased, particularly in posterior brain regions.[48] But there are also reports of significantly reduced LGI in central structures of the brain (e.g., precentral and postcentral gyrus),[49] and in inferior frontal and medial parieto-occipital brain regions.[50] There is also a study in ASD reporting LGI increases in childhood and decreases during adolescence.[51] Hence, no consensus has been reached whether local gyrification is increased or decreased in ASD; and how this depends on the trajectory of brain maturation (for a systematic review, see Refs. 52).

In summary, the autistic brain differs in multiple aspects of cortical neuroanatomy, which are summarized schematically in Fig. 2. These neuroanatomical atypicalities affect multiple areas of the brain that are functionally linked to ASD symptoms and traits.

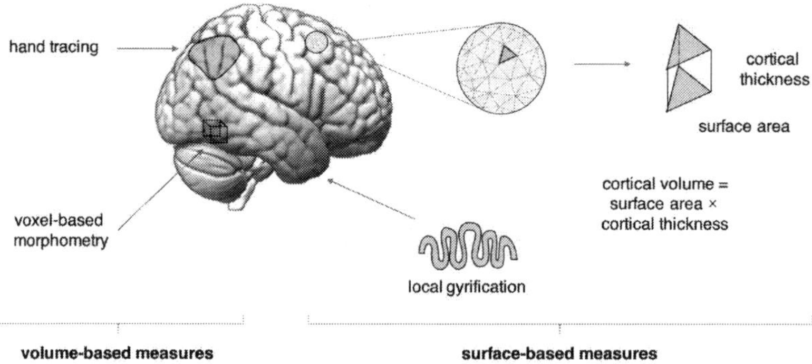


FIG. 2 Volume- and surface-based measures of neuroanatomy. Commonly used approaches include volume-based measures (e.g., derived from hand-tracing and voxel-based morphometry) as well as surface-based measures (e.g., cortical volume, surface area, cortical thickness, and measures of cortical folding, such as local gyrification).

# The regional neuroanatomy of ASD

## Gray matter atypicalities

In addition to global neuroanatomical perturbations across a variety of neuroanatomical features, studies have also uncovered regional differences within large-scale neural systems that have been linked functionally to core symptoms and associated traits in ASD.

For instance, studies in children and adults with ASD have reported neuroanatomical differences in temporal lobe structures (e.g., the superior temporal sulcus and fusiform[53,54]) associated with "social perception."[55] Similarly, studies have found brain structural differences in orbitofrontal,[56] frontoparietal, and anterior and posterior cingulate regions, as well as the amygdala (reviewed, e.g., in Ref. 57), which are thought to form part of the neural circuitry linking social perception to emotion, motivation, and cognition.[55]

The amygdala in particular has been identified as a key region in ASD. A study in toddlers, for example, reported volumetric increases in the amygdala in those individuals who later received a diagnosis of ASD; and amygdala volume was correlated with social and communication impairments.[58] Studies in autistic children have reported not only greater amygdala volume, but also an enhanced rate of growth, compared to neurotypical controls.[21] Last, in adolescents and adults with autism, amygdala volume was lower compared to neurotypicals; and correlated with mentalizing ability (i.e., the ability to attend to mental states in oneself and others).[59] Combined, these findings implicate the amygdala in the neuropathology of autism across development; and highlight its potential relevance to ASD core symptoms in the social domain.

Another region implicated in ASD is the striatum—a part of the basal ganglia that includes the caudate, putamen, and nucleus accumbens. Neuroanatomical differences in the striatum have also been linked to ASD core symptoms, including restricted and repetitive patterns of interests and behaviors. Studies in children, adolescents, and young adults, for instance, have reported caudate enlargement in ASD compared to neurotypicals.[20] In (young) adults with ASD, volume of both the caudate and putamen further correlated positively with repetitive behavior scores.[60] Moreover, in autistic children, the caudate growth rate was increased compared to neurotypicals; and this faster growth correlated with more severe repetitive symptoms.[61,62] Another (cortical) region that has been linked to restricted and repetitive symptoms is the superior parietal lobule, where reduced volume was observed in autistic adults.[63] Thus, autistic individuals may also display atypical brain structure (and structural development) in cortical and subcortical regions linked to ASD core symptoms in the nonsocial domain.

Last, another brain region that has been highlighted as atypical in ASD is the cerebellum. However, while studies in young children with ASD have reported reduced volume of the cerebellum in general[64] and the vermis (lobe VI–VII) in particular,[64,65] there may exist significant intragroup heterogeneity; and findings remain inconclusive.

In sum, there is robust evidence for structural differences across age in multiple brain regions (the regions mentioned above are depicted in Fig. 3) that are considered essential for complex cognitive functions including those implicated in ASD. However, it is important to note that these regional differences are not unique to ASD; and it remains unclear if and how they contribute to symptoms in this condition. For instance, while the caudate has been implicated in restricted and repetitive behavior in ASD,[61,62] (neuroanatomically atypical) frontostriatal circuitry has also been suggested to mediate obsessive and compulsive behaviors in conditions such as obsessive compulsive disorder.[66,67] Similarly, previous studies have observed volumetric anomalies in the temporal lobe[53,54] and striatum[20,61,62] not only in ASD,[53,54] but also in the frequently cooccurring epilepsy.[68] Future studies are therefore required to examine the association between these (overlapping) neuroanatomical and clinical phenotypes; and whether disease mechanisms in these conditions involve distinct and/or shared genetic and molecular pathways.

## White matter atypicalities

The large-scale neural systems implicated in ASD may be characterized not only by regional differences, but also by atypical structural connections between these regions. Accordingly, differences in structural brain

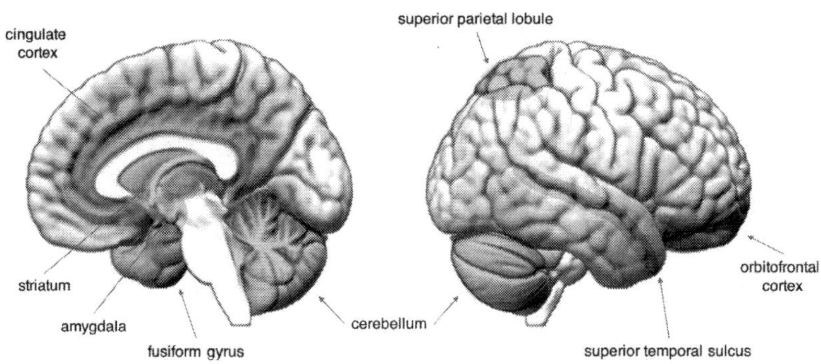


FIG. 3 Regional brain structure (gray matter) in ASD. This schematic highlights several brain regions that have been implicated in ASD, including cortical (orbitofrontal cortex, cingulate cortex, superior temporal sulcus, fusiform gyrus, superior parietal lobule) and subcortical (amygdala, striatum) regions; and the cerebellum.

connectivity have been observed in ASD, e.g., in systems underlying socio-emotional processing,[69] restricted and repetitive patterns of behavior,[70] mentalizing/theory of mind,[71] language,[72] and motor[73] processing.

In particular, several studies have reported macrostructural (volumetric) white matter differences in ASD. For instance, using VBM, McAlonan et al. observed reduced white matter in autistic children (compared to neurotypicals) in the left internal capsule, the fornices, and the cerebellum.[22] Additionally, a wealth of research has provided evidence for microstructural white matter anomalies, such as atypical measures of structural "integrity," across the brain in ASD.[74] Specifically, in children and young adults with ASD, studies have consistently reported decreased fractional anisotropy in the corpus callosum, cingulum, and several white matter tracts connecting temporal lobe regions; and these reductions are often accompanied by increases in mean and radial diffusivity.[74,75] Notably, white matter structural differences have also been associated with ASD core symptoms; for instance, in children with ASD, reduced fractional anisotropy in prefrontal white matter tracts correlated negatively with social impairments.[76]

Thus, ASD is characterized by a wealth of widespread white matter atypicalities, which may further relate to (core) symptoms in this condition. However, like gray matter differences, white matter differences in ASD are not unique to this condition. For instance, a recent study identified an overlap in white matter atypicalities in the corpus callosum between children with autism and children with attention-deficit/hyperactivity disorder.[77] Also, how white matter and gray matter anomalies interact remains poorly understood. For example, it remains unclear if and how white matter pathology contributes to or results from altered gray matter. Finally, the contribution of white matter anomalies to symptomatology remains poorly understood. In sum, future studies are required to elucidate the role of white matter atypicality in the disease mechanisms and clinical phenotype of ASD.

## Neuropathology

In contrast to the wealth of research focusing on macrostructural atypicalities in ASD, relatively few studies have examined microstructure. This is largely because such studies mostly rely on postmortem tissue, which is difficult to obtain and susceptible to confounds (e.g., through methodological approaches, cause of death, comorbidities, etc.). Consequently, findings from postmortem studies remain scarce and largely heterogeneous. Nonetheless, there is converging evidence that ASD is accompanied by several cytoarchitectural differences. One of the first qualitative neuropathological studies in ASD consistently identified coarseness and poor lamination in the anterior cingulate cortex across six autistic individuals.[78] A subsequent study further revealed cortical dysgenesis (i.e., disordered development) in autism.[79] Specifically, findings included greater neuronal density and numbers of neurons in the molecular layer, irregular lamination patterns, and ectopic gray matter (e.g., larger numbers of neurons in the white matter) in ASD compared to neurotypicals.[79] These findings of atypical neurodevelopment have since been replicated, and it is now widely accepted that ASD is accompanied by atypical neurogenesis, disrupted neural migration, dysplasia, and heterotopia in multiple brain regions.[80] Following these initial observations of atypical development of the cortical microstructure, Casanova et al. (2002) reported abnormalities in the structure of so-called "minicolumns," the smallest organizational unit of the brain.[81] In a seminal paper, the authors investigated cell column morphological features in the prefrontal cortex and temporal lobe. In autism, minicolumns were found to be more numerous, smaller, and less compact relative to the typically developing brain.[81] These observations have since been replicated and extended. For instance, examining a broader age range and additional brain regions, a recent study supplied further evidence for alterations in minicolumnar organization, including in primary sensory regions and especially at a younger age.[82] Investigating microstructure at greater detail, Courchesne et al. (2011) further demonstrated that, in prefrontal cortex, autistic individuals showed greater numbers of neurons, albeit no differences in neuronal size[83]; and there is emerging evidence that the number of glia cells may also be atypically increased in ASD.[84] The atypical number, growth, and organization of both neurons and glia cells are also reflected in altered cell pattering in autism. For example, this includes irregularities at the gray-white matter boundary (i.e., a lack of a clear distinction between the cortical layer VI and the underlying white matter) in the frontal, temporal, and parietal lobe.[85] Notably, these histological findings have recently been replicated by a number of in vivo neuroimaging studies.[86,87]

In conclusion, while studies in ASD have identified multiple neuropathological differences across brain regions and age, the field remains in its relative infancy. Nonetheless, efforts focused on the acquisition, sharing, and systematic and quantitative analysis of higher-quality and more numerous samples hold great promise in better understanding the neuropathology of ASD.[57]

## Neuroanatomical heterogeneity

Notably, neuroanatomy, like most features in this condition, varies significantly across the autism spectrum. Sources of variability include intrasubject/within-subject heterogeneity (i.e., where individuals change in neuroanatomy across development[41]) and intersubject heterogeneity, where neuroanatomical measures vary between individuals, e.g., based on the individual's sex,[37,88] age, intelligence,[37] cooccurring conditions,[89] and/or differences in clinical symptom profiles, etc.[90] This heterogeneity represents a significant challenge both for research into the neurobiological mechanisms of ASD and in clinical settings. Moreover, traditional studies have primarily examined autism using case-control studies that test for differences at the group level (i.e., based on mean differences). However, this approach may mask effects at the individual level and, consequently, hinder our ability to understand autism pathophysiology, to link neurobiological and clinical phenotypes, and to discover and validate (pharmacological) interventions. Thus, parsing the heterogeneity of ASD is a crucial step toward a better understanding of ASD disease mechanisms, and the development of targeted (precision medicine) treatment approaches. Fortunately, a growing body of research is addressing this issue.

For example, an increasing number of studies are implementing multivariate machine learning approaches, such as support vector machines (SVM; supervised learning models). These can be used to classify data, e.g., predict group membership for cases (or more biologically homogeneous subgroups within ASD) and controls. Using multivariate pattern classification analysis, it was possible, e.g., to distinguish between children with ASD and neurotypicals with an accuracy of 90% based on gray matter in frontotemporal default mode regions.[91] Similarly, using a whole-brain SVM approach, Ecker et al. examined the potential of neuroanatomy to predict ASD in adults.[92] The authors found that spatially distributed patterns of neuroanatomical anomalies, including in frontal, limbic, and cerebellar regions, helped discriminate between autistic and neurotypical adults with a specificity of 86% (using gray matter) and 68% (using white matter). Thus, data-driven approaches may be useful not only to identify neuroanatomical atypicalities in ASD, but also to distinguish between cases and controls; and this may have future applications, e.g., in aiding the diagnostic process. However, it is increasingly recognized that, due to the significant heterogeneity within ASD, the accurate distinction between cases and controls becomes more difficult with increasing participant numbers.[93]

More recent studies have therefore begun to use machine learning to search for subgroups within the autism spectrum. For instance, a recent study conducted data-driven subtyping of neuroanatomical markers of cortical organization in a multisite sample of male children and adults.[94] The authors identified robust neuroanatomical ASD subgroups that also displayed distinct clinical profiles (e.g., including difficulties in social interaction).[94] Similarly, Zabihi et al. recently performed subtyping in female and male children, adolescents, and adults with and without ASD.[95] Based on measures of CT, the authors identified five autism subgroups, which differed in brain structure and also displayed distinct loadings onto symptoms and polygenic risk.[95] Thus, machine learning applied to brain structure (and other data modalities) within ASD may help uncover previously unknown "biotypes" within this condition, which may inform future research both into disease mechanisms and potential treatments.

Additionally, studies are increasingly implementing statistical approaches, such as normative modeling, that target individual rather than (sub)group effects. For instance, a study in children, adolescents, and adults with and without ASD examined autistic individuals' deviation from the neurotypical developmental trajectory of voxel-wise CT.[95] The authors not only discovered widespread differences in ASD, but these also correlated with the severity of repetitive behaviors.[95] Similarly, using a measure of voxel-wise gray matter lateralization, a recent study by Floris et al. found that autistic individuals displayed highly individualized patterns of extreme deviations from the neurotypical mean, which further correlated with (social) symptom severity.[96] Together, these observations highlight the potential of individual-level statistics in studying brain structure in greater detail and linking neuroanatomy to other (e.g., clinical) phenotypes.

Combined, studies addressing (brain structural) heterogeneity in ASD have provided promising insights into our ability to stratify the ASD population into meaningful subgroups. However, existing research also highlights the need for larger and more heterogeneous feature-rich and deeply phenotyped datasets.[97] Fortunately, several international research initiatives aimed at addressing this need are currently underway (e.g., Refs. 98,99).

## References


1. Pringle B, Colpe LJ, Blumberg SJ, Avila RM, Kogan MD. Diagnostic history and treatment of school-aged children with autism spectrum disorder and special health care needs. *NCHS Data Brief.* 2012;(97):1–8.
2. Lord C, Bishop S, Anderson D. Developmental trajectories as autism phenotypes. *Am J Med Genet C: Semin Med Genet.* 2015;169(2):198–208.
3. Bourgeron T. Current knowledge on the genetics of autism and propositions for future research. *C R Biol.* 2016;339(7–8):300–307.
4. Karimi P, Kamali E, Mousavi SM, Karahmadi M. Environmental factors influencing the risk of autism. *J Res Med Sci.* 2017;22:27.
5. Schumann CM, Nordahl CW. Bridging the gap between MRI and postmortem research in autism. *Brain Res.* 2011;1380:175–186.
6. Harisinghani MG, O'Shea A, Weissleder R. Advances in clinical MRI technology. *Sci Transl Med.* 2019;11(523).
7. Bailey A, Luthert P, Bolton P, Le Couteur A, Rutter M, Harding B. Autism and megalencephaly. *Lancet.* 1993;341(8854):1225–1226.
8. Lainhart JE, Piven J, Wzorek M, et al. Macrocephaly in children and adults with autism. *J Am Acad Child Adolesc Psychiatry.* 1997;36(2):282–290.
9. Fombonne E, Roge B, Claverie J, Courty S, Fremolle J. Microcephaly and macrocephaly in autism. *J Autism Dev Disord.* 1999;29(2):113–119.

10. Hazlett HC, Poe M, Gerig G, et al. Magnetic resonance imaging and head circumference study of brain size in autism: birth through age 2 years. *Arch Gen Psychiatry.* 2005;62(12):1366–1376.
11. Courchesne E, Karns CM, Davis HR, et al. Unusual brain growth patterns in early life in patients with autistic disorder: an MRI study. *Neurology.* 2001;57(2):245–254.
12. Nordahl CW, Lange N, Li DD, et al. Brain enlargement is associated with regression in preschool-age boys with autism spectrum disorders. *Proc Natl Acad Sci U S A.* 2011;108(50):20195–20200.
13. Courchesne E. Abnormal early brain development in autism. *Mol Psychiatry.* 2002;7(Suppl 2):S21–S23.
14. Schumann CM, Bloss CS, Barnes CC, et al. Longitudinal magnetic resonance imaging study of cortical development through early childhood in autism. *J Neurosci.* 2010;30(12):4419–4427.
15. Lange N, Travers BG, Bigler ED, et al. Longitudinal volumetric brain changes in autism spectrum disorder ages 6-35 years. *Autism Res.* 2015;8(1):82–93.
16. Carper RA, Courchesne E. Localized enlargement of the frontal cortex in early autism. *Biol Psychiatry.* 2005;57(2):126–133.
17. Gogtay N, Giedd JN, Lusk L, et al. Dynamic mapping of human cortical development during childhood through early adulthood. *Proc Natl Acad Sci U S A.* 2004;101(21):8174–8179.
18. Luyster R, Gotham K, Guthrie W, et al. The Autism Diagnostic Observation Schedule-toddler module: a new module of a standardized diagnostic measure for autism spectrum disorders. *J Autism Dev Disord.* 2009;39(9):1305–1320.
19. Hazlett HC, Gu H, Munsell BC, et al. Early brain development in infants at high risk for autism spectrum disorder. *Nature.* 2017;542(7641):348–351.
20. Langen M, Durston S, Staal WG, Palmen SJ, van Engeland H. Caudate nucleus is enlarged in high-functioning medication-naive subjects with autism. *Biol Psychiatry.* 2007;62(3):262–266.
21. Nordahl CW, Scholz R, Yang X, et al. Increased rate of amygdala growth in children aged 2 to 4 years with autism spectrum disorders: a longitudinal study. *Arch Gen Psychiatry.* 2012;69(1):53–61.
22. McAlonan GM, Cheung V, Cheung C, et al. Mapping the brain in autism. A voxel-based MRI study of volumetric differences and intercorrelations in autism. *Brain.* 2005;128(Pt 2):268–276.
23. Ecker C, Suckling J, Deoni SC, et al, MRC AIMS Consortium. Brain anatomy and its relationship to behavior in adults with autism spectrum disorder: a multicenter magnetic resonance imaging study. *Arch Gen Psychiatry.* 2012;69(2):195–209. https://doi.org/10.1001/archgenpsychiatry.2011.1251. 22310506.
24. Fischl B, Dale AM. Measuring the thickness of the human cerebral cortex from magnetic resonance images. *Proc Natl Acad Sci U S A.* 2000;97(20):11050–11055.
25. Panizzon MS, Fennema-Notestine C, Eyler LT, et al. Distinct genetic influences on cortical surface area and cortical thickness. *Cereb Cortex.* 2009;19(11):2728–2735.
26. Pontious A, Kowalczyk T, Englund C, Hevner RF. Role of intermediate progenitor cells in cerebral cortex development. *Dev Neurosci.* 2008;30(1–3):24–32.
27. Armstrong E, Schleicher A, Omran H, Curtis M, Zilles K. The ontogeny of human gyrification. *Cereb Cortex.* 1995;5(1):56–63.
28. Dahnke R, Gaser C. *Surface and Shape Analysis. Brain Morphometry.* Springer; 2018:51–73.
29. Schaer M, Cuadra MB, Tamarit L, Lazeyras F, Eliez S, Thiran JP. A surface-based approach to quantify local cortical gyrification. *IEEE Trans Med Imaging.* 2008;27(2):161–170.
30. Mak-Fan KM, Taylor MJ, Roberts W, Lerch JP. Measures of cortical grey matter structure and development in children with autism spectrum disorder. *J Autism Dev Disord.* 2012;42(3):419–427.

31. Hardan AY, Muddasani S, Vemulapalli M, Keshavan MS, Minshew NJ. An MRI study of increased cortical thickness in autism. *Am J Psychiatry.* 2006;163(7):1290–1292.
32. Hadjikhani N, Joseph RM, Snyder J, Tager-Flusberg H. Anatomical differences in the mirror neuron system and social cognition network in autism. *Cereb Cortex.* 2006;16(9):1276–1282.
33. Hyde KL, Samson F, Evans AC, Mottron L. Neuroanatomical differences in brain areas implicated in perceptual and other core features of autism revealed by cortical thickness analysis and voxel-based morphometry. *Hum Brain Mapp.* 2010;31(4):556–566.
34. Scheel C, Rotarska-Jagiela A, Schilbach L, et al. Imaging derived cortical thickness reduction in high-functioning autism: key regions and temporal slope. *NeuroImage.* 2011;58(2):391–400.
35. Wallace GL, Dankner N, Kenworthy L, Giedd JN, Martin A. Age-related temporal and parietal cortical thinning in autism spectrum disorders. *Brain.* 2010;133(Pt 12):3745–3754.
36. Khundrakpam BS, Lewis JD, Kostopoulos P, Carbonell F, Evans AC. Cortical thickness abnormalities in autism spectrum disorders through late childhood, adolescence, and adulthood: a large-scale MRI study. *Cereb Cortex.* 2017;27(3):1721–1731.
37. Bedford SA, Park MTM, Devenyi GA, et al. Large-scale analyses of the relationship between sex, age and intelligence quotient heterogeneity and cortical morphometry in autism spectrum disorder. *Mol Psychiatry.* 2020;25(3):614–628.
38. Raznahan A, Shaw P, Lalonde F, et al. How does your cortex grow? *J Neurosci.* 2011;31(19):7174–7177.
39. Zielinski BA, Prigge MB, Nielsen JA, et al. Longitudinal changes in cortical thickness in autism and typical development. *Brain.* 2014;137(Pt 6):1799–1812.
40. Wallace GL, Eisenberg IW, Robustelli B, et al. Longitudinal cortical development during adolescence and young adulthood in autism spectrum disorder: increased cortical thinning but comparable surface area changes. *J Am Acad Child Adolesc Psychiatry.* 2015;54(6):464–469.
41. Hazlett HC, Poe MD, Gerig G, et al. Early brain overgrowth in autism associated with an increase in cortical surface area before age 2 years. *Arch Gen Psychiatry.* 2011;68(5):467–476.
42. Ecker C, Ginestet C, Feng Y, et al. Brain surface anatomy in adults with autism: the relationship between surface area, cortical thickness, and autistic symptoms. *JAMA Psychiat.* 2013;70(1):59–70.
43. Ecker C, Shahidiani A, Feng Y, et al. The effect of age, diagnosis, and their interaction on vertex-based measures of cortical thickness and surface area in autism spectrum disorder. *J Neural Transm (Vienna).* 2014;121(9):1157–1170.
44. Piven J, Berthier ML, Starkstein SE, Nehme E, Pearlson G, Folstein S. Magnetic resonance imaging evidence for a defect of cerebral cortical development in autism. *Am J Psychiatry.* 1990;147(6):734–739.
45. Hardan AY, Jou RJ, Keshavan MS, Varma R, Minshew NJ. Increased frontal cortical folding in autism: a preliminary MRI study. *Psychiatry Res.* 2004;131(3):263–268.
46. Levitt JG, Blanton RE, Smalley S, et al. Cortical sulcal maps in autism. *Cereb Cortex.* 2003;13(7):728–735.
47. Auzias G, Viellard M, Takerkart S, et al. Atypical sulcal anatomy in young children with autism spectrum disorder. *Neuroimage Clin.* 2014;4:593–603.
48. Wallace GL, Robustelli B, Dankner N, Kenworthy L, Giedd JN, Martin A. Increased gyrification, but comparable surface area in adolescents with autism spectrum disorders. *Brain.* 2013;136(Pt 6):1956–1967.
49. Libero LE, DeRamus TP, Deshpande HD, Kana RK. Surface-based morphometry of the cortical architecture of autism spectrum disorders: volume, thickness, area, and gyrification. *Neuropsychologia.* 2014;62:1–10.
50. Schaer M, Ottet MC, Scariati E, et al. Decreased frontal gyrification correlates with altered connectivity in children with autism. *Front Hum Neurosci.* 2013;7:750.

51. Kohli JS, Kinnear MK, Fong CH, Fishman I, Carper RA, Muller RA. Local cortical gyrification is increased in children with autism spectrum disorders, but decreases rapidly in adolescents. *Cereb Cortex.* 2019;29(6):2412–2423.
52. Gharehgazlou A, Freitas C, Ameis SH, et al. Cortical gyrification morphology in individuals with ASD and ADHD across the lifespan: a systematic review and meta-analysis. *Cereb Cortex.* 2020;31:2653–2669.
53. Patriquin MA, DeRamus T, Libero LE, Laird A, Kana RK. Neuroanatomical and neurofunctional markers of social cognition in autism spectrum disorder. *Hum Brain Mapp.* 2016;37(11):3957–3978.
54. Pelphrey K, Adolphs R, Morris JP. Neuroanatomical substrates of social cognition dysfunction in autism. *Ment Retard Dev Disabil Res Rev.* 2004;10(4):259–271.
55. Adolphs R. The neurobiology of social cognition. *Curr Opin Neurobiol.* 2001;11(2):231–239.
56. Girgis RR, Minshew NJ, Melhem NM, Nutche JJ, Keshavan MS, Hardan AY. Volumetric alterations of the orbitofrontal cortex in autism. *Prog Neuro-Psychopharmacol Biol Psychiatry.* 2007;31(1):41–45.
57. Amaral DG, Schumann CM, Nordahl CW. Neuroanatomy of autism. *Trends Neurosci.* 2008;31(3):137–145.
58. Schumann CM, Barnes CC, Lord C, Courchesne E. Amygdala enlargement in toddlers with autism related to severity of social and communication impairments. *Biol Psychiatry.* 2009;66(10):942–949.
59. Radeloff D, Ciaramidaro A, Siniatchkin M, et al. Structural alterations of the social brain: a comparison between schizophrenia and autism. *PLoS One.* 2014;9(9), e106539.
60. Hollander E, Anagnostou E, Chaplin W, et al. Striatal volume on magnetic resonance imaging and repetitive behaviors in autism. *Biol Psychiatry.* 2005;58(3):226–232.
61. Langen M, Bos D, Noordermeer SD, Nederveen H, van Engeland H, Durston S. Changes in the development of striatum are involved in repetitive behavior in autism. *Biol Psychiatry.* 2014;76(5):405–411.
62. Qiu T, Chang C, Li Y, et al. Two years changes in the development of caudate nucleus are involved in restricted repetitive behaviors in 2-5-year-old children with autism spectrum disorder. *Dev Cogn Neurosci.* 2016;19:137–143.
63. Watanabe T, Lawson RP, Wallden YSE, Rees G. A neuroanatomical substrate linking perceptual stability to cognitive rigidity in autism. *J Neurosci.* 2019;39(33):6540–6554.
64. Webb SJ, Sparks BF, Friedman SD, et al. Cerebellar vermal volumes and behavioral correlates in children with autism spectrum disorder. *Psychiatry Res.* 2009;172(1):61–67.
65. Scott JA, Schumann CM, Goodlin-Jones BL, Amaral DG. A comprehensive volumetric analysis of the cerebellum in children and adolescents with autism spectrum disorder. *Autism Res.* 2009;2(5):246–257.
66. Pauls DL, Abramovitch A, Rauch SL, Geller DA. Obsessive-compulsive disorder: an integrative genetic and neurobiological perspective. *Nat Rev Neurosci.* 2014;15(6):410–424.
67. Atmaca M, Yildirim H, Ozdemir H, Tezcan E, Poyraz AK. Volumetric MRI study of key brain regions implicated in obsessive-compulsive disorder. *Prog Neuro-Psychopharmacol Biol Psychiatry.* 2007;31(1):46–52.
68. Dabbs K, Jones J, Seidenberg M, Hermann B. Neuroanatomical correlates of cognitive phenotypes in temporal lobe epilepsy. *Epilepsy Behav.* 2009;15(4):445–451.
69. Ameis SH, Catani M. Altered white matter connectivity as a neural substrate for social impairment in autism spectrum disorder. *Cortex.* 2015;62:158–181.
70. Blackmon K, Ben-Avi E, Wang X, et al. Periventricular white matter abnormalities and restricted repetitive behavior in autism spectrum disorder. *Neuroimage Clin.* 2016;10:36–45.
71. Kana RK, Libero LE, Hu CP, Deshpande HD, Colburn JS. Functional brain networks and white matter underlying theory-of-mind in autism. *Soc Cogn Affect Neurosci.* 2014;9(1):98–105.

72. Ecker C, Suckling J, Deoni SC, et al. Brain anatomy and its relationship to behavior in adults with autism spectrum disorder: a multicenter magnetic resonance imaging study. *Arch Gen Psychiatry.* 2012;69(2):195–209.
73. Mostofsky SH, Burgess MP, Gidley Larson JC. Increased motor cortex white matter volume predicts motor impairment in autism. *Brain.* 2007;130(Pt 8):2117–2122.
74. Travers BG, Adluru N, Ennis C, et al. Diffusion tensor imaging in autism spectrum disorder: a review. *Autism Res.* 2012;5(5):289–313.
75. Shukla DK, Keehn B, Lincoln AJ, Muller RA. White matter compromise of callosal and subcortical fiber tracts in children with autism spectrum disorder: a diffusion tensor imaging study. *J Am Acad Child Adolesc Psychiatry.* 2010;49(12):1269–1278. 78 e1–2.
76. Noriuchi M, Kikuchi Y, Yoshiura T, et al. Altered white matter fractional anisotropy and social impairment in children with autism spectrum disorder. *Brain Res.* 2010;1362:141–149.
77. Aoki Y, Yoncheva YN, Chen B, et al. Association of white matter structure with autism spectrum disorder and attention-deficit/hyperactivity disorder. *JAMA Psychiat.* 2017;74(11):1120–1128.
78. Kemper TL, Bauman ML. The contribution of neuropathologic studies to the understanding of autism. *Neurol Clin.* 1993;11(1):175–187.
79. Bailey A, Luthert P, Dean A, et al. A clinicopathological study of autism. *Brain.* 1998;121(Pt 5):889–905.
80. Wegiel J, Kuchna I, Nowicki K, et al. The neuropathology of autism: defects of neurogenesis and neuronal migration, and dysplastic changes. *Acta Neuropathol.* 2010;119(6):755–770.
81. Casanova MF, Buxhoeveden DP, Switala AE, Roy E. Minicolumnar pathology in autism. *Neurology.* 2002;58(3):428–432.
82. McKavanagh R, Buckley E, Chance SA. Wider minicolumns in autism: a neural basis for altered processing? *Brain.* 2015;138(Pt 7):2034–2045.
83. Courchesne E, Mouton PR, Calhoun ME, et al. Neuron number and size in prefrontal cortex of children with autism. *JAMA.* 2011;306(18):2001–2010.
84. Menassa DA, Sloan C, Chance SA. Primary olfactory cortex in autism and epilepsy: increased glial cells in autism. *Brain Pathol.* 2017;27(4):437–448.
85. Avino TA, Hutsler JJ. Abnormal cell patterning at the cortical gray-white matter boundary in autism spectrum disorders. *Brain Res.* 2010;1360:138–146.
86. Bletsch A, Schafer T, Mann C, et al. Atypical measures of diffusion at the gray-white matter boundary in autism spectrum disorder in adulthood. *Hum Brain Mapp.* 2020;42:467–484.
87. Andrews DS, Avino TA, Gudbrandsen M, et al. In vivo evidence of reduced integrity of the gray-white matter boundary in autism spectrum disorder. *Cereb Cortex.* 2017;27(2):877–887.
88. Lai MC, Lombardo MV, Suckling J, et al. Biological sex affects the neurobiology of autism. *Brain.* 2013;136(Pt 9):2799–2815.
89. Hazlett HC, Poe MD, Lightbody AA, et al. Teasing apart the heterogeneity of autism: same behavior, different brains in toddlers with fragile X syndrome and autism. *J Neurodev Disord.* 2009;1(1):81–90.
90. Chen H, Uddin LQ, Guo X, et al. Parsing brain structural heterogeneity in males with autism spectrum disorder reveals distinct clinical subtypes. *Hum Brain Mapp.* 2019;40(2):628–637.
91. Uddin LQ, Menon V, Young CB, et al. Multivariate searchlight classification of structural magnetic resonance imaging in children and adolescents with autism. *Biol Psychiatry.* 2011;70(9):833–841.
92. Ecker C, Rocha-Rego V, Johnston P, et al. Investigating the predictive value of whole-brain structural MR scans in autism: a pattern classification approach. *NeuroImage.* 2010;49(1):44–56.
93. Wolfers T, Floris DL, Dinga R, et al. From pattern classification to stratification: towards conceptualizing the heterogeneity of autism spectrum disorder. *Neurosci Biobehav Rev.* 2019;104:240–254.

94. Hong SJ, Valk SL, Di Martino A, Milham MP, Bernhardt BC. Multidimensional neuroanatomical subtyping of autism spectrum disorder. *Cereb Cortex.* 2018;28(10):3578–3588.
95. Zabihi M, Oldehinkel M, Wolfers T, et al. Dissecting the heterogeneous cortical anatomy of autism spectrum disorder using normative models. *Biol Psychiatry Cogn Neurosci Neuroimaging.* 2019;4(6):567–578.
96. Floris DL, Wolfers T, Zabihi M, et al. Atypical brain asymmetry in autism-A candidate for clinically meaningful stratification. *Biol Psychiatry Cogn Neurosci Neuroimaging.* 2020;6:802–812.
97. Lombardo MV, Lai MC, Baron-Cohen S. Big data approaches to decomposing heterogeneity across the autism spectrum. *Mol Psychiatry.* 2019;24(10):1435–1450.
98. Murphy D, Spooren W. EU-AIMS: a boost to autism research. *Nat Rev Drug Discov.* 2012;11(11):815–816.
99. Thompson PM, Stein JL, Medland SE, et al. The ENIGMA consortium: large-scale collaborative analyses of neuroimaging and genetic data. *Brain Imaging Behav.* 2014;8(2):153–182.

CHAPTER

# 6

# Brain function and brain connectivity in autism

*Julie A. Trapani*[a], *Haley M. Bednarz*[a], *and Rajesh K. Kana*[b]

[a]Department of Neuropsychology, Children's Healthcare of Atlanta & Emory University School of Medicine, Atlanta, GA, United States, [b]Department of Psychology, The Center for Innovative Research in Autism, University of Alabama, Tuscaloosa, AL, United States

## Introduction

The underlying etiology of autism spectrum disorder (ASD) is complex, and the exact causes of the disorder are unknown. There are likely many different pathways of interacting biological and environmental factors[1,2] that result in the development of ASD,[3] and this likely contributes to the widespread heterogeneity of symptom presentation within the autism spectrum. Despite its complex etiology, it is well-understood that the downstream impact of these factors is altered development and functioning of the brain in ASD, leading to differences in sociocognitive aspects and behavior. Brain differences in ASD have been studied at multiple levels, including differences at the cellular (e.g., altered pruning, overactive glial cells, fewer Purkinje cells in the cerebellum, and differences in cellular organization) and structural (e.g., accelerated growth in brain volume, decreased corpus callosum volume, etc.) levels as reviewed in other chapters in this book. We now shift our attention to studies of brain function (e.g., activation and connectivity) and the currently established *functional* markers of ASD. This chapter focuses on the evidence for altered brain function and connectivity, its diagnostic utility, and its contribution to the conceptualization and treatment of ASD.

The advent of functional neuroimaging has made it possible to study brain function in vivo in both health and disease. A variety of noninvasive


https://doi.org/10.1016/B978-0-12-816393-1.00003-8

functional neuroimaging techniques allow researchers to understand brain function (Box 6.1). In the context of neurodevelopmental disorders, functional magnetic resonance imaging (fMRI) is particularly useful for several reasons: (1) fMRI allows for brain processes to be examined at a more direct level (compared to inferring brain function secondary to performance on cognitive tasks); (2) Certain types of functional neuroimaging

BOX 6.1

### Techniques of measuring functional brain activation

Since the emergence of modern neuroimaging methods nearly three decades ago, research investigating functional activation (i.e., brain regions that are activated during specific cognitive tasks) has dominated in the study of atypical mechanisms underlying cognitive, social, linguistic, and perceptual functions in people with ASD. Here, we briefly review a few concepts related to functional activation studies.

**Functional magnetic resonance imaging (fMRI) basics.** Functional Magnetic Resonance Imaging (fMRI) is among the most frequently employed methods for estimating neuronal activity and localizing brain function. Neurons require energy in the form of oxygen and glucose to fire. When a cluster of neurons are recruited for a cognitive task, there is a greater demand for oxygen, resulting in increased blood flow to that region of the brain. MRI is able to capture these changes in blood flow due to the molecular structure of hemoglobin, an oxygen-carrying protein found in red blood cells: *deoxygenated* hemoglobin has greater magnetic properties than *oxygenated* hemoglobin. These differences, detected using fMRI, are used to measure brain activity and localize it to certain regions of the brain. Blood-oxygen-level-dependent (BOLD) signal is the most common metric derived from fMRI and reflects this series of complex changes in blood flow.

**fMRI experimental designs.** Some fMRI experiments have participants complete an activity in the scanner to capture patterns of brain activation that underlie certain cognitive, emotional, or behavioral states (commonly referred to as *task-based fMRI*). These designs typically involve comparing an active *task condition*, which targets a specific cognitive process (e.g., attention, memory, etc.), to a *nontask condition*, also referred to as *control* or *baseline* condition. Even at rest, the brain remains active as it must maintain ongoing processes such as respiration, sensory processing, and general conscious awareness. Thus, it is important for experimenters to disentangle brain activation patterns that

BOX 6.1 *(cont'd)*

are related to the task itself, versus unrelated brain activation patterns. Through statistical analyses, researchers compare, or *contrast*, the average hemodynamic response elicited by the task condition and nontask condition. For example, Baron-Cohen et al.[10] conducted a social cognition fMRI study in which participants viewed photographs of people's eyes. In the *active task* condition, participants indicated what the person in the photograph might be thinking or feeling (inference-making). In the *control* condition, participants indicated whether the person in the photograph was male or female. This allowed for the neural processes underlying inference-making to be dissociated from other processes that are not of interest, such as visual processing and motor response via button press.

**fMRI group designs.** Lastly, neuroimaging research investigating altered brain functioning within the ASD population often involves comparing participants with ASD to a "typically developing" (TD) group to determine how neurologic functions are altered in ASD. Within the ASD literature, TD samples often include individuals of similar age and sex that do not have a history of ASD. Additionally, many studies often exclude participants from the TD group if they report certain developmental (e.g., ADHD), cognitive (e.g., intellectual disability, learning disability), or mood/psychiatric conditions (e.g., bipolar disorder, schizophrenia).

can capture brain function *during specific tasks* (e.g., social tasks, cognitive tasks) to specifically target the brain differences that underlie behaviors in ASD; (3) Imaging is noninvasive and can be used to study early development among children with ASD; and (4) It has the potential to eventually be integrated into a clinical/medical setting to aid diagnosis should a biomarker be identified. This last point has been at the forefront of ASD brain research. Specifically, there is great interest in the ability of functional neuroimaging techniques to identify objective biomarkers that could improve the clinical identification, diagnosis, and treatment of ASD.[4–9] A potential avenue is that neuroimaging could be used to identify infants at high-risk for developing ASD so that targeted interventions could be implemented earlier (*risk biomarker*). Additionally, neuroimaging could improve the efficiency, sensitivity, and accuracy of diagnosing ASD (*diagnostic biomarker*). Identification of a biomarker could also make the diagnosis of ASD more widely available in areas that have less access to the highly specialized multidisciplinary teams that are often required to make the differential diagnosis. Finally, a biomarker could be used to predict the progression of ASD, as well as an individual's response to treatment (*prognostic biomarker*). Thus, identifying a biomarker for ASD would have important implications and has been a central focus of many functional neuroimaging studies. However, there are many challenges associated with identifying a reliable brain biomarker for ASD, which will be described in this chapter.

This chapter will (1) review the pivotal findings of atypical brain region activation in ASD, (2) introduce brain connectivity and how it is measured, (3) review findings and promising implications of functional connectivity research in ASD, (4) discuss the disrupted connectivity hypothesis as a neural model of ASD, and finally (5) discuss future directions and clinical implications of this work.

## Functional activation in ASD

Neuroimaging techniques, most commonly fMRI, have highlighted several brain regions that commonly show altered activation (typically *hypo-*, or *under-activation*) among groups with ASD. It is important to note at the outset that many brain regions have been implicated in fMRI activation studies of ASD, with some inconsistent findings across studies. A number of factors likely contribute to this inconsistency, including smaller sample sizes of initial fMRI studies,[11] the heterogeneity of ASD population in terms of symptom presentation and underlying etiology,[12] differences in experimental design and data analysis approaches, exclusion/inclusion criteria for the study,[13] etc. Metaanalyses (statistical analysis that combines/integrates the results of multiple scientific studies) have been very helpful in summarizing the findings and in informing our current scientific understanding of brain activation–based inferences in ASD.[14–16] A few of the relatively more consistent findings to date are reviewed here.

One of the most widely studied brain regions in the ASD literature is the fusiform gyrus (FG) and its subregion fusiform face area (FFA), well-documented in its specialization for face processing. The FFA is located within the ventral occipitotemporal cortex, and is part of the human visual system uniquely specialized for face processing; fMRI tasks consistently reveal activation in this region in response to viewing faces.[17,18] Following established behavioral studies of deficient face-processing in ASD, Schultz and colleagues[19] were among the first to report significant findings of altered brain activation in FG in adolescents and adults with ASD on a face discrimination task. While a group of typically developing (TD) control participants exhibited functional activation in the right FG, individuals with ASD did not; instead, they demonstrated increased activation in the inferior temporal gyri (ITG), a brain region known to be involved in object recognition. These results suggested that individuals with ASD may process faces in a similar manner to how TD individuals process objects, which was suspected to be driven by the limited experience (or expertise) of individuals with ASD for face processing. Subsequent studies and adaptations replicated these findings, revealing consistent hypoactivation in the FFA on face recognition tasks and ultimately bolstering the neurocognitive models underlying altered face processing in ASD.[16,20,21] As the quest for reliable ASD biomarkers continues, it should be noted that altered neural responses in the FFA are theorized to be a consequence of social deficits in ASD and not a *cause*. The limited activation in the FFA in individuals with ASD likely reflects downstream effects driven by limited practice and experience in face processing due to reduced motivation to look at faces.[22] This hypothesis is further supported by research findings of brain activation in the FFA in response to viewing stimuli with which one has great familiarity or expertise, such as car and bird experts demonstrating greater activation in response to photographs of their respective expertise compared to everyday objects.[23]

Along with FFA, the posterior superior temporal sulcus (pSTS) is also implicated in social processing in ASD. Located in the temporal lobe, the pSTS plays a central role in theory-of-mind, voice perception, and processing biological motion.[24] Pelphrey and colleagues[25] posit that aberrant activity in the right pSTS is central to the overall neural disruption of the social brain observed in ASD. Compared to TD individuals, their research suggests that this region is not uniquely specialized for processing biological motion or inferring intentions in young adults with ASD. Research investigating social perception in siblings of individuals with ASD also reveal abnormal neural functioning in the pSTS, despite no clinically significant behavioral symptoms.[26] Further, several studies have documented the relationships between hypoactivation in the pSTS and deficits in joint attention (shared attention on a common object or event),[27] an early behavioral symptom noted in ASD.

The amygdala is another brain region implicated in the neurobiology of ASD. The amygdala is part of the limbic system, located deep within the medial temporal lobe, and plays a central role in emotion processing. The amygdala has consistently emerged in research investigating the "social brain"[28] and aberrant functional activation of amygdala has been noted across neuropsychiatric conditions. Within ASD research, fMRI studies have revealed hypoactivation in the amygdala on social tasks.[10] On a theory-of-mind task that required the inference of mental states of others, Baron-Cohen and colleagues found that the amygdala was not activated in individuals with ASD, but was activated in healthy control individuals. The amygdala has also been implicated for its involvement in face processing, with both hyperactivation[22] and hypoactivation documented.[29,30] It is theorized that these differences in activation are driven by a mixture of difficulties in social processing and anxiety; social difficulties tend to be associated with amygdala hypoactivation, while increased anxiety is related to hyperactivation in the amygdala.[31] Lastly, these functional differences are consistent with the abnormal structural developmental trajectory of the amygdala in ASD, including reduced volume and neuronal count.[32]

The cerebellum has been one of the earliest and most consistent brain regions found to be implicated in the neurobiology of ASD.[33] Initial studies identified the cerebellum's role in coordinating voluntary motor patterns[34–36]; however, more recent research has made it evident that the cerebellum is involved in many aspects of cognitive, emotional, and social functioning.[37–40] In fact, the cerebellum has been conceptualized as a "co-processor," such that it integrates information from various regions of the brain to smoothly coordinate motor patterns, language, social interactions, among many other diverse functions.[41,42] In this way, the cerebellum has been an interesting brain region to study in the context of ASD, given that that the presentation of ASD includes multiple symptoms (i.e., social-communication impairment, restrictive-repetitive behaviors) that could potentially be explained by cerebellar involvement in modulating multiple cognitive processes. Several earlier fMRI investigations found altered activation of the cerebellum during motor tasks.[43–45] For example, Allen and Courchesne[43] observed hyperactivation of the cerebellum during a motor task, but hypoactivation during a visual attention task. Additionally, differences in cerebellar activation have been reported during emotional processing, attention, executive functioning, language, among other tasks.[46]

As illustrated above, multiple brain regions have been found to have altered activation in ASD. However, findings across studies have been inconsistent and have not resulted in a reliable fMRI biomarker. For example, there are some studies investigating face processing in ASD that have documented typical activation in the FFA.[47,48] Such studies point to face processing difficulty in ASD to be a more perceptual issue than social. In addition, isolating altered brain functioning in ASD to a single brain region may be simplistic. The FFA activation differences may be reflective of disrupted core and extended brain networks of face processing. It is difficult to explain the heterogeneous symptoms of ASD (e.g., social-communication deficits, stereotyped behaviors, executive function deficits, sometimes intellectual disability) with the implication of one brain region alone. Ultimately, the existing literature on focal region–based investigations has been inadequate in fully understanding the neurobiology of the disorder and for holding any promise as a potential clinical biomarker. In recent years, neuroimaging research has largely shifted to examining the brain at a *network* level rather than a *local* level which offers a more comprehensive and nuanced understanding of brain functioning.

## Functional connectivity

Localization of function is certainly clinically meaningful. However, brain regions hardly function in isolation. Ultimately, neurological functions occur through interactive processes across connected brain regions, forming systems and networks. These processes are cognitively and computationally taxing, and thus require efficient allocation of neural resources for optimal functioning. The human brain is organized to meet these demands through a delicate balance of functional specialization and functional integration.[49] Functional specialization should sound familiar, as we have just discussed a few brain areas that are specialized for certain functions (e.g., FFA for face processing). Functional integration refers to how the specialized regions communicate and cooperate to accomplish a task. These principles can be demonstrated through classic motor tasks, such as finger tapping of the right hand: fMRI results provide evidence for a clear neural motor map, with increased activation in the precentral gyrus in the left hemisphere and right hemisphere cerebellum activation.[50] The precentral gyrus, also referred to as the primary motor cortex, is specialized for executing voluntary motor movements. Meanwhile, the cerebellum receives information from other parts of the brain to regulate motor movement. The functional integration of these brain regions (and likely additional regions, such as the premotor cortex with involvement in motor planning) is what results in effective task completion. The balance between specialization and integration begins early in brain development, with brain regions becoming anatomically segregated across the cortex and connections forming across these regions through integration.[51] As ASD is a neurodevelopmental disorder with notable disruptions in early brain development (see Chapters 5 and 7), a compelling line of research points to disruptions in functional specialization and functional integration within this disorder that may ultimately lead to clinical symptoms.[52]

So, how is functional integration measured? Information travels throughout the brain via axons along white matter tracts. *Structural connectivity* explains how information flows along these white matter tracts. *Functional connectivity* refers to how activity across brain regions may be coordinated through neurons that are firing in sync with one another. Neuropsychologist Donald Hebb's theory of learning expands on concepts of connectivity and long-term potentiation, indicating that neural networks become stronger with repetition/coactivation. This concept is famously summarized with the phrase *"neurons that fire together, wire together."*[53] As far as measuring these constructs, current metrics of structural connectivity are anatomical (DWI: Diffusion Weighted Imaging), while functional connectivity is measured through a correlation of time series of local activation across brain regions (fMRI, MEG, EEG, TMS). Simultaneous activation is sometimes referred to as *coactivation*. One of the most common ways of measuring functional connectivity is through functional connectivity MRI (fcMRI). The specific methodology of fcMRI depends on the underlying constructs to be investigated. As briefly introduced earlier in this chapter, task-based fMRI allows researchers to understand which parts of the brain are activated by a certain task or cognitive process; task-based fcMRI allows researchers to investigate which of these brain regions work together in synchronization to accomplish this task. Another common metric is *resting-state connectivity*, which refers to the functional connectivity when participants are at rest in the MRI scanner. For these studies, participants are typically instructed to lie awake in the scanner and not think about anything in particular. The BOLD signal changes are analyzed to identify intrinsic and synchronous fluctuations in functional activity between brain regions. These studies provide insights into different brain networks including the Default Mode Network (DMN). Müller[54] put it best when describing ASD as a "distributed disorder" that is best characterized neurobiologically by understanding disruptions at the network and system level. Functional connectivity has been consistently identified as a promising avenue for understanding ASD.[55] Specific patterns of altered functional connectivity offer a potential neurobiological theory underlying the clinical presentation of ASD.

## Functional connectivity in ASD

### Underconnectivity in ASD

The first evidence of altered functional connectivity in ASD was the result of a Positron Emission Tomography (PET) study that found under-connectivity between frontal and parietal regions of the brain in the ASD group.[56] One of the earliest and influential fMRI investigations of brain connectivity in ASD revealed under-connectivity among core language areas (i.e., Wernicke's and Broca's areas) during a sentence comprehension task.[57] In the years since, task-based fcMRI has consistently revealed alterations in brain connectivity across tasks that tap into a myriad of psychological domains that are impacted in ASD, including cognitive, social, language, visuospatial, and motor functioning.[58,59] These alterations in connectivity are thought to largely reflect less efficient allocation of neural resources across brain regions.[60] Although the underlying cognitive processes and brain regions vary across studies, a consistent pattern that has emerged is cortical underconnectivity between frontal and other cortical and subcortical regions.[61–64] The most common pattern to emerge is underconnectivity between frontal and posterior brain areas.[65] Cortical underconnectivity is also well documented in resting state connectivity studies, demonstrating reduced synchronization in the DMN when the brain is not cognitively engaged in a task.[66–68]

The findings of neural underconnectivity in ASD are hypothesized to underlie the broad deficits in "higher-order" functions that require the integration of multiple cognitive skills. For example, successful and efficient social processing requires functional integration between multiple regions involved in domains such as face processing and theory-of-mind (e.g., FFA, amygdala, STS, posterior cingulate cortex, precuneus, etc.).[69–71] Aberrant functional connectivity between these regions is well-documented in the literature,[58] suggesting less efficient neural integration and communication in ASD.

## Overconnectivity in ASD

There is also evidence of *overconnectivity* in ASD, particularly between neighboring cortical and subcortical regions.[72,73] In conceptualizing these findings, overconnectivity at the *local level* is also considered to be disruptive to functioning. Overconnectivity may reflect hyperspecialization of lower-level cognitive processes, or an increased communication between brain regions that may not be best suited for effective cognition or task completion.[74] This inefficiency in processing could be related to early differences in brain development, including impaired synaptic pruning and early brain overgrowth. Anatomical investigations reveal differences in white matter development in a subset of children with ASD.[75] Postmortem studies of infants and toddlers with ASD have revealed significantly increased neuronal counts in the prefrontal cortex compared to TD controls,[76] as well as smaller and more numerous cortical minicolumns within the frontal and temporal lobes.[77] These findings converge to suggest that early brain overgrowth and macrocephaly could be driven by overproduction of neurons and white matter tracts, ultimately driving local overconnectivity and wiring brain regions to "talk to themselves."

## Implications of differences in connectivity

Research investigations have begun to establish relationships between the strength of brain connectivity and symptom severity in ASD. Several studies have found that scores on the Autism Diagnostic Observation Schedule (ADOS) and the Autism Diagnostic Interview-Revised (ADI-R), the gold standard diagnostic assessments for ASD, are correlated with specific patterns of functional connectivity.[78–82] For example, Weng and colleagues[82] found that in adolescents with ASD, symptom severity in the domains of social skills and RRBs were associated with underconnectivity within in the DMN, while impairments in verbal and nonverbal communication were associated with overconnectivity of certain regions. These differences in connectivity are more notable during adolescence than adulthood, suggesting that the developmental trajectories of this disorder may be critical for understanding symptom presentation. Overall, behavioral symptom presentation has been linked to altered connectivity in ASD and provides additional clues for the underlying neuropathology of this disorder.

The developmental and causal relationships between underconnectivity and overconnectivity are not yet well understood. Maximo and colleagues[59] described an overconnected local network as a "peninsula," with long-distance connectivity constrained due to its isolation and limited access to other regions. A possible compensatory strategy adopted by the developing brain is to communicate with the neighboring regions it *does* have access to.[60] It is also possible that the findings of under- and overconnectivity in ASD are related to one another, such that overconnectivity of local brain regions may prevent the formation of long-distance connections, or potentially, the lack of integrative long-distance brain connectivity may result in a greater emphasis of neural processing at the local level.[58] The large consensus in the literature is not to characterize either as consequential or causal, but to consider findings of either to be representative of the general disruptions in connectivity, which provides continued support for ASD as a disorder of distributed neurobiological disruptions.

## Overview of disrupted connectivity hypothesis

An integrated theory that accounts for the neurobiological disruption and ultimately the heterogeneous behavioral presentation in ASD is *the disrupted connectivity hypothesis*. Primary disruptions in connectivity, or underconnectivity, are reported between the frontal cortex and other areas of the brain. The frontal cortex is vital for higher-order cognitive skills, including social processing, language, and executive functions—all of which are found to be impacted in ASD. Aberrant projections from the prefrontal cortex can account for the wide variety of presentation across and within these cognitive processes, and a possible adaptation may be local overconnectivity. These functional differences are also supported by well-documented anatomical differences. For example, the structural integrity of white matter pathways, or the communication tracts between neurons within the brain, are reduced in ASD.[83] Further, disruptions in connectivity between frontal and posterior regions also correlate with corpus callosum size, providing additional support for the relationship between functional connectivity and the structural integrity of white matter pathways. Based on the convergence of functional connectivity findings and anatomical studies of differences in brain development, ASD has been broadly characterized as a disorder of brain network organization.[84]

Relationships have also been drawn between the disrupted connectivity hypothesis and cognitive theories of ASD. For example, the weak central coherence (WCC) hypothesis proposes a detail-focused cognitive style within ASD, with limited ability to see the "big picture" or context and greater processing of small details.[85] This pattern of WCC has been conceptualized as emerging from disruptions to functional connectivity,[60,78] such that higher-order cognitive skills are disrupted (underconnectivity) and lower-level features are overemphasized (overconnectivity) in ASD and that this pattern is driven by compensatory development in neural circuitry.

A future direction in this line of research is focused attention on illuminating the neurodevelopmental trajectories in ASD. There is overwhelming evidence of atypical brain development and maturation in ASD. Alterations in connectivity could be driven by delayed and disrupted brain development. In typical development, white matter volume and structural integrity increases with age and is suspected to represent increases in long-range connectivity established through repetition and learning.[86] One of the patterns of atypical brain maturation in ASD is early brain overgrowth, marked by overgrowth of white matter in young children and reduced white matter in adolescence and adulthood.[52] Along those lines, much of the research investigating children under 12 years of age report increased functional connectivity, while studies of adolescents and adults report reduced functional connectivity.[87] Despite these findings, there are few longitudinal studies that investigate nuanced connectivity patterns across the lifespan, in both typical development and in individuals with ASD. The use of multimodal neuroimaging may provide the layered tools to detect these nuanced differences. Many studies utilize a singular neuroimaging modality, primarily fMRI and fcMRI. Continued methodological investigation of the links between approaches is warranted to promote convergence of findings across previous studies and within future study design. Further, there is ongoing discussion within the neuroimaging community about what these varying metrics of functional connectivity truly measure, such as differences at the cellular level versus differences in informational processing efficiency.[65,88] Clarifying these points will impact the inferences drawn from aberrant functional connectivity in ASD and other neurologic conditions.

## Clinical implications

As described at the beginning of this chapter, a number of studies have sought to identify neural biomarkers to aid in the diagnosis and treatment of ASD. Additionally, researchers have begun to explore other avenues for translating fMRI research to clinical practice, such as integrating fMRI with cognitive and behavioral intervention/treatment to monitor neural changes across time. Such intervention-based fMRI studies target brain plasticity and use intense training to change the brain activation and connectivity to facilitate improvement in behavioral functions. While plenty of promises lie in the quest for neuroimaging-based biomarkers of autism, neuroimaging methods are not without their limitations. See Box 6.2 for a brief review of the barriers that have limited the clinical translatability of fMRI findings to date.

BOX 6.2

## Methodological limitations

There has been great difficulty in replicating and generalizing the findings of functional connectivity studies in ASD,[13,89–91] which has led to a closer examination of fMRI experimental techniques. For example, there is concern regarding the nefarious effects of head motion on fMRI findings. Children[92–94] and individuals with ASD and related developmental disorders[13] commonly have greater difficulty remaining still in the MRI scanner. Greater levels of head motion during scanning has been associated with artifactual findings, including decreased long-distance functional connectivity and increased short-distance connectivity.[95,96] This has led to concerns that findings of altered functional connectivity in ASD may be attributed at least in part to greater levels of head motion in this group.[68,97] Researchers have increasingly adopted behavioral (e.g., practice mock scanning sessions)[93,98,99] and computational methods[95,100–105] to control for head motion; however, there is evidence that many traditional motion correction techniques do not completely remove the influence of head motion.[101]

Smaller sample size and limited diversity of symptom severity significantly limit the generalizability of findings to the broader ASD population. MRI studies are costly and technical, posing logistical limitations for data acquisition and impacting the feasibility of gathering large datasets. Further, the traditional MRI environment is not inherently suitable for individuals with difficulties with receptive language and comprehension of instruction, emotion dysregulation, repetitive behaviors, and differences in sensory processing. For these reasons, many research studies utilizing fMRI selectively recruit high-functioning individuals with ASD. Unfortunately, this limits the ability to study and understand the true spectrum of neurobiological underpinnings in this disorder. Nordahl and colleagues[106] proposed specific adaptations to the MRI environment utilizing applied behavioral analysis (ABA) principles that yielded significant successful data acquisition in individuals with ASD and comorbid intellectual disability. Resting-state fMRI, which does not require comprehension of a task, may also be an important tool for examining samples of low-functioning individuals.[107] Further, there is also clear direction for addressing the limitations of smaller sample sizes in research this population. Study replications and data sharing are increasing in popularity, with repositories such as the Autism Brain Imaging Data Exchange (ABIDE) allowing researchers across settings to pool their data.[108] This shows great promise for overcoming the challenges associated with small sample size and site-specific data collection methods (e.g., scanner, analysis pipeline) that may also influence results.[89]

## Functional connectivity as a potential biomarker?

A number of studies have utilized the disrupted connectivity model of ASD as the basis for identifying neural markers that could improve the diagnostic process. Studies have found that ASD severity and behavioral symptom presentation are associated with altered brain connectivity.[80] Additionally, fMRI studies of corpus callosum size and structural integrity of white matter tracts in high-risk infants revealed reliable prediction of which individuals will later receive a diagnosis of ASD,[109] suggesting that aberrant differences in connectivity are present early and may be a sensitive predictor for downstream behavioral impacts. Several studies have utilized task-based functional connectivity[110–112] and more commonly, resting-state connectivity[7,113–120] to classify and differentiate participants with ASD from TD (and sometimes other populations).

A recent review of MRI biomarker studies found that classifier performance (e.g., accuracy, sensitivity, specificity) was variable across studies, with inconsistencies at least partly due to differences in participant age, classifier use, and sample size (e.g., greater classification accuracy found with smaller sample sizes).[7] Additionally, ASD is highly comorbid with other developmental disorders and conditions that have similar genetic factors (e.g., attention-deficit/hyperactivity disorder (ADHD), Tourette's syndrome, anxiety)[121,122] and it is unclear what a biomarker would look like in the context of comorbid conditions (e.g., would multiple biomarkers be present? Would a different biomarker be present?).[13] Current research demonstrates overlap in disruptions in functional connectivity between individuals with ASD and ADHD,[123] which poses a barrier for the clinical utility of this feature as a sensitive biomarker. With regards to medical comorbidities, it is well documented that individuals with ASD are at increased risk for seizures and epilepsy.[124] While this serves as additional evidence for the disruption to neural circuitry in ASD, it also offers another difficulty in terms of isolating specific patterns of disruption that are unique to ASD. An effective biomarker would need to identify the presence of ASD and also differentiate it from other comorbid conditions. Ultimately, classifier performance is not yet at the level that it can be employed clinically. Continued investigations of the unique patterns of neural circuitry across these conditions are needed in order to operationalize functional connectivity in a clinical setting.

In addition to supporting classification and diagnosis, there is evidence that neuroimaging could also serve as a unique assessment tool to monitor response to treatment.[125,126] This research indicates that response to behavioral interventions also have the potential to "normalize" brain function and connectivity, and lend further support that disruptions to these networks could be the driver of symptom presentation. A worthwhile direction for future research is to identify specific profiles of brain function and connectivity to determine which interventions may be best suited for certain individuals.

## Conclusions

Technological advances in recent decades have allowed for functional neuroimaging to play a key role in elucidating neural differences in the ASD brain. While research investigating functional activation in ASD has been abundant and illuminating, the literature investigating brain regions at the local level has been inconsistent and inadequate for fully understanding the neural underpinnings of ASD. In recent years, neuroimaging research has largely shifted to examining the brain at a *network* level. Functional connectivity research has lent way to the disrupted connectivity hypothesis, which postulates that ASD is a distributed disorder marked by inefficiencies in the way the brain communicates and synchronizes activity. In particular, there is cortical *underconnectivity* of long-distance connections, coupled with local *overconnectivity*. The pursuit of sensitive and accessible biomarkers remains at the forefront of research efforts, and the utilization of disruptions in functional connectivity is emerging as a potential future tool for assessing risk, classifying symptom presentation, and determining treatment response and prognostic status.

## References

1. Chaste P, Leboyer M. Autism risk factors: genes, environment, and gene-environment interactions. *Dialogues Clin Neurosci.* 2012;14(3):281–292.
2. Tordjman S, Somogyi E, Coulon N, et al. Gene×environment interactions in autism spectrum disorders: role of epigenetic mechanisms. *Front Psych.* 2014;5:53.
3. Oron O, Elliott E. Delineating the common biological pathways perturbed by ASD's genetic etiology: lessons from network-based studies. *Int J Mol Sci.* 2017;18(4):828.
4. Anderson GM. Autism biomarkers: challenges, pitfalls and possibilities. *J Autism Dev Disord.* 2015;45(4):1103–1113.
5. Li D, Karnath H-O, Xu X. Candidate biomarkers in children with autism spectrum disorder: a review of MRI studies. *Neurosci Bull.* 2017;33(2):219–237.
6. Loth E, Spooren W, Ham LM, et al. Identification and validation of biomarkers for autism spectrum disorders. *Nat Rev Drug Discov.* 2016;15(1):70.
7. Uddin LQ, Dajani DR, Voorhies W, Bednarz H, Kana RK. Progress and roadblocks in the search for brain-based biomarkers of autism and attention-deficit/hyperactivity disorder. *Transl Psychiatry.* 2017;7(8):e1218.
8. Voineagu I, Yoo HJ. Current progress and challenges in the search for autism biomarkers. *Dis Markers.* 2013;35(1):55.
9. Walsh P, Elsabbagh M, Bolton P, Singh I. In search of biomarkers for autism: scientific, social and ethical challenges. *Nat Rev Neurosci.* 2011;12(10):603–612.
10. Baron-Cohen S, Ring HA, Bullmore ET, Wheelwright S, Ashwin C, Williams SCR. The amygdala theory of autism. *Neurosci Biobehav Rev.* 2000;24(3):355–364.
11. Turner BO, Paul EJ, Miller MB, Barbey AK. Small sample sizes reduce the replicability of task-based fMRI studies. *Commun Biol.* 2018;1(1):62.

12. Lombardo MV, Lai M-C, Baron-Cohen S. Big data approaches to decomposing heterogeneity across the autism spectrum. *Mol Psychiatry.* 2019;24(10):1435–1450.
13. Bednarz HM, Kana RK. Advances, challenges, and promises in pediatric neuroimaging of neurodevelopmental disorders. *Neurosci Biobehav Rev.* 2018;90:50–69.
14. Anagnostou E, Taylor M. Review of neuroimaging in autism spectrum disorders: what have we learned and where we go from here. *Mol Autism.* 2011;2:4.
15. Minshew NJ, Keller TA. The nature of brain dysfunction in autism: functional brain imaging studies. *Curr Opin Neurol.* 2010;23(2):124–130.
16. Philip RCM, Dauvermann MR, Whalley HC, Baynham K, Lawrie SM, Stanfield AC. A systematic review and meta-analysis of the fMRI investigation of autism spectrum disorders. *Neurosci Biobehav Rev.* 2012;36(2):901–942.
17. Kanwisher N, McDermott J, Chun MM. The fusiform face area: a module in human extrastriate cortex specialized for face perception. Published online, 1997;17:4302–4311. 10.
18. Sergent J, Ohta S, MacDonald B. Functional neuroanatomy of face and object processing: a positron emission tomography study. *Brain.* 1992;115(1):15–36.
19. Schultz RT, Gauthier I, Klin A, et al. Abnormal ventral temporal cortical activity during face discrimination among individuals with autism and Asperger syndrome. *Arch Gen Psychiatry.* 2000;57(4):331–340.
20. Hubl D, Bölte S, Feineis-Matthews S, et al. Functional imbalance of visual pathways indicates alternative face processing strategies in autism. *Neurology.* 2003;61(9):1232–1237.
21. Pierce K, Müller RA, Ambrose J, Allen G, Courchesne E. Face processing occurs outside the fusiform "face area" in autism: evidence from functional MRI. *Brain J Neurol.* 2001;124(Pt 10):2059–2073.
22. Dalton KM, Nacewicz BM, Johnstone T, et al. Gaze fixation and the neural circuitry of face processing in autism. *Nat Neurosci.* 2005;8(4):519–526.
23. Gauthier I, Skudlarski P, Gore JC, Anderson AW. Expertise for cars and birds recruits brain areas involved in face recognition. *Nat Neurosci.* 2000;3(2):191–197.
24. Zilbovicius M, Meresse I, Chabane N, Brunelle F, Samson Y, Boddaert N. Autism, the superior temporal sulcus and social perception. *Trends Neurosci.* 2006;29(7):359–366.
25. Pelphrey KA, Shultz S, Hudac CM, Wyk BCV. Research review: constraining heterogeneity: the social brain and its development in autism spectrum disorder. *J Child Psychol Psychiatry.* 2011;52(6):631–644.
26. Spencer MD, Holt RJ, Chura LR, et al. A novel functional brain imaging endophenotype of autism: the neural response to facial expression of emotion. *Transl Psychiatry.* 2011;1(7), e19.
27. Redcay E, Dodell-Feder D, Mavros PL, et al. Atypical brain activation patterns during a face-to-face joint attention game in adults with autism spectrum disorder. *Hum Brain Mapp.* 2013;34(10):2511–2523.
28. Skuse D, Morris J, Lawrence K. The amygdala and development of the social brain. *Ann N Y Acad Sci.* 2003;1008:91–101.
29. Corbett BA, Carmean V, Ravizza S, et al. A functional and structural study of emotion and face processing in children with autism. *Psychiatry Res.* 2009;173(3):196–205.
30. Critchley HD, Daly EM, Bullmore ET, et al. The functional neuroanatomy of social behaviour: changes in cerebral blood flow when people with autistic disorder process facial expressions. *Brain.* 2000;123(11):2203–2212.
31. Herrington JD, Miller JS, Pandey J, Schultz RT. Anxiety and social deficits have distinct relationships with amygdala function in autism spectrum disorder. *Soc Cogn Affect Neurosci.* 2016;11(6):907–914.
32. Avino TA, Barger N, Vargas MV, et al. Neuron numbers increase in the human amygdala from birth to adulthood, but not in autism. *Proc Natl Acad Sci U S A.* 2018;115(14):3710–3715.
33. Fatemi SH, Aldinger KA, Ashwood P, et al. Consensus paper: pathological role of the cerebellum in autism. *Cerebellum.* 2012;11(3):777–807.

34. Houk JC, Buckingham JT, Barto AG. Models of the cerebellum and motor learning. *Behav Brain Sci.* 1996;19:368–383.
35. Ito M. Mechanisms of motor learning in the cerebellum. *Brain Res.* 2000;886(1–2):237–245. Published online.
36. Llinás R, Welsh JP. On the cerebellum and motor learning. *Curr Opin Neurobiol.* 1993;3(6):958–965.
37. Overwalle FV. Cerebellar areas dedicated to social cognition? A comparison of meta-analytic and connectivity results. 2015;10:337–344.
38. Stoodley CJ. The cerebellum and cognition: evidence from functional imaging studies. *Cerebellum.* 2012;11(2):352–365.
39. Van Overwalle F, Baetens K, Mariën P, Vandekerckhove M. Social cognition and the cerebellum: a meta-analysis of over 350 fMRI studies. *Neuroimage.* 2014;86:554–572.
40. Van Overwalle F, Mariën P. Functional connectivity between the cerebrum and cerebellum in social cognition: a multi-study analysis. *Neuroimage.* 2016;124:248–255.
41. D'Angelo E, Casali S. Seeking a unified framework for cerebellar function and dysfunction: from circuit operations to cognition. *Front Neural Circuits.* 2013;6:116.
42. Ito M. Control of mental activities by internal models in the cerebellum. *Nat Rev Neurosci.* 2008;9(4):304–313.
43. Allen G, Courchesne E. Differential effects of developmental cerebellar abnormality on cognitive and motor functions in the cerebellum: an fMRI study of autism. *Am J Psychiatry.* 2003;160(2):262–273.
44. Allen G, Müller R-A, Courchesne E. Cerebellar function in autism: functional magnetic resonance image activation during a simple motor task. *Biol Psychiatry.* 2004;56(4):269–278.
45. Müller R-A, Cauich C, Rubio MA, Mizuno A, Courchesne E. Abnormal activity patterns in premotor cortex during sequence learning in autistic patients. *Biol Psychiatry.* 2004;56(5):323–332.
46. Becker EBE, Stoodley CJ. Autism spectrum disorder and the cerebellum. In: *International Review of Neurobiology.* Vol 113. Elsevier; 2013:1–34.
47. Hadjikhani N, Joseph RM, Snyder J, et al. Activation of the fusiform gyrus when individuals with autism spectrum disorder view faces. *Neuroimage.* 2004;22(3):1141–1150.
48. Pierce K, Haist F, Sedaghat F, Courchesne E. The brain response to personally familiar faces in autism: findings of fusiform activity and beyond. *Brain J Neurol.* 2004;127(Pt 12):2703–2716.
49. Tononi G, Edelman GM, Sporns O. Complexity and coherency: integrating information in the brain. *Trends Cogn Sci.* 1998;2(12):474–484.
50. Mattay VS, Weinberger DR. Organization of the human motor system as studied by functional magnetic resonance imaging. *Eur J Radiol.* 1999;30(2):105–114.
51. Friston KJ. Functional and effective connectivity: a review. *Brain Connect.* 2011;1(1):13–36.
52. Courchesne E. Abnormal early brain development in autism. *Mol Psychiatry.* 2002;7(Suppl 2):S21–S23.
53. Shatz CJ. The developing brain. *Sci Am.* 1992;267(3):60–67.
54. Müller R-A. The study of autism as a distributed disorder. *Ment Retard Dev Disabil Res Rev.* 2007;13(1):85–95.
55. Maximo JO, Cadena EJ, Kana RK. The implications of brain connectivity in the neuropsychology of autism. *Neuropsychol Rev.* 2014;24(1):16–31.
56. Horwitz B. The cerebral metabolic landscape in autism: intercorrelations of regional glucose utilization. *Arch Neurol.* 1988;45(7):749.
57. Just MA, Cherkassky VL, Keller TA, Minshew NJ. Cortical activation and synchronization during sentence comprehension in high-functioning autism: evidence of underconnectivity. *Brain.* 2004;127(8):1811–1821.
58. Kana RK, Libero LE, Moore MS. Disrupted cortical connectivity theory as an explanatory model for autism spectrum disorders. *Phys Life Rev.* 2011;8(4):410–437.

59. Maximo JO, Cadena EJ, Kana RK. The implications of brain connectivity in the neuropsychology of autism. *Neuropsychol Rev.* 2014;24(1):16–31.
60. Belmonte MK, Cook EH, Anderson GM, et al. Autism as a disorder of neural information processing: directions for research and targets for therapy. *Mol Psychiatry.* 2004;9(7):646–663.
61. Anderson JS, Druzgal TJ, Froehlich A, et al. Decreased interhemispheric functional connectivity in autism. *Cereb Cortex.* 2011;21(5):1134–1146.
62. Kana RK, Keller TA, Minshew NJ, Just MA. Inhibitory control in high-functioning autism: decreased activation and underconnectivity in inhibition networks. *Biol Psychiatry.* 2007;62(3):198–206.
63. Kana RK, Keller TA, Cherkassky VL, Minshew NJ, Just MA. Atypical frontal-posterior synchronization of theory of mind regions in autism during mental state attribution. *Soc Neurosci.* 2009;4(2):135–152.
64. Vasa RA, Mostofsky SH, Ewen JB. The disrupted connectivity hypothesis of autism spectrum disorders: time for the next phase in research. *Biol Psychiatry Cogn Neurosci Neuroimaging.* 2016;1(3):245–252.
65. Just MA, Keller TA, Malave VL, Kana RK, Varma S. Autism as a neural systems disorder: a theory of frontal-posterior underconnectivity. *Neurosci Biobehav Rev.* 2012;36(4):1292–1313.
66. Cherkassky VL, Kana RK, Keller TA, Just MA. Functional connectivity in a baseline resting-state network in autism. *Neuroreport.* 2006;17(16):1687–1690.
67. Kennedy DP, Courchesne E. The intrinsic functional organization of the brain is altered in autism. *Neuroimage.* 2008;39(4):1877–1885.
68. Tyszka JM, Kennedy DP, Paul LK, Adolphs R. Largely typical patterns of resting-state functional connectivity in high-functioning adults with autism. *Cereb Cortex.* 2014;24(7):1894–1905.
69. Adolfi F, Couto B, Richter F, et al. Convergence of interoception, emotion, and social cognition: a twofold fMRI meta-analysis and lesion approach. *Cortex.* 2017;88:124–142.
70. Tso IF, Rutherford S, Fang Y, Angstadt M, Taylor SF. The "social brain" is highly sensitive to the mere presence of social information: an automated meta-analysis and an independent study. Hayasaka S, ed *PLoS One.* 2018;13(5), e0196503.
71. van Veluw SJ, Chance SA. Differentiating between self and others: an ALE meta-analysis of fMRI studies of self-recognition and theory of mind. *Brain Imaging Behav.* 2014;8(1):24–38.
72. Cerliani L, Mennes M, Thomas RM, Di Martino A, Thioux M, Keysers C. Increased functional connectivity between subcortical and cortical resting-state networks in autism spectrum disorder. *JAMA Psychiat.* 2015;72(8):767–777.
73. Maximo JO, Kana RK. Aberrant "deep connectivity" in autism: a cortico-subcortical functional connectivity magnetic resonance imaging study. *Autism Res.* 2019;12(3):384–400.
74. Noonan SK, Haist F, Müller R-A. Aberrant functional connectivity in autism: evidence from low-frequency BOLD signal fluctuations. *Brain Res.* 2009;1262:48–63.
75. Herbert MR, Ziegler DA, Deutsch CK, et al. Dissociations of cerebral cortex, subcortical and cerebral white matter volumes in autistic boys. *Brain J Neurol.* 2003;126(Pt 5):1182–1192.
76. Courchesne E, Campbell K, Solso S. Brain growth across the life span in autism: age-specific changes in anatomical pathology. *Brain Res.* 2011;1380:138–145.
77. Casanova MF, Buxhoeveden DP, Switala AE, Roy E. Minicolumnar pathology in autism. *Neurology.* 2002;58(3):428–432.
78. Just MA, Cherkassky VL, Keller TA, Kana RK, Minshew NJ. Functional and anatomical cortical underconnectivity in autism: evidence from an FMRI study of an executive function task and corpus callosum morphometry. *Cereb Cortex.* 2007;17(4):951–961.
79. Lee PS, Yerys BE, Della Rosa A, et al. Functional connectivity of the inferior frontal cortex changes with age in children with autism spectrum disorders: a fcMRI study of response inhibition. *Cereb Cortex.* 2009;19(8):1787–1794.

80. Liu X, Huang H. Alterations of functional connectivities associated with autism spectrum disorder symptom severity: a multi-site study using multivariate pattern analysis. *Sci Rep.* 2020;10(1):4330.
81. Monk CS, Peltier SJ, Wiggins JL, et al. Abnormalities of intrinsic functional connectivity in autism spectrum disorders. *Neuroimage.* 2009;47(2):764–772.
82. Weng S-J, Wiggins JL, Peltier SJ, et al. Alterations of resting state functional connectivity in the default network in adolescents with autism spectrum disorders. *Brain Res.* 2010;1313:202–214.
83. Travers BG, Adluru N, Ennis C, et al. Diffusion tensor imaging in autism spectrum disorder: a review. *Autism Res.* 2012;5(5):289–313.
84. Rudie JD, Shehzad Z, Hernandez LM, et al. Reduced functional integration and segregation of distributed neural systems underlying social and emotional information processing in autism spectrum disorders. *Cereb Cortex.* 2012;22(5):1025–1037.
85. Frith U. *Autism: Explaining the Enigma.* Blackwell Publishing; 2003.
86. Uddin LQ, Supekar KS, Ryali S, Menon V. Dynamic reconfiguration of structural and functional connectivity across core neurocognitive brain networks with development. *J Neurosci.* 2011;31(50):18578–18589.
87. Uddin LQ, Supekar K, Menon V. Reconceptualizing functional brain connectivity in autism from a developmental perspective. *Front Hum Neurosci.* 2013;7:458.
88. Bourgeron T. From the genetic architecture to synaptic plasticity in autism spectrum disorder. *Nat Rev Neurosci.* 2015;16(9):551–563.
89. He Y, Byrge L, Kennedy DP. Nonreplication of functional connectivity differences in autism spectrum disorder across multiple sites and denoising strategies. *Hum Brain Mapp.* 2020;41(5):1334–1350.
90. King JB, Prigge MBD, King CK, et al. Generalizability and reproducibility of functional connectivity in autism. *Mol Autism.* 2019;10(1):27.
91. Nair S. Local resting state functional connectivity in autism: site and cohort variability and the effect of eye status. *Brain Imaging Behav.* 2018;12:168–179. Published online.
92. Bookheimer SY. Methodological issues in pediatric neuroimaging. *Ment Retard Dev Disabil Res Rev.* 2000;6(3):161–165.
93. Poldrack RA, Paré-Blagoev EJ, Grant PE. Pediatric functional magnetic resonance imaging: progress and challenges. *Top Magn Reson Imaging.* 2002;13(1):61–70.
94. Thomas KM, King SW, Franzen PL, et al. A developmental functional MRI study of spatial working memory. *Neuroimage.* 1999;10(3):327–338.
95. Power JD, Barnes KA, Snyder AZ, Schlaggar BL, Petersen SE. Spurious but systematic correlations in functional connectivity MRI networks arise from subject motion. *Neuroimage.* 2012;59(3):2142–2154.
96. Van Dijk KRA, Sabuncu MR, Buckner RL. The influence of head motion on intrinsic functional connectivity MRI. *Neuroimage.* 2012;59(1):431–438.
97. Deen B, Pelphrey K. Perspective: brain scans need a rethink. *Nature.* 2012;491(7422):S20.
98. Kana RK, Murdaugh DL, Libero LE, et al. Probing the brain in autism using fMRI and diffusion tensor imaging. *J Vis Exp.* 2011;55, e3178.
99. De Amorim e Silva CJT, Mackenzie A, Hallowell LM, Stewart SE, Ditchfield MR. Practice MRI: reducing the need for sedation and general anaesthesia in children undergoing MRI. *Australas Radiol.* 2006;50(4):319–323.
100. Caballero-Gaudes C, Reynolds RC. Methods for cleaning the BOLD fMRI signal. *Neuroimage.* 2017;154:128–149.
101. Ciric R, Rosen AFG, Erus G, et al. Mitigating head motion artifact in functional connectivity MRI. *Nat Protoc.* 2018;13(12):2801–2826.
102. Parkes L, Fulcher B, Yücel M, Fornito A. An evaluation of the efficacy, reliability, and sensitivity of motion correction strategies for resting-state functional MRI. *Neuroimage.* 2018;171:415–436.

103. Power JD, Mitra A, Laumann TO, Snyder AZ, Schlaggar BL, Petersen SE. Methods to detect, characterize, and remove motion artifact in resting state fMRI. *Neuroimage.* 2014;84:320–341.
104. Power JD, Schlaggar BL, Petersen SE. Recent progress and outstanding issues in motion correction in resting state fMRI. *Neuroimage.* 2015;105:536–551.
105. Satterthwaite TD, Ciric R, Roalf DR, Davatzikos C, Bassett DS, Wolf DH. Motion artifact in studies of functional connectivity: characteristics and mitigation strategies. *Hum Brain Mapp.* 2019;40:2033–2051.
106. Nordahl CW, Mello M, Shen AM, et al. Methods for acquiring MRI data in children with autism spectrum disorder and intellectual impairment without the use of sedation. *J Neurodev Disord.* 2016;8:1–10.
107. Li G, Rossbach K, Jiang W, Du Y. Resting-state brain activity in Chinese boys with low functioning autism spectrum disorder. *Ann Gen Psychiatry.* 2018;17(1):47.
108. Di Martino A, Yan C-G, Li Q, et al. The autism brain imaging data exchange: towards a large-scale evaluation of the intrinsic brain architecture in autism. *Mol Psychiatry.* 2014;19(6):659–667.
109. Wolff JJ, Gerig G, Lewis JD, et al. Altered corpus callosum morphology associated with autism over the first 2 years of life. *Brain.* 2015;138(7):2046–2058.
110. Deshpande G, Libero LE, Sreenivasan KR, Deshpande HD, Kana RK. Identification of neural connectivity signatures of autism using machine learning. *Front Hum Neurosci.* 2013;7:670.
111. Murdaugh DL, Shinkareva SV, Deshpande HR, Wang J, Pennick MR, Kana RK. Differential deactivation during mentalizing and classification of autism based on default mode network connectivity. *PLoS One.* 2012;7(11), e50064.
112. Libero LE, DeRamus TP, Lahti AC, Deshpande G, Kana RK. Multimodal neuroimaging based classification of autism spectrum disorder using anatomical, neurochemical, and white matter correlates. *Cortex.* 2015;66:46–59.
113. Abraham A, Milham MP, Di Martino A, et al. Deriving reproducible biomarkers from multi-site resting-state data: an autism-based example. *Neuroimage.* 2017;147:736–745.
114. Anderson JS, Nielsen JA, Froehlich AL, et al. Functional connectivity magnetic resonance imaging classification of autism. *Brain J Neurol.* 2011;134(Pt 12):3742–3754.
115. Chen CP, Keown CL, Jahedi A, et al. Diagnostic classification of intrinsic functional connectivity highlights somatosensory, default mode, and visual regions in autism. *NeuroImage: Clinical.* 2015;8:238–245.
116. Liu J, Sheng Y, Lan W, Guo R, Wang Y, Wang J. Improved ASD classification using dynamic functional connectivity and multi-task feature selection. *Pattern Recogn Lett.* 2020;138:82–87.
117. Nielsen JA, Zielinski BA, Fletcher PT, et al. Multisite functional connectivity MRI classification of autism: ABIDE results. *Front Hum Neurosci.* 2013;7:599.
118. Plitt M, Barnes KA, Martin A. Functional connectivity classification of autism identifies highly predictive brain features but falls short of biomarker standards. *NeuroImage: Clinical.* 2015;7:359–366.
119. Uddin LQ, Supekar K, Lynch CJ, et al. Salience network–based classification and prediction of symptom severity in children with autism. *JAMA Psychiat.* 2013;70(8):869–879.
120. Yahata N, Morimoto J, Hashimoto R, et al. A small number of abnormal brain connections predicts adult autism spectrum disorder. *Nat Commun.* 2016;7(1):11254.
121. Lichtenstein P, Carlström E, Råstam M, Gillberg C, Anckarsäter H. The genetics of autism spectrum disorders and related neuropsychiatric disorders in childhood. *Am J Psychiatry.* 2010;167(11):1357–1363.
122. Ronald A, Simonoff E, Kuntsi J, Asherson P, Plomin R. Evidence for overlapping genetic influences on autistic and ADHD behaviours in a community twin sample. *J Child Psychol Psychiatry.* 2008;49(5):535–542.

123. Bathelt J, Caan M, Geurts H. *More Similarities Than Differences Between ADHD and ASD in Functional Brain Connectivity.* PsyArXiv; 2020, DOI:10.31234/osf.io/4tfmn.
124. Ballaban-Gil K, Tuchman R. Epilepsy and epileptiform EEG: association with autism and language disorders. *Ment Retard Dev Disabil Res Rev.* 2000;6(4):300–308.
125. Calderoni S, Billeci L, Narzisi A, Brambilla P, Retico A, Muratori F. Rehabilitative interventions and brain plasticity in autism spectrum disorders: focus on MRI-based studies. *Front Neurosci.* 2016;10:139.
126. Murdaugh DL, Maximo JO, Kana RK. Changes in intrinsic connectivity of the brain's reading network following intervention in children with autism. *Hum Brain Mapp.* 2015;36(8):2965–2979.

CHAPTER

# 7

# White matter microstructure in autism

*Michael Connaughton[a], Erik O'Hanlon[a], and Jane McGrath[a,b]*

[a]Psychiatry, Trinity College, Dublin, Ireland, [b]Consultant Child and Adolescent Psychiatrist, ADMiRE, Linn Dara CAMHS, Health Service Executive, Dublin, Ireland

## Introduction

Neuroimaging research has demonstrated numerous abnormalities in brain structure and function in ASD, from which a number of theories of altered cortical connectivity in ASD have emerged.[1–7] Together, these theories hold that core social and cognitive features of ASD are underpinned by abnormal interregional brain connectivity. This idea is compelling as it could unify a number of the current neuropsychological theories about the etiology of ASD. For example, disrupted neural connectivity in ASD could contribute to restricted and repetitive behavior (the executive dysfunction hypothesis[8]), social and communication deficits (the empathizing-systemizing theory[9]), weak central coherence (the weak central coherence theory[10,11]), and superior perceptual function (the enhanced perceptual functioning theory[12]).

Brain "functional connectivity" and "structural connectivity" have been investigated in ASD, and these studies have provided accumulating evidence for the theory of abnormal cortical connectivity. Functional connectivity refers to the coordination of processing, or communication, between brain regions and can be measured using a variety of approaches including functional magnetic resonance imaging (fMRI), Positron Emission Tomography (PET), electroencephalography (EEG), magnetoencephalography (MEG), and regional homogeneity (ReHo) analyses. A growing body of literature suggests that functional connectivity abnormalities in


https://doi.org/10.1016/B978-0-12-816393-1.00012-9

ASD are widespread, affect multiple cognitive functions, and can be characterized by both reduced[4] and increased[13] patterns of connectivity. The pathophysiology of this abnormal functional connectivity is poorly understood, but it may arise from disrupted organization of white matter in inter- and intrahemispheric tracts.

Structural connectivity is a term referring to the micro- and macrostructural organization of white matter (the nerve fibers) of the brain. Brain anatomical data, using a variety of measurement techniques including structural MRI, postmortem histological analysis, and in particular DW-MRI, has revealed a number of abnormalities in ASD that are suggestive of disrupted structural connectivity. Findings of accelerated early brain growth, white matter enlargement, and atypical structural organization of white matter are all abnormalities that could compromise connections between brain regions in ASD and lead to disrupted structural connectivity. The majority of DW-MRI studies in children, adolescents, and adults with ASD have reported reduced organization of white matter microstructure, although affected white matter tracts vary significantly between studies.[14] In parallel with neuroimaging research, genetic studies have identified numerous susceptibility genes for ASD. Many of these risk variants appear to impact functionally on neural connectivity including synaptogenesis, neuronal motility, and axon guidance.[15]

DW-MRI is a technique that allows the noninvasive, in vivo examination of white matter tissue microstructure, or structural connectivity, in the human brain.[16–18] Since the first DW-MRI study of ASD in 2004, the literature regarding the microstructural properties of white matter in ASD has expanded rapidly. This chapter provides an overview of studies that have investigated white matter microstructure in ASD. In the first section, an introduction to DW-MRI and commonly used diffusion measures is provided. In the following sections, the methods of voxel-based (whole-brain and region of interest), tractography and connectomics analyses are described, and the key findings from studies using these approaches in ASD are summarized.

## Introduction to diffusion-weighted MRI (DW-MRI)

### Physics of DW-MRI

DW-MRI allows for the in vivo examination of the underlying architectural organization of white matter tracts through measurement of the restricted diffusion of water molecules in tissue.[16,17,19,20] When water molecule diffusion is not impeded by any barriers such as cell membranes, the diffusion occurs equally in all directions. In such a situation, if diffusion from one particular point is measured, the water molecules will diffuse

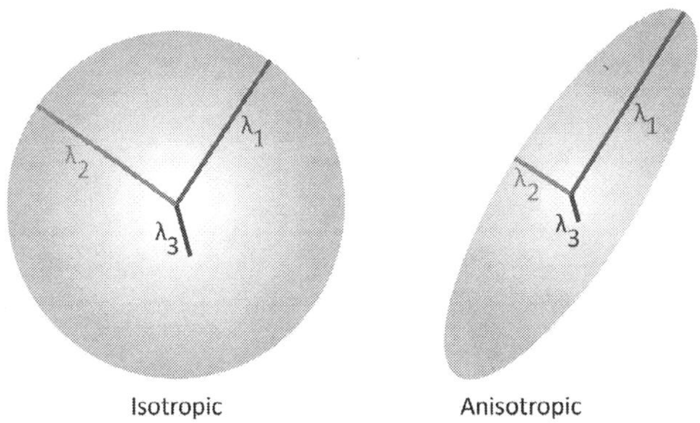


**FIG. 1** Isotropic and anisotropic diffusion including the three eigenvalues (λ1, λ2, and λ3).

away from this central point in a sphere. This type of unhindered water diffusion is called "isotropic." In body tissue however, there are numerous barriers to the diffusion of water molecules (e.g., cell membranes or axonal myelin sheaths in brain white matter). When the diffusing water molecules meet such a barrier, the "sphere" of diffusion will be disrupted, and diffusion becomes uneven. In this case, when measuring diffusion from a particular point, the mobility of the water molecules from the origin will now have a shape different to a sphere. This shape is often modeled as an ellipsoid, and the diffusion is termed "anisotropic" (see Fig. 1). In white matter, the axonal myelin sheaths act as the principle barrier to the diffusion of water molecules. Bundles of axons allow parallel diffusion of water molecules along the orientation of the fibers, but restrict perpendicular diffusion. It is this phenomenon that permits DW-MRI to distinguish white matter tracts in the brain. In major white matter tracts, where there are many bundles of myelinated axons clustered together, a high degree of anisotropic diffusion is expected.

## Measures of white matter microstructural organization

DW-MRI allows measurement of a number of diffusivity indices that relate to the microstructural organization of brain white matter.[18,21] The most common indices reported in studies using tradition diffusion tensor modeling are fractional anisotropy (FA), mean diffusivity (MD), radial diffusivity (RD) and axial diffusivity (AD). FA is a ratio, where a value of "0" refers to a perfect sphere with pure isotropic diffusion, and a value of "1" refers to ideal linear diffusion. Typically, white matter tracts have an FA greater than 0.2. The measurement of the degree of anisotropy provides information about the structural integrity of the white matter; in conditions where the structure of the axon is disrupted, for example inflammation/trauma/tumor, the barrier to diffusion will be reduced, and anisotropy will be less than expected. Hence, directional change (increases or decreases) in FA is thought to be associated with disrupted organization of white matter fiber tracts.

Reduced FA may reflect demyelination, axonal damage, or loss of white matter coherence.[18,21–24] Conversely, increased FA may reflect increased myelination of white matter fibers, increased numbers of myelinated fibers, smaller axonal diameter, or reduced neural branches within the MRI voxel.[25,26] Increased FA could also be artifactual, resulting from excessive partial volume averaging from multiple, differently oriented, fibers within a voxel[25,27,28] and may indicate the presence of more complex fiber orientations with increased crossing fibers. In such a case, it is feasible that a nondisease-related reduction in FA could be observed in localized regions with multiple fiber bundles intersecting. It is therefore important to contextualize the directionality of FA change because reduced FA is not a blanket identification of diseased or damaged white matter tissue.

While FA is very sensitive to microstructural changes, it is not very specific about the type of change. It has been suggested that to better characterize the tissue microstructure, diffusion measures of axial diffusivity, radial diffusivity, and mean diffusivity should be measured in conjunction with FA.[18] The ellipsoid resulting from anisotropic diffusion of water molecules in tissue can be deconstructed into three principle eigenvalues ($\lambda1$, $\lambda2$ and $\lambda3$). The largest eigenvalue ($\lambda1$) is referred to as axial diffusivity and represents diffusion parallel to the axonal direction. Radial diffusivity (calculated by $(\lambda2+\lambda3)/2$) reflects diffusion perpendicular to the white matter tracts. Reduced axial diffusivity may indicate altered axonal integrity and increased radial diffusivity is generally accepted to be a sensitive marker for demyelination.[29] These values are thought to allow detection of subtle structural abnormalities that cannot be detected by FA.[18] Mean diffusivity (calculated by $(\lambda1+\lambda2+\lambda3)/3)$) is a scalar value which refers to the total magnitude of diffusion in a voxel regardless of direction. An increase in mean diffusivity is thought to reflect edema, demyelination and axonal loss.[18,30] Generalized fractional anisotropy (GFA) is derived from higher order diffusion models such as Q-ball and is similar to FA, providing information about the level of white matter microstructural organization based on diameter, packing density, directional coherence and myelination of axons.[31]

## Voxel-based analyses research in ASD

The majority of the earlier studies (2004–10) that used DW-MRI to investigate white matter pathology in ASD explored whole-brain white matter using voxel-based analysis. Voxel-based analysis is a technique that compares local-voxel-wise differences across either the whole-brain or a predefined region of interest (ROI).

In the first published DW-MRI study in ASD, Barnea-Goraly et al. performed a whole-brain voxel-based analysis of DW-MRI data and found reduced FA in a number of frontal and temporal brain regions that have been implicated in social cognition and theory of mind tasks including the fusiform gyrus, amygdala, superior temporal sulcus, temporoparietal junction, prefrontal cortex and anterior cingulate.[32] Since then, voxel-based studies have provided strong evidence for aberrant white matter microstructure in ASD, characterized by reduced FA in frontal regions,[32–41] temporal regions,[32–35,37,38,41–44] occipital regions,[33,34,42] and the cingulate gyrus.[32,37,45]

In addition, voxel-based studies have reported abnormal white matter microstructure in a large number of major white matter tracts in ASD including in the corpus callosum,[33,36–38,41,46–50] superior longitudinal fasciculus,[36,37,48] inferior longitudinal fasciculus,[51–53] inferior fronto-occipital fasciculus and arcuate fasciculus,[53] cingulum bundle,[33,53] uncinate fasciculus,[48,53] fornix,[48] cerebellar peduncles,[38,49] internal capsule,[33,38,47,49] external capsule,[42] and corticospinal tracts.[36]

## Tract-based spatial statistics (TBSS) research in ASD

Although the voxel-based analyses of DW-MRI data have revealed disruption of white matter throughout the brain in ASD, there is significant heterogeneity in methodologies and participants, and it is difficult to identify a common underlying pattern of neuropathology across all studies.[54] In addition, this typical whole-brain and region of interest voxel-by-voxel approach to analysis of diffusion-weighted data is limited by misalignment and arbitrarily applied smoothing parameters, which can produce abnormal results.[55,56] An analytic approach called Tract-based Spatial Statistics (TBSS) (http://www.fmrib.ox.ac.uk/fsl/tbss/) was specifically designed to resolve some of the methodological issues associated with whole-brain and ROI voxel-wise analyses of diffusion weighted data. TBSS is an automated, observer-independent method that performs voxel-wise comparisons of diffusion properties of white matter. There are a number of benefits associated with this method. It includes a method of reliable registration of subjects to a common space by projecting all subjects' FA data onto a mean FA tract skeleton. It avoids the use of a smoothing kernel. It minimizes partial volume effects and it uses permutation statistics that are not dependent on a normal distribution of data. It has been suggested that the data-driven approach of TBSS may be particularly useful in a disorder like ASD, for which regional patterns of brain abnormalities are not fully determined.[57]

TBSS studies have consistently reported atypical white matter organization in both children and adults with ASD. In children with ASD, disrupted white matter microstructure, typically characterized by reduced FA, increased MD or increased RD, has been reported in white matter in including temporal[58,59] and parietal brain regions,[59] as well as in specific white matter tracts including the corpus callosum,[54,57,59–69] cingulum bundle,[57,60,62,66,69,70] arcuate fasciculus,[71] uncinate fasciculus,[62,63,65,66,70,72] superior longitudinal fasciculus,[57,60,65–67,69,70,73,74] inferior longitudinal fasciculus,[54,57,60,62,65–67,69–71,73] inferior fronto-occipital fasciculus,[54,57,62,65,70–73] corona radiata,[64,69] forceps major and minor,[70] thalamic radiations,[57,62–65,67,69,70] corticospinal tract,[57,59,62,65,66,72] internal capsule,[57,59,69] brainstem,[69] and cerebellum.[59]

In contrast with the relatively consistent finding of reduced microstructural organization of white matter in children and adolescents with ASD, increased FA has been reported in many studies of infants and young children (<4 years). In this younger population, increased FA has been observed in frontal tracts,[75] corpus callosum,[75–78] superior longitudinal fasciculus,[76,78] inferior longitudinal fasciculus, inferior fronto-occipital fasciculus, corticospinal tract,[76] cingulum bundle,[78] and brain stem tracts.[76,77] Studies of children aged 4–14 years have also reported increased FA in frontal regions,[79,80] inferior fronto-occipital fasciculus and areas of the optic radiation,[81] supplementary motor area,[80] corpus callosum, internal and external capsule, arcuate fasciculus,[82] cingulum and cerebellum.[79,80]

TBSS studies of adults with ASD have reported widespread reduction in white matter organization with reduced FA in brain regions such as frontal, temporal, parietal, and occipital white matter[83] as well as major white matter tracts such as the corona radiata,[84] thalamic radiation,[84–86] internal capsule,[84] external capsule,[84] corpus callosum,[83,87,88] fornix,[84] stria terminalis,[84] sagittal stratum,[84] superior fronto-occipital fasciculus,[84] superior longitudinal fasciculus,[84,86] uncinate fasciculus,[84,86] cingulum,[84,86,87] arcuate fasciculus,[87] brain stem tracts,[84] cerebral peduncles,[84] external capsule,[87] and the corticospinal tract,[84] although some studies have failed to find a difference in white matter microstructure between adults with ASD.[62,89,90]

In summary, the results of this large number of TBSS studies suggest that white matter organization is disrupted in numerous major white matter tracts in ASD, but despite the homogeneity of the TBSS analytic method and the relative similarity of participants in the majority of these studies, results do not provide a clear picture of common underlying neuropathology. It is possible that the discrepancies in results from these TBSS studies are a consequence of the use of different DW-MRI acquisition protocols and preprocessing methodologies.[91]

## Tractography research in ASD

Although voxel-based studies are informative about overall changes in white matter, they are unable to provide information about the microstructural organization of specific white matter tracts connecting brain regions. A technique that can partially overcome the limitations of traditional voxel-based approaches to DW-MRI analysis is diffusion tensor imaging (DTI) based tractography.[92–95] DTI-based tractography is an analytic process that essentially uses the orientation of the diffusion profile to reconstruct the trajectories of white matter fiber bundles. With advances in fiber-tracking software, it is possible to perform virtual in vivo dissections of white matter tracts, visualize white matter pathways and measure microstructural organization within specific white-matter tracts in the human brain.[16] The diffusion tractography approach revolutionized the ability to investigate specific white matter connections in the brain and how their structure relates to brain function, behavior, and disease.

A number of DTI tractography studies have reported abnormalities of specific white matter tracts in individuals with ASD. There is evidence of disruption of white matter micro- and macrostructure in a number of major inter- and intrahemispheric tracts including the corpus callosum, uncinate fasciculus, cingulum, arcuate fasciculus, inferior fronto-occipital fasciculus, inferior longitudinal fasciculus, superior longitudinal fasciculus, fornix, internal capsule, anterior thalamic radiation and fronto-striatal tracts, which are discussed in detail below.

### Corpus callosum

Structural MRI studies have consistently reported reduction in the volume of the corpus callosum (CC) in ASD.[96,97] The results of diffusion tractography studies that have isolated the CC are quite mixed, however, and provide an unclear picture of the pathology. Several studies of children and adolescents with ASD have reported reduced FA[98–101] and reduced GFA[102] in the CC; however, some have not reported any abnormality in WM microstructure of this tract.[48,103] Adults with ASD have also showed disrupted CC microstructure in some research[87] but other studies have failed to find any difference.[104] Studies of infants and young children aged 6 months,[105] $<2.5$ years,[106] and $<4$ years[78] have reported increased FA. This finding revealed greater white matter organization in infants and young children with ASD, but reduced organization in older children and adults in in keeping with a theory that the developmental trajectory of white matter in ASD is atypical. This is discussed in more detail later in this chapter.

Other white matter abnormalities identified in the CC in ASD imply compromise of macrostructural organization. Reduced volume of the CC,[68,107] a reduction in interhemispheric frontal streamlines,[68] increased length and fiber density of the CC[99] and shorter average fiber length in the forceps major[108] have been reported in ASD.

## Uncinate fasciculus

Results from diffusion tractography studies that have examined the uncinate fasciculus (UF) in ASD are quite mixed and, as for the corpus callosum, no clear picture of the underlying pathology has emerged. Reduced FA in the UF has been reported in studies of children[48,99] and young adults.[109] Elevated MD has also been identified in this tract in both children[110] and adults with ASD,[87] but 6-month-old infants who subsequently developed ASD had higher FA in the UF than neurotypical controls.[105]

From a macro-structural perspective, a reduced number of streamlines, which is a possible surrogate of tract volume,[110] increased left lateralization of volume, as measured by the number of streamlines and number of voxels,[104] and increased curvature at the fronto-temporal junction[111] has been reported in the UF in ASD. A number of other studies have failed to find any difference in WM microstructure in the UF in infants (12–24 months[105]), in children[98,103,112] and in adults with ASD.[104]

## Cingulum

A study of very young children with ASD (mean age 3.2 years) found increased FA in the cingulum,[78] whereas reduced FA was found in studies of older children aged 5 years,[99] 7–13 years,[112,113] 18 years,[114] and also in adults.[87] Increased MD and RD of the cingulum have been reported in children and adolescents with ASD.[115] Structurally, findings of increased number of streamlines in right and left cingulum in adults with ASD[110] and increased fiber density in left cingulum in young children with ASD[99] have been reported.

## Arcuate fasciculus

Reduced FA[48,99,116] and increased MD[117] and RD[87] of the arcuate fasciculus (AF) have been reported in individuals with ASD, though not in all studies.[118] Reduced left lateralization,[102,119,120] increased curvature[111] and increased tract volume of the AF[116] have been described in ASD.

## Inferior fronto-occipital fasciculus

Relative to controls, reduced FA in the right inferior fronto-occipital fasciculus (IFOF) was reported in children and young adults with ASD aged 15–20 years[118] and increased left lateralization of volume was reported in this tract in adults with ASD.[104] A number of other studies did not observe any abnormalities of this tract.[98,99,110,112]

## Inferior longitudinal fasciculus

Reduced FA and increased RD in the inferior longitudinal fasciculus (ILF) was described in one study of individuals aged 11–18 years with ASD,[121] but not in a number of others.[98,103,104,110,112] Increased FA in the inferior longitudinal fasciculus was reported in 6-month-old infants with ASD (but not 12- or 24-month-olds[105]). Increased left lateralization of ILF tract volume[104] and increased number of streamlines in the ILF[110] have been reported in ASD.

## Superior longitudinal fasciculus

Atypical white matter microstructure of the superior longitudinal fasciculus (SLF) has been reported, but as for other major white matter tracts, the results have been mixed. Reduced FA was reported in the SLF in children and adults with a mean age of 20 in one study,[122] yet another study of children and adults with a similar mean age reported an increase in FA in this tract.[64] Increased number of streamlines[123] in the SLF has also been observed but other studies have reported no abnormalities of this tract in ASD.[98,103]

## Internal capsule and anterior thalamic radiation

Infants with ASD showed increased FA at 6 months but reduced FA at 24 months in the anterior and posterior limb of the internal capsule (IC) and reduced FA at 12 and 24 months in the left anterior thalamic radiation (ATR) relative to controls.[105] Increased MD and RD of thalamic white matter tracts, was observed in young children (<36 months)[124] and adolescents.[125] Another study of older children and young adults found no differences in white matter microstructure in the ATR.[103] An increase in FA was reported in the left fornix in infants (6 months) who developed ASD but as for other major white matter tracts, there was no between-group difference in FA at 12 and 24 months,[105] nor was there a difference in FA in this tract in older children (6–13 years) with ASD.[48,112]

## Other white matter tracts

Reduced white matter microstructural organization characterized by reduced FA or increased MD has been described in a number of other white matter tracts in individuals with ASD including in the fronto-striatal tracts,[126] but not,[127] the corticospinal tract,[128] intrainsular and thalamocortical tracts,[129] short intracerebellar fibers,[130] in hippocampo-fusiform and amygdalo-fusiform pathways,[131] in white matter tracts connecting the amygdala with the cortex[132] in fiber tracts between the inferior frontal lobe and fusiform gyrus, inferior frontal lobe and medial temporal gyrus[133] and the putamen and frontal cortex.[126]

## Higher-order models of diffusion tractography

In the earlier years of DW-MRI analysis, the diffusion tensor model was the most commonly used framework to relate the diffusion signal to the direction of the fibers in early tractography research.[94,134] In voxels that contain "crossing" fibers where there is more than one coherently oriented fiber population, however, the diffusion tensor model is lacking.[135–139] It is now known that voxels containing crossing fibers occur very frequently throughout the white matter[140–142] and this has profound implications for tractography based on diffusion tensor imaging, and tensor-derived scalar measures.[140,143] In regions of crossing fibers, measures derived from the tensor model such as FA and MD are not reliable[143,144] and the interpretation of these measures is ambiguous.[140] In addition, in voxels with crossing fibers the diffusion tensor model cannot accurately describe the orientation of the fibers, and therefore, the underlying orientation of the white matter tracts cannot be reliably estimated. Tractography algorithms that rely on the diffusion tensor model will produce unreliable results in regions containing multiple fiber orientations.[145–147]

In order to overcome the limitations of the diffusion tensor model, more complex diffusion reconstruction schemes have been developed. These include constrained spherical deconvolution (CSD), diffusion kurtosis imaging (DKI), Q-ball, diffusion spectrum imaging (DSI), and fixel-based analyses (FBA). These analyses estimate the fiber orientation distribution function (fODF) for CSD, or diffusion orientation distribution function (dODF) for DSI and Q-ball, a parameter that can describe the direction of diffusion in voxels with multiple crossing fibers. These higher order-models overcome partial volume effects associated with the diffusion tensor model and facilitate accurate estimation of diffusion measures and fiber-tracking through regions of complex fiber architecture.[141,148,149]

Diffusion metrics derived from the use of these higher order models have been shown to have increased accuracy and yield clinically relevant information that cannot be obtained when using the DTI model.[150]

## Constrained spherical deconvolution (CSD)

Using CSD-based tractography, studies of children and young adults with ASD have reported reduced FA in the right inferior fronto-occipital fasciculus[118] and in white matter tracts between the occipital lobe and caudate, and occipital lobe and thalamus in children and young adults with ASD.[118] Increased FA has been reported in the inferior longitudinal fasciculus in adults with ASD[72] and increased FA of a component of superior longitudinal fasciculus (SLF II) and greater linear diffusion co-efficient (CL) of left SLF I and right SLF II was also reported in a CSD-based tractography study of children and young adults with ASD.[64]

## Diffusion spectrum imaging (DSI)

Research using DSI tractography found reduced GFA values in the corpus callosum,[102,151,152] right dorsal cingulum bundle,[153] left parieto-ponto-cerebellar tract,[154] superior longitudinal fasciculus,[155] frontal aslant tracts,[155] right arcuate fasciculus,[151] and bilateral frontoparietal tracts connecting the pars opercularis and supramarginal gyrus.[152]

## Diffusion kurtosis imaging (DKI)

The small numbers of studies that have used DKI have reported abnormalities in white matter microstructure in a number of tracts in adults and children with ASD. Reduced axial kurtosis, a diffusion metric that provides information about the level of organization of white matter, has been reported in the body and splenium of the corpus callosum in adults with ASD.[156] Significantly reduced faxon, a diffusion metric reflecting axon caliber and density, and reduced intraaxonal diffusivity (D axon) was observed in adults with ASD in a large number of white matter tracts, including the corpus callosum,[157,158] corticospinal tracts, superior and inferior longitudinal fasciculus, and inferior fronto-occipital fasciculus.[157]

## Q-ball

Q-ball tractography has been used to investigate white matter properties of the dentatorubrothalamic pathway in children with ASD and described reduced FA win white matter tracts originating in all four subdivisions of the dentate nucleus of the cerebellum.[159]

## Fixel-based

One fixel-based analysis reported that children and young adults with ASD showed reduced fiber density (FD) suggesting decreased axonal count, in the corpus callosum, bilateral inferior fronto-occipital fasciculus, right arcuate fasciculus, right uncinate fasciculus, as well as in global white matter.[160] A second fixel-based analysis found no significant differences in white matter micro- and macrostructure between adults with ASD and neurotypical controls; however, when stratified by sex, females with ASD had reduced FD in the corpus callosum relative to controls.[161]

## Connectomics

The term "connectomics" refers to the mapping and study of the network of neural connections in the brain.[162] Studies using a connectomics approach have provided novel insights into the neural pathophysiology of ASD. In connectomics research, the brain is modeled as a network which is defined as a set of nodes (gray matter regions) linked by connections known as edges (white matter tracts). The strength or weakness between each node is calculated and used to indicate the presence or absence of brain interconnections. This connection profile is then topographically represented to meaningfully identify brain circuits with highly correlated brain regions, and to detail characteristics of the anatomical white matter tracts describing features such as density and size.

Graph theory is a mathematical algorithm used for the assessment and representation of the human brain connectome. In general, the framework represents brain architecture as a set of nodes or cortical regions and the links between them which are representative of the white matter fiber pathways or tracts in the brain. Graph theory builds a matrix to represent the brain network where matrix rows represent the nodes and matrix columns represent the connectivity between a node and every other node in the defined network. In this way, the connectivity matrix (CM) is built and used to investigate structural connectivity. A variety of measures can be extrapolated from this technique which provide information on properties of the whole-brain network, subnetworks of the brain, and "rich-club analysis."

### Whole-brain network analysis

Graph theory analysis suggests that individuals with ASD display abnormal structural connectivity in both whole-brain and functionally distinct networks. Rudie and colleagues (2013) found reduced integrity of short- and long-range white matter tracts in ASD. However, they also found increased fiber count in the ASD group. With age, global efficiency was found to decrease in individuals with ASD suggesting that in ASD network efficiency does not appropriately transition from a local to a distributed pattern as is seen during development in a neurotypical brain.[163] Dean and colleagues (2016) found significantly less coherence in white matter microstructure in children with ASD, characterized by reduced mean clustering coefficient (a measure of how well-connected a given node is to its neighbors[164]), reduced global efficiency (a measure of a network's overall ability for integrated processing and information processing[165]), reduced local efficiency (a measure of the average global efficiency of a selected network module[165,166]; and reduced mean degree (a measure of the network's overall density[166]) in the ASD group.[167] A network with low global and local efficiency can be viewed as one that inefficiently transfers information both globally and locally in a network.[168] Li and colleagues (2018) found individuals with ASD had significantly different global topological profiles of white matter networks compared to controls with decreased characteristic path length, increased global efficiency, and increased clustering coefficient. The authors suggest that the findings of significantly altered topological profiles suggest hyperconnectivity in the brain of children with ASD.[169] Although the results of global efficiency were mixed, graph theory whole- brain network analysis suggests hyperconnectivity in individuals with ASD accompanied by reduced network organization, which may lead to suboptimal information transfer across brain regions.

## Subnetwork analysis

The analysis of subnetworks enables researchers to investigate how specific functional brain regions are integrated into the brain.[170] In a study of Wernicke's area (speech comprehension) and Broca's area (speech motor control), children with ASD displayed reduced local clustering coefficient,[171] a finding that suggests that these areas are less interconnected with the surrounding regions. This study also reported that in the ASD group, Wernicke's area was associated with reduced betweenness centrality, a measure of how important a given brain region is for the efficiency of the network.[171] This implies that Wernicke's area was less integrated into the network in individuals with ASD.

Network analyses of the basal ganglia have also identified atypical connectivity in ASD. Adults with ASD were observed to have increased centrality of the right caudate, implying that the right caudate was more central to information transfer in ASD compared with controls.[72] Children with ASD were reported to have increased nodal efficiency, a measure of the local connections of nodes, in the basal ganglia.[169]

Structural network disconnectivity has also been described in the temporal pole[72] and in the fronto-parietal network.[172] A longitudinal analysis using whole-brain structural connectomes found a reduction in structural connectivity of the fronto-parietal network in ASD during adolescence and adulthood.[172] Greater fronto-parietal connectivity at baseline predicted a lower ASD symptom load at follow up, suggesting that in ASD, adaptive neuronal pruning in the fronto-parietal network between late childhood to early adulthood influences improvements in symptoms.[172]

## Rich-club analysis

Rich-club analysis examines the links between identified highly connected hubs or subnetworks and evaluates associated efficiency or brain optimization. The highly connected hub "nodes" are thought to indicate a higher level of functional specification resulting in optimized or more efficient communication routes. Rich-club architecture refers to a neural network where highly connected nodes (gray matter) within a connectome (the human brain), tend to connect with other highly connected nodes; such architecture is characteristic in a neurotypical brain. The presence or absence of rich-club architecture provides information about the organization, efficiency, and robustness of the brain's structural connectivity network.[173–176] Once the rich-club is defined, analysis is conducted to measure both the level of rich club organization and connectedness, information that provides insight into the neural efficiency of the network.[176] Rich-club analysis can provide information into how psychiatric disorders affect brain topology, as disruption to this rich-club architecture is associated with suboptimal brain function and several psychiatric disorders.

Children with ASD were found to display similar regions of rich-club architecture to neurotypical children; however, there were significant differences in the connectedness of these rich-club regions.[177] The ASD group showed higher connectivity than controls inside the rich-club network, but not outside the rich-club network. The increased connectivity in ASD was characterized by an increased number of connections (white matter fibers) but not an increase in GFA, suggesting a unique correlate corresponding to hyperconnectivity seen inside these highly connected brain regions.[177] Significant differences in rich-club organization were also reported in adolescents with ASD relative to typically developing controls, whereby the typical age-related increase in efficiency of rich-club networks was not seen in ASD[178] This relative anatomical immaturity seen in adolescents with ASD was correlated with the severity of ASD social symptoms.[178] The findings of these two rich-club studies suggest that although individuals with ASD display rich-club architecture there are significant differences to the connectedness and development of these networks. Connectomics studies in ASD have highlighted abnormalities in global and local network topology, less coherent white matter microstructure organization and reduced integration of networks, all findings that support the theory of neural disconnectivity in the condition.

# Behavioral consequences of disrupted structural connectivity in ASD

There appear to be significant behavioral consequences of disrupted structural connectivity in ASD; however, many studies have not investigated correlation between white matter organization and behavioral measures (see Ref.[14] for review). In addition, very few studies report correlation analysis of the same behavioral measure and diffusion metrics in the same white matter tract and at present, there is no consensus on the overall impact white matter pathology has on core features of ASD or specific behavioral measures.

Several studies have explored the relationship between white matter organization and ASD symptom severity. Increased severity of restricted and repetitive behaviors was correlated with reduced FA in left precentral gyrus and posterior brain regions,[34] right frontal regions,[35] right anterior cingulate cortex,[45] right body of the corpus callosum, right superior longitudinal fasciculus,[64] uncinate fasciculus, inferior longitudinal fasciculus, inferior front-occipital fasciculus, corticospinal tract, and the anterior thalamic radiation.[90] Restricted and repetitive behaviors contributing to ASD diagnosis at 2 years old were significantly associated with increased FA in the genu of the corpus callosum during infancy.[179] More severe restricted repetitive behaviors have also been associated with a reduction in the number of tracts in the forceps minor and body of the corpus callosum,[104] reduced number of streamlines of the left arcuate fasciculus,[87] reduced rightward asymmetry of local network efficiency[180] and lateralization of white matter pathways.[181] Greater social-communicative deficits have been correlated with reduced FA in regions of the corpus callosum,[34,64,160] uncinate fasciculus,[48,63,109] superior longitudinal fasciculus,[48,73] inferior longitudinal fasciculus, inferior fronto-occipital fasciculus,[73] anterior thalamic radiation,[63,64] left and right fornix,[48] fronto-striatal white matter,[34] anterior corona radiata,[64] forceps major,[108] right hemisphere parieto-frontal tracts,[182] fronto- and temporo-thalamic tracts,[183] cerebellar peduncle,[130] the dorsolateral prefrontal cortex,[37] and temporal regions.[34]

Greater social-communication impairment has also been associated with increased volume and fiber density of the uncinate fasciculus and arcuate fasciculus[99] and a reduction in the number of streamlines of the left uncinate fasciculus.[87] Reduced axial kurtosis in white matter tracts related to social-emotional processing (uncinate fasciculus, inferior longitudinal fasciculus, inferior fronto-occipital fasciculus and superior longitudinal fasciculus) was also associated with greater severity of ASD symptoms.[156] Some studies however have found no relationship between ASD symptomatology and white matter measures.[41,46,49,66,69,70,85,107,112,184–187]

Reduced organization of white matter microstructure in ASD (typically reported as reduced FA or GFA, increased MD or increased RD) has also been correlated with a variety of behavioral measures including lower IQ scores,[39,43,46,98,131] poorer language functioning,[41,43,51,120,123,188,189] lower adaptive behavior scores,[43,159] atypical visuospatial processing,[118] reduced processing speed,[157] faster spatial recognition memory,[153] poorer face-[131] and emotion-recognition,[132] increased dysregulation,[190] impairment in attention switching,[132] worse executive functioning,[114] increased response times in a pictorial problem-solving task,[191] slower movement time,[192] and greater levels of sensory sensitivity[88] and tactile defensiveness.[52]

## Developmental trajectories of white matter in ASD

Results from a large body of literature suggest that developmental trajectory of the brain is atypical in ASD. Structural MRI studies and head circumference studies have provided accumulating evidence that there are two phases of early brain growth pathology in ASD; a period of exceptionally rapid head growth during the first year of life followed by the slowing or arrest of growth during early childhood[193–197] with global differences typically resolved by adulthood.[198] Increased early brain volume in ASD appears to be driven mainly by disproportionate enlargement of white matter.[194,199] The underlying neurobiology of this overgrowth is unknown. One theory holds that it may result from an excess of neurons in key frontal and temporal regions that mediate higher-order cognitive functions. The excess of neurons may be the result of a reduction in the normal process of synaptic pruning and apoptosis that occurs in the first 2 years of life or it may be due to excessive glial proliferation.[196] Although the abnormal brain growth trajectory in ASD does not necessarily imply abnormal structural connectivity, there is some evidence to suggest that acceleration of brain growth may lead to different optimal connectivity patterns,[200] see Ref.[201] for review. Larger brains tend to rely more on local than long- distance connections in part because of conduction delays and increased cellular costs.[202] Therefore, in ASD, accelerated early brain growth may lead to greater reliance on local short-range neural connectivity and reduced reliance on global long-range connectivity.

In neurotypical children and adolescents, increasing age is correlated with an increase in white matter density and organization as evidenced by an increase in FA and a reduction in MD and RD.[203] Results from a large number of DW-MRI studies have reported atypical age-related changes in white matter microstructure in ASD suggesting that in individuals with ASD, this typical pattern of white matter maturation is not followed.[57]

Relative to controls, infants and very young children with ASD have shown increased FA in the frontal lobe,[34,35] temporal lobe[35,191] and occipital lobe[34] as well as in major white matter tracts including radiate white matter,[204] uncinate fasciculus,[133] the corpus callosum, cingulum,[78,205] and superior longitudinal fasciculus.[78] A large prospective study that examined white matter fiber tract organization from 6 to 24 months in infants who were at high-risk of developing ASD[105] showed that there was abnormal development of white matter in the children who developed ASD; relative to controls, FA was increased at 6 months, but reduced at 24 months in a number of major white matter tracts.[105]

In children and adolescents with ASD, the neurotypical increase in FA and reduction in MD and RD appears to reverse, with lower FA and higher MD and RD reported in many diffusion MRI studies, although there is significant heterogeneity about the specific brain regions and white matter tracts that are affected. In young people with ASD, the expected age- associated increases in FA were not seen in major white matter tracts including the corpus callosum,[50,57] cingulum,[57,103,112,114] arcuate fasciculus,[79] uncinate fasciculus,[90] superior longitudinal fasciculus, inferior longitudinal fasciculus, inferior fronto-occipital fasciculus,[57,62,90,103] internal capsule, anterior thalamic radiation,[57,90] thalamus and posterior limb of the internal capsule[206] and corticospinal tract.[57,90] Atypical age-related development of MD and RD have also been reported with findings of increased MD[30,74,103,207] and RD[49] in children with ASD relative to controls.

In older adolescents and adults, fewer differences in diffusion measures have been observed.[132,208] Some studies have reported that differences in white matter microstructure appeared to normalize in adulthood,[62,206] although other studies have shown that lower FA[87] and higher MD and RD persists in adults with ASD relative to controls.[209]

Overall, the evidence is strongly suggestive of an atypical trajectory of white matter development in ASD; however, the relationship between age and microstructural organization of white matter remains unclear. While some studies have reported a stronger association between age and white matter development in ASD,[60,62,64,84,90,206] others have suggested that this relationship is stronger in neurotypical controls.[57,77,79,209] These differences may reflect differences in study methods including sample size, inclusion of males and females, and technical processes including motion correction.[90] Further well-controlled longitudinal studies in large sample sizes are required.

## Brain asymmetry/lateralization in ASD

The organizational principal of brain lateralization proposes that the two hemispheres of the human brain display significant structural asymmetries and differ in their functional specialization.[210] Functionally, leftward lateralization is involved in language and motor skills and rightward lateralization is involved in spatial perceptual abilities.[211] Core symptoms of ASD are associated with impairments in left hemisphere skills such as language, social-communication and motor function, but right hemisphere functions such as visuospatial processing appear to be less affected.[212] This has led to a theory that disrupted hemispheric lateralization contributes to the pathophysiology in ASD.[210,212–216]

Structural neuroimaging research has provided support for this theory of atypical brain asymmetry in ASD. A mega-analysis conducted using the large ENIGMA consortium ASD dataset demonstrated reduced asymmetry of cortical thickness in ASD in medial frontal, orbitofrontal, cingulate and inferior temporal regions.[217] Another study using two other large ASD imaging datasets reported atypical right- and leftward gray matter asymmetry, which was associated with both language delay and ASD symptom severity.[216]

Many DW-MRI studies have reported atypical lateralization of white matter in ASD. Children and adults with ASD have shown increased leftward asymmetry compared with neurotypical controls in whole-brain white matter,[114] Broca's area,[181] and a number of white matter tracts including the arcuate fasciculus,[117,119,218] though not[120] posterior thalamic radiation,[186] corona radiata,[186] and superior longitudinal fasciculus.[123] In contrast, reduced leftward asymmetry in ASD has been reported in the corticospinal tract,[128] uncinate fasciculus[102] and cingulum bundle.[102] Increased rightward asymmetry has been observed in both children and adults with ASD in several white matter tracts including the frontal radiate white matter, anterior corona radiata, internal capsule,[186] and superior longitudinal fasciculus.[64] On a network level, connectomics research reported reduced rightward asymmetry of network efficiencies with increased age in a neurotypical control group, but not in the ASD group.[180] Together these studies suggest that structural brain asymmetry is abnormal is ASD, with widespread differences across the brain in both gray and white matter.

## Gray-white matter boundary in ASD

There has been increasing interest in examining the architecture of superficial white matter to probe local connectivity in ASD. Superficial white matter is located beneath the gray-white matter boundary and is mainly comprised of short-range association fibers. Studies have reported reduced FA and increased MD in superficial white matter in the frontal, temporal and parietal lobes (Refs.[30,40,57,219,220] (reduced GFA)), and disrupted microstructure of superficial white matter has been associated with atypical functional connectivity[221] and symptom severity.[220,221] Atypical diffusion within superficial white matter also appears to be modulated by sex and depends on the cortical region as well as the depth the white matter is sampled at.[219] Histological features that may contribute to the disrupted diffusion reported in neuroimaging studies include differences in the density and thickness of myelinated axons,[222–224] and an excess of interstitial neurons in the superficial white matter.[225]

## White matter sex differences in ASD

ASD is more prevalent in males than females but the underlying biological reasons for this are poorly understood. Atypical sexual dimorphism in white matter of children[70,226] and adults[53,227] with ASD has been observed in diffusion imaging studies.

In preschool children with ASD (3–5 years), females with ASD had higher MD, AD and RD than controls in the corpus callosum; however, males with ASD did not show any differences in corpus callosum microstructure compared with controls.[226] In slightly older children and young adults with ASD (4–21 years), females with ASD displayed significant reductions in FA across association (cingulum bundle, uncinate fasciculus, superior longitudinal fasciculus, inferior longitudinal fasciculus, inferior fronto-occipital fasciculus), projection (anterior thalamic radiation, corticospinal tract), and commissural (forceps major and minor) tracts compared to typically developing females, but no differences in white matter microstructure were reported for males with ASD compared with controls.[70]

In adults with ASD, Beacher and colleagues (2012) found significant interactions between sex and diagnosis in total white matter volume and FA in the corpus callosum, cingulum and corona radiata in ASD. FA in these tracts was higher for males than females in controls, but not in those with ASD, indicating an absence of neurotypical sexual dimorphism.[227]

Similarly, Zeestraten and colleagues reported that compared with controls, males with ASD were observed to have reduced FA in frontal white matter tracts including the cingulum, uncinate fasciculus, arcuate fasciculus, and inferior fronto-occipital fasciculus, but this effect was not found in females with ASD.[53]

More recently, studies investigating the neural correlates of the sex disparity in ASD using DW-MRI have demonstrated that the sex-by-ASD diagnosis interaction appears to be modulated by white matter connectivity of the lateral temporal lobe, temporo-parietal junction and medial parietal lobe[228] and corpus callosum.[76,161] In the corpus callosum, one study reported that adult females with ASD had increased white matter organization compared with sex-matched controls, whereas males with ASD had reduced white matter organization compared to sex-matched controls.[76] A second study reported that adult females with ASD have reduced fiber density and cross-section in the corpus callosum, a finding that was absent in males with ASD.[161]

Overall, these findings suggest that in ASD the impact of sex on white matter organization is different in children and adults. Compared with males, female children with ASD appear to have reduced organization of white matter.[70,226] In adulthood, the pattern appears to reverse, with male adults with ASD showing reduced white matter organization compared with females.[53,76,227] There is, however, not a clear pattern of the impact of sex on white matter organization, with some studies reporting no difference between males and females,[89] or a seemingly opposite pattern of difference.[161] It has been suggested that these mixed results may be due to differences in study methods (sample size, age, and neuroimaging processing) and there is a need for future research to incorporate strict methodology, group matching, and neuroimaging data quality control.[70]

## Conclusion

White matter microstructure in ASD has been extensively investigated using a variety of diffusion MRI approaches. There is a large body of research that has reported atypical organization of white matter microstructure in diverse brain regions and white matter tracts. Disrupted organization of white matter structure has been associated with ASD severity as well as with a variety of other behavioral measures, although further studies are needed to investigate the links between atypical structural connectivity and the ASD phenotype. The developmental trajectory of white matter is abnormal in ASD, atypical lateralization of white matter has been reported in many studies, and sex appears to influence microstructural organization of white matter. Overall, studies of brain white matter microstructure support the theory of disconnectivity in ASD and suggest that disorganization of white matter microstructure is a core pathophysiological feature of the condition.

## References

1. Brock J, et al. The temporal binding deficit hypothesis of autism. *Dev Psychopathol.* 2002;14(2):209–224.
2. Frith C. What do imaging studies tell us about the neural basis of autism? *Novartis Found Symp.* 2003;251:149–166. discussion 166-76, 281-97.
3. Belmonte MK, et al. Autism and abnormal development of brain connectivity. *J Neurosci.* 2004;24(42):9228–9231.
4. Just MA, et al. Cortical activation and synchronization during sentence comprehension in high-functioning autism: evidence of underconnectivity. *Brain.* 2004;127(Pt 8):1811–1821.
5. Courchesne E, Pierce K. Why the frontal cortex in autism might be talking only to itself: local over-connectivity but long-distance disconnection. *Curr Opin Neurobiol.* 2005;15(2):225–230.
6. Just MA, et al. Functional and anatomical cortical underconnectivity in autism: evidence from an FMRI study of an executive function task and corpus callosum morphometry. *Cereb Cortex.* 2007;17(4):951–961.
7. Kana RK, Libero LE, Moore MS. Disrupted cortical connectivity theory as an explanatory model for autism spectrum disorders. *Phys Life Rev.* 2011;8(4):410–437.
8. Turner M. Annotation: repetitive behaviour in autism: a review of psychological research. *J Child Psychol Psychiatry.* 1999;40(6):839–849.
9. Baron-Cohen S. The extreme male brain theory of autism. *Trends Cogn Sci.* 2002;6(6):248–254.
10. Frith U, Happé F. Autism: beyond "theory of mind". *Cognition.* 1994;50(1–3):115–132.
11. Happé F, Frith U. The weak coherence account: detail-focused cognitive style in autism spectrum disorders. *J Autism Dev Disord.* 2006;36(1):5–25.

12. Mottron L, et al. Enhanced perceptual functioning in autism: an update, and eight principles of autistic perception. *J Autism Dev Disord.* 2006;36(1):27–43.
13. Monk CS, et al. Abnormalities of intrinsic functional connectivity in autism spectrum disorders. *NeuroImage.* 2009;47(2):764–772.
14. Rane P, et al. Connectivity in autism: a review of MRI connectivity studies. *Harv Rev Psychiatry.* 2015;23(4):223–244.
15. Geschwind DH. Genetics of autism spectrum disorders. *Trends Cogn Sci.* 2011;15(9):409–416.
16. Catani M, de Schotten MT. A diffusion tensor imaging tractography atlas for virtual in vivo dissections. *Cortex.* 2008;44(8):1105–1132.
17. Stieltjes B, et al. Diffusion tensor imaging and axonal tracking in the human brainstem. *NeuroImage.* 2001;14(3):723–735.
18. Alexander AL, et al. Diffusion tensor imaging of the brain. *Neurotherapeutics.* 2007;4(3):316–329.
19. Basser PJ, Jones DK. Diffusion-tensor MRI: theory, experimental design and data analysis—a technical review. *NMR Biomed.* 2002;15(7–8):456–467.
20. Jones DK, Leemans A. Diffusion tensor imaging. *Methods Mol Biol.* 2011;711:127–144.
21. Basser PJ, Pierpaoli C. Microstructural and physiological features of tissues elucidated by quantitative-diffusion-tensor MRI. *J Magn Reson B.* 1996;111(3):209–219.
22. Basser PJ. Inferring microstructural features and the physiological state of tissues from diffusion-weighted images. *NMR Biomed.* 1995;8(7–8):333–344.
23. Werring DJ, et al. Diffusion tensor imaging can detect and quantify corticospinal tract degeneration after stroke. *J Neurol Neurosurg Psychiatry.* 2000;69(2):269–272.
24. Zhang Y, Burock MA. Diffusion tensor imaging in Parkinson's disease and parkinsonian syndrome: a systematic review. *Front Neurol.* 2020;11:1091.
25. Beaulieu C. The basis of anisotropic water diffusion in the nervous system—a technical review. *NMR Biomed.* 2002;15(7–8):435–455.
26. Hoeft F, et al. More is not always better: increased fractional anisotropy of superior longitudinal fasciculus associated with poor visuospatial abilities in Williams syndrome. *J Neurosci.* 2007;27(44):11960–11965.
27. Le Bihan D. Molecular diffusion, tissue microdynamics and microstructure. *NMR Biomed.* 1995;8(7-8):375–386.
28. Schwartz ED, Hackney DB. Diffusion-weighted MRI and the evaluation of spinal cord axonal integrity following injury and treatment. *Exp Neurol.* 2003;184(2):570–589.
29. Song SK, et al. Demyelination increases radial diffusivity in corpus callosum of mouse brain. *NeuroImage.* 2005;26(1):132–140.
30. Peterson D, et al. Left-hemispheric microstructural abnormalities in children with high-functioning autism spectrum disorder. *Autism Res.* 2015;8(1):61–72.
31. Tuch DS. Q-ball imaging. *Magn Reson Med.* 2004;52(6):1358–1372.
32. Barnea-Goraly N, et al. White matter structure in autism: preliminary evidence from diffusion tensor imaging. *Biol Psychiatry.* 2004;55(3):323–326.
33. Bloemen OJ, et al. White matter integrity in Asperger syndrome: a preliminary diffusion tensor magnetic resonance imaging study in adults. *Autism Res.* 2010;3(5):203–213.
34. Cheung C, et al. White matter fractional anisotrophy differences and correlates of diagnostic symptoms in autism. *J Child Psychol Psychiatry.* 2009;50(9):1102–1112.
35. Ke X, et al. White matter impairments in autism, evidence from voxel-based morphometry and diffusion tensor imaging. *Brain Res.* 2009;1265:171–177.
36. Mueller S, et al. Convergent findings of altered functional and structural brain connectivity in individuals with high functioning autism: a multimodal MRI study. *PLoS One.* 2013;8(6).
37. Noriuchi M, et al. Altered white matter fractional anisotropy and social impairment in children with autism spectrum disorder. *Brain Res.* 2010;1362:141–149.

38. Ogur T, Boyunaga OL. Relation of behavior problems with findings of cranial diffusion tensor MRI and MR spectroscopy in autistic children. *Int J Clin Exp Med.* 2015;8(4):5621–5630.
39. Pardini M, et al. White matter reduced streamline coherence in young men with autism and mental retardation. *Eur J Neurol.* 2009;16(11):1185–1190.
40. Sundaram SK, et al. Diffusion tensor imaging of frontal lobe in autism spectrum disorder. *Cereb Cortex.* 2008;18(11):2659–2665.
41. Abdel Razek A, Mazroa J, Baz H. Assessment of white matter integrity of autistic preschool children with diffusion weighted MR imaging. *Brain and Development.* 2014;36(1):28–34.
42. Ingalhalikar M, et al. DTI based diagnostic prediction of a disease via pattern classification. *Med Image Comput Comput Assist Interv.* 2010;13(Pt 1):558–565.
43. Lange N, et al. Atypical diffusion tensor hemispheric asymmetry in autism. *Autism Res.* 2010;3(6):350–358.
44. Lee PS, et al. Atypical neural substrates of embedded figures task performance in children with autism spectrum disorder. *NeuroImage.* 2007;38(1):184–193.
45. Thakkar KN, et al. Response monitoring, repetitive behaviour and anterior cingulate abnormalities in autism spectrum disorders (ASD). *Brain.* 2008;131(9):2464–2478.
46. Alexander AL, et al. Diffusion tensor imaging of the corpus callosum in Autism. *Neuroimage.* 2007;34(1):61–73.
47. Keller TA, Kana RK, Just MA. A developmental study of the structural integrity of white matter in autism. *Neuroreport.* 2007;18(1):23–27.
48. Poustka L, et al. Fronto-temporal disconnectivity and symptom severity in children with autism spectrum disorder. *World J Biol Psychiatry.* 2012;13(4):269–280.
49. Shukla DK, et al. White matter compromise of callosal and subcortical fiber tracts in children with autism spectrum disorder: a diffusion tensor imaging study. *J Am Acad Child Adolesc Psychiatry.* 2010;49(12):1269–1278.e12782.
50. Travers BG, et al. Atypical development of white matter microstructure of the corpus callosum in males with autism: a longitudinal investigation. *Mol Autism.* 2015;6(1).
51. Mills BD, et al. White matter microstructure correlates of narrative production in typically developing children and children with high functioning autism. *Neuropsychologia.* 2013;51(10):1933–1941.
52. Pryweller JR, et al. White matter correlates of sensory processing in autism spectrum disorders. *Neuroimage Clin.* 2014;6:379–387.
53. Zeestraten EA, et al. Sex differences in frontal lobe connectivity in adults with autism spectrum conditions. *Transl Psychiatry.* 2017;**7**(4).
54. Jou RJ, et al. Structural neural phenotype of autism: preliminary evidence from a diffusion tensor imaging study using tract-based spatial statistics. *AJNR Am J Neuroradiol.* 2011;32(9):1607–1613.
55. Jones DK, et al. The effect of filter size on VBM analyses of DT-MRI data. *Neuroimage.* 2005;26(2):546–554.
56. Smith SM, et al. Tract-based spatial statistics: voxelwise analysis of multi-subject diffusion data. *NeuroImage.* 2006;31(4):1487–1505.
57. Shukla DK, Keehn B, Müller RA. Tract-specific analyses of diffusion tensor imaging show widespread white matter compromise in autism spectrum disorder. *J Child Psychol Psychiatry.* 2011;52(3):286–295.
58. Kana R. Multimodal neuroimaging markers of autism spectrum disorders. *Biol Psychiatry.* 2014;75(9):139S–140S.
59. Walker L, et al. Diffusion tensor imaging in young children with autism: biological effects and potential confounds. *Biol Psychiatry.* 2012;72(12):1043–1051.
60. Ameis SH, et al. Impaired structural connectivity of socio-emotional circuits in autism spectrum disorders: a diffusion tensor imaging study. *PLoS One.* 2011;6(11), e28044.

61. Aoki Y, et al. Association of white matter structure with autism spectrum disorder and attention-deficit/hyperactivity disorder. *JAMA Psychiatry.* 2017;74(11):1120–1128.
62. Bakhtiari R, et al. Differences in white matter reflect atypical developmental trajectory in autism: a tract-based spatial statistics study. *NeuroImage Clin.* 2012;1(1):48–56.
63. Cheon KA, et al. Involvement of the anterior thalamic radiation in boys with high functioning autism spectrum disorders: a diffusion tensor imaging study. *Brain Res.* 2011;1417:77–86.
64. Fitzgerald J, Gallagher L, McGrath J. Widespread disrupted white matter microstructure in autism spectrum disorders. *J Autism Dev Disord.* 2019;49(7):2664–2674.
65. Itahashi T, et al. Linked alterations in gray and white matter morphology in adults with high-functioning autism spectrum disorder: a multimodal brain imaging study. *NeuroImage Clin.* 2015;7:155–169.
66. Jou RJ, et al. White matter abnormalities in autism and unaffected siblings. *J Neuropsychiatry Clin Neurosci.* 2016;28(1):49–55.
67. Roine U, et al. Increased coherence of white matter fiber tract organization in adults with asperger syndrome: a diffusion tensor imaging study. *Autism Res.* 2013;6(6):642–650.
68. Schaer M, et al. Decreased frontal gyrification associated with altered connectivity in children with autism. *Biol Psychiatry.* 2013;73(9):87S–88S.
69. Vogan VM, et al. Widespread white matter differences in children and adolescents with autism spectrum disorder. *J Autism Dev Disord.* 2016;46(6):2138–2147.
70. Lei J, et al. Altered neural connectivity in females, but not males with autism: preliminary evidence for the female protective effect from a quality-controlled diffusion tensor imaging study. *Autism Res.* 2019;12(10):1472–1483.
71. Hrdlicka M, et al. Diffusion tensor imaging and tractography in autistic, dysphasic, and healthy control children. *Neuropsychiatr Dis Treat.* 2019;15:2843–2852.
72. Roine U, et al. Abnormal wiring of the connectome in adults with high-functioning autism spectrum disorder. *Mol Autism.* 2015;6(1).
73. Im WY, et al. Impaired white matter integrity and social cognition in high-function autism: diffusion tensor imaging study. *Psychiatry Investig.* 2018;15(3):292–299.
74. Lisiecka DM, et al. Developmental white matter microstructure in autism phenotype and corresponding endophenotype during adolescence. *Transl Psychiatry.* 2015;5(3), e529.
75. Solso S, et al. Diffusion tensor imaging provides evidence of possible axonal overconnectivity in frontal lobes in autism spectrum disorder toddlers. *Biol Psychiatry.* 2016;79(8):676–684.
76. Andrews DS, et al. A diffusion-weighted imaging tract-based spatial statistics study of autism spectrum disorder in preschool-aged children. *J Neurodev Disord.* 2019;11(1):32.
77. Ouyang M, et al. Atypical age-dependent effects of autism on white matter microstructure in children of 2-7 years. *Hum Brain Mapp.* 2016;37(2):819–832.
78. Weinstein M, et al. Abnormal white matter integrity in young children with autism. *Hum Brain Mapp.* 2011;32(4):534–543.
79. Cheng Y, et al. Atypical development of white matter microstructure in adolescents with autism spectrum disorders. *NeuroImage.* 2010;50(3):873–882.
80. Ellmore TM, et al. Tract-based spatial statistics reveal altered relationship between non-verbal reasoning abilities and white matter integrity in autism spectrum disorder. *J Int Neuropsychol Soc.* 2013;19(6):723–728.
81. Bode MK, et al. White matter in autism spectrum disorders—evidence of impaired fiber formation. *Acta Radiol.* 2011;52(10):1169–1174.
82. Billeci L, et al. White matter connectivity in children with autism spectrum disorders: a tract-based spatial statistics study. *BMC Neurol.* 2012;12.
83. Gibbard CR, et al. White matter microstructure correlates with autism trait severity in a combined clinical-control sample of high-functioning adults. *NeuroImage Clin.* 2013;3:106–114.

84. Kleinhans NM, et al. Age-related abnormalities in white matter microstructure in autism spectrum disorders. *Brain Res.* 2012;1479:1–16.
85. Haigh SM, et al. Reduced white matter integrity and deficits in neuropsychological functioning in adults with autism spectrum disorder. *Autism Res.* 2020;13(5):702–714.
86. Perkins TJ, et al. Increased left hemisphere impairment in high-functioning autism: a tract based spatial statistics study. *Psychiatry Res Neuroimaging.* 2014.
87. Catani M, et al. Frontal networks in adults with autism spectrum disorder. *Brain.* 2016;139(Pt 2):616–630.
88. Ohta H, et al. White matter alterations in autism spectrum disorder and attention-deficit/hyperactivity disorder in relation to sensory profile. *Mol Autism.* 2020;**11**(1).
89. Kirkovski M, et al. Diffusion tensor imaging reveals no white matter impairments among adults with autism spectrum disorder. *Psychiatry Res.* 2015;233(1):64–72.
90. Thompson A, et al. Age-related differences in white matter diffusion measures in autism spectrum condition. *Mol Autism.* 2020;11(1).
91. Keedwell PA, et al. Cingulum white matter in young women at risk of depression: the effect of family history and anhedonia. *Biol Psychiatry.* 2012;72(4):296–302.
92. Basser PJ, et al. In vivo fiber tractography using DT-MRI data. *Magn Reson Med.* 2000;44(4):625–632.
93. Conturo TE, et al. Tracking neuronal fiber pathways in the living human brain. *Proc Natl Acad Sci U S A.* 1999;96(18):10422–10427.
94. Mori S, van Zijl PC. Fiber tracking: principles and strategies—a technical review. *NMR Biomed.* 2002;15(7-8):468–480.
95. Jones DK, et al. Non-invasive assessment of axonal fiber connectivity in the human brain via diffusion tensor MRI. *Magn Reson Med.* 1999;42(1):37–41.
96. Frazier TW, Hardan AY. A meta-analysis of the corpus callosum in autism. *Biol Psychiatry.* 2009;66(10):935–941.
97. Stanfield AC, et al. Towards a neuroanatomy of autism: a systematic review and meta-analysis of structural magnetic resonance imaging studies. *Eur Psychiatry.* 2008;23(4):289–299.
98. Kato Y, et al. White matter tract-cognitive relationships in children with high- functioning autism spectrum disorder. *Psychiatry Investig.* 2019;16(3):220–233.
99. Kumar A, et al. Alterations in frontal lobe tracts and corpus callosum in young children with autism spectrum disorder. *Cereb Cortex.* 2010;20(9):2103–2113.
100. Libero LE, et al. Multimodal neuroimaging based classification of autism spectrum disorder using anatomical, neurochemical, and white matter correlates. *Cortex.* 2015;66:46–59.
101. Nickel K, et al. Altered white matter integrity in adults with autism spectrum disorder and an IQ >100: a diffusion tensor imaging study. *Acta Psychiatr Scand.* 2017;135(6):573–583.
102. Lo YC, et al. The loss of asymmetry and reduced interhemispheric connectivity in adolescents with autism: a study using diffusion spectrum imaging tractography. *Psychiatry Res.* 2011;192(1):60–66.
103. Karahanoğlu FI, et al. Diffusion-weighted imaging evidence of altered white matter development from late childhood to early adulthood in autism spectrum disorder. *Neuroimage Clin.* 2018;19:840–847.
104. Thomas C, et al. The anatomy of the callosal and visual-association pathways in high-functioning autism: a DTI tractography study. *Cortex.* 2011;47(7):863–873.
105. Wolff JJ, et al. Differences in white matter fiber tract development present from 6 to 24 months in infants with autism. *Am J Psychiatry.* 2012;169(6):589–600.
106. Fingher N, et al. Toddlers later diagnosed with autism exhibit multiple structural abnormalities in temporal corpus callosum fibers. *Cortex.* 2017;97:291–305.
107. Hong S, et al. Detecting abnormalities of corpus callosum connectivity in autism using magnetic resonance imaging and diffusion tensor tractography. *Psychiatry Res.* 2011;194(3):333–339.

108. Hanaie R, et al. Abnormal corpus callosum connectivity, socio-communicative deficits, and motor deficits in children with autism spectrum disorder: a diffusion tensor imaging study. *J Autism Dev Disord.* 2014;44(9):2209–2220.
109. Samson AC, et al. White matter structure in the uncinate fasciculus: implications for socio-affective deficits in autism spectrum disorder. *Psychiatry Res Neuroimaging.* 2016;255:66–74.
110. Pugliese L, et al. The anatomy of extended limbic pathways in Asperger syndrome: a preliminary diffusion tensor imaging tractography study. *NeuroImage.* 2009;47(2):427–434.
111. Jeong JW, et al. Sharp curvature of frontal lobe white matter pathways in children with autism spectrum disorders: tract-based morphometry analysis. *AJNR Am J Neuroradiol.* 2011;32(9):1600–1606.
112. Li Y, et al. A fiber tractography study of social-emotional related fiber tracts in children and adolescents with autism spectrum disorder. *Neurosci Bull.* 2017;33(6):722–730.
113. Ameis SH, et al. Altered cingulum bundle microstructure in autism spectrum disorder. *Acta Neuropsychiatr.* 2013;25(5):275–282.
114. Ikuta T, et al. Abnormal cingulum bundle development in autism: a probabilistic tractography study. *Psychiatry Res Neuroimaging.* 2014;221(1):63–68.
115. Hau J, et al. The cingulum and cingulate U-fibers in children and adolescents with autism spectrum disorders. *Hum Brain Mapp.* 2019;40(11):3153–3164.
116. Zhang L, et al. Arcuate fasciculus in autism spectrum disorder toddlers with language regression. *Open Med.* 2018;13(1):90–95.
117. Roberts TPL, et al. Left hemisphere diffusivity of the arcuate fasciculus: influences of autism spectrum disorder and language impairment. *Am J Neuroradiol.* 2014;35(3):587–592.
118. McGrath J, et al. Abnormal functional connectivity during visuospatial processing is associated with disrupted organisation of white matter in autism. *Eur Child Adolesc Psychiatry.* 2013;22(2):S110–S111.
119. Fletcher PT, et al. Microstructural connectivity of the arcuate fasciculus in adolescents with high-functioning autism. *NeuroImage.* 2010;51(3):1117–1125.
120. Joseph RM, et al. Structural asymmetries of language-related gray and white matter and their relationship to language function in young children with ASD. *Brain Imaging Behav.* 2014;8(1):60–72.
121. Boets B, et al. Alterations in the inferior longitudinal fasciculus in autism and associations with visual processing: a diffusion-weighted MRI study. *Mol Autism.* 2018;9(1).
122. Libero LE, et al. White matter diffusion of major fiber tracts implicated in autism spectrum disorder. *Brain Connect.* 2016;6(9):691–699.
123. Verly M, et al. Structural and functional underconnectivity as a negative predictor for language in autism. *Hum Brain Mapp.* 2014;35(8):3602–3615.
124. Conti E, et al. High angular resolution diffusion imaging in a child with autism spectrum disorder and comparison with his unaffected identical twin. *Funct Neurol.* 2015;30(3):203–208.
125. Nair A, et al. Regional specificity of aberrant thalamocortical connectivity in autism. *Hum Brain Mapp.* 2015;36(11):4497–4511.
126. Langen M, et al. Fronto-striatal circuitry and inhibitory control in autism: findings from diffusion tensor imaging tractography. *Cortex.* 2012;48(2):183–193.
127. Delmonte S, et al. Functional and structural connectivity of frontostriatal circuitry in autism spectrum disorder. *Front Hum Neurosci.* 2013;7:430.
128. Carper RA, et al. Corticospinal tract anatomy and functional connectivity of primary motor cortex in autism. *J Am Acad Child Adolesc Psychiatry.* 2015;54(10):859–867.
129. Failla MD, et al. Intrainsular connectivity and somatosensory responsiveness in young children with ASD. *Mol Autism.* 2017;8(1):25.
130. Catani M, et al. Altered cerebellar feedback projections in Asperger syndrome. *Neuroimage.* 2008;41(4):1184–1191.

131. Conturo TE, et al. Neuronal fiber pathway abnormalities in autism: an initial MRI diffusion tensor tracking study of hippocampo-fusiform and amygdalo-fusiform pathways. *J Int Neuropsychol Soc.* 2008;14(6):933–946.
132. Gibbard CR, et al. Structural connectivity of the amygdala in young adults with autism spectrum disorder. *Hum Brain Mapp.* 2018;39(3):1270–1282.
133. Sahyoun CP, et al. Neuroimaging of the functional and structural networks underlying visuospatial vs. linguistic reasoning in high-functioning autism. *Neuropsychologia.* 2010;48(1):86–95.
134. Basser PJ, Mattiello J, LeBihan D. MR diffusion tensor spectroscopy and imaging. *Biophys J.* 1994;66(1):259–267.
135. Alexander DC, Barker GJ, Arridge SR. Detection and modeling of non-Gaussian apparent diffusion coefficient profiles in human brain data. *Magn Reson Med.* 2002;48(2):331–340.
136. Frank LR. Characterization of anisotropy in high angular resolution diffusion-weighted MRI. *Magn Reson Med.* 2002;47(6):1083–1099.
137. Tournier J-D, Mori S, Leemans A. Diffusion tensor imaging and beyond. *Magn Reson Med.* 2011;65(6):1532.
138. Tuch DS, et al. High angular resolution diffusion imaging reveals intravoxel white matter fiber heterogeneity. *Magn Reson Med.* 2002;48(4):577–582.
139. Wedeen V, et al. Mapping fiber orientation spectra in cerebral white matter with Fourier-transform diffusion MRI. In: *Proceedings of the 8th Annual Meeting of ISMRM, Denver;* 2000.
140. Jeurissen B, et al. Investigating the prevalence of complex fiber configurations in white matter tissue with diffusion magnetic resonance imaging. *Hum Brain Mapp.* 2013;34(11):2747–2766.
141. Tournier J-D, et al. Resolving crossing fibres using constrained spherical deconvolution: validation using diffusion-weighted imaging phantom data. *NeuroImage.* 2008;42(2):617–625.
142. Vos SB, et al. Partial volume effect as a hidden covariate in DTI analyses. *Neuroimage.* 2011;55(4):1566–1576.
143. Vos SB, et al. The influence of complex white matter architecture on the mean diffusivity in diffusion tensor MRI of the human brain. *NeuroImage.* 2012;59(3):2208–2216.
144. Jones DK, Cercignani M. Twenty-five pitfalls in the analysis of diffusion MRI data. *NMR Biomed.* 2010;23(7):803–820.
145. Behrens TE, et al. Probabilistic diffusion tractography with multiple fibre orientations: what can we gain? *NeuroImage.* 2007;34(1):144–155.
146. Jeurissen B, et al. Probabilistic fiber tracking using the residual bootstrap with constrained spherical deconvolution. *Hum Brain Mapp.* 2011;32(3):461–479.
147. Pierpaoli C, et al. Water diffusion changes in Wallerian degeneration and their dependence on white matter architecture. *NeuroImage.* 2001;13(6 Pt 1):1174–1185.
148. Tournier J-D, Calamante F, Connelly A. Robust determination of the fibre orientation distribution in diffusion MRI: non-negativity constrained super-resolved spherical deconvolution. *NeuroImage.* 2007;35(4):1459–1472.
149. Tournier JD, et al. Direct estimation of the fiber orientation density function from diffusion-weighted MRI data using spherical deconvolution. *NeuroImage.* 2004;23(3):1176–1185.
150. Van Hecke WEL, Sunaert S. *Diffusion Tensor Imaging: A Practical Handbook.* New York: Springer-Verlag; 2016.
151. Chiang HL, et al. Different neural substrates for executive functions in youths with ADHD a diffusion spectrum imaging tractography study. *Psychol Med.* 2016;46(6):1225–1238.
152. Chien HY, et al. Altered cortical thickness and tract integrity of the mirror neuron system and associated social communication in autism spectrum disorder. *Autism Res.* 2015;8(6):694–708.

153. Chien HY, Gau SSF, Isaac Tseng WY. Deficient visuospatial working memory functions and neural correlates of the default-mode network in adolescents with autism spectrum disorder. *Autism Res.* 2016;9(10):1058–1072.
154. Lin CW, et al. Alterations in white matter microstructure and regional volume are related to motor functions in boys with autism spectrum disorder. *Prog Neuro-Psychopharmacol Biol Psychiatry.* 2019;90:76–83.
155. Lo YC, et al. Reduced tract integrity of the model for social communication is a neural substrate of social communication deficits in autism spectrum disorder. *J Child Psychol Psychiatry.* 2017;58(5):576–585.
156. Hattori A, et al. White matter alterations in adult with autism spectrum disorder evaluated using diffusion kurtosis imaging. *Neuroradiology.* 2019;61(12):1343–1353.
157. Lazar M, et al. Axonal deficits in young adults with high functioning autism and their impact on processing speed. *NeuroImage Clin.* 2014;4:417–425.
158. Sui YV, et al. Diffusional kurtosis imaging of the corpus callosum in autism. *Mol Autism.* 2018;9(1):1–12.
159. Jeong J-W, et al. Altered white matter structure of the dentatorubrothalamic pathway in children with autistic spectrum disorders. *Cerebellum.* 2012;11(4):957–971.
160. Dimond D, et al. Reduced white matter fiber density in autism spectrum disorder. *Cereb Cortex.* 2019;29(4):1778–1788.
161. Kirkovski M, et al. Fixel based analysis reveals atypical white matter micro- and macrostructure in adults with autism spectrum disorder: an investigation of the role of biological sex. *Front Integr Neurosci.* 2020;14.
162. Sporns O, Tononi G, Kötter R. The human connectome: a structural description of the human brain. *PLoS Comput Biol.* 2005;1(4), e42.
163. Rudie JD, et al. Altered functional and structural brain network organization in autism. *NeuroImage Clin.* 2013;2(1):79–94.
164. Tijms BM, et al. Alzheimer's disease: connecting findings from graph theoretical studies of brain networks. *Neurobiol Aging.* 2013;34(8):2023–2036.
165. Bullmore E, Sporns O. The economy of brain network organization. *Nat Rev Neurosci.* 2012;13(5):336–349.
166. Rubinov M, Sporns O. Complex network measures of brain connectivity: uses and interpretations. *NeuroImage.* 2010;52(3):1059–1069.
167. Dean DC, et al. Investigating the microstructural correlation of white matter in autism spectrum disorder. *Brain Connect.* 2016;6(5):415–433.
168. Ginestet CE, et al. Brain network analysis: separating cost from topology using cost-integration. *PLoS One.* 2011;6(7), e21570.
169. Li SJ, et al. Alterations of white matter connectivity in preschool children with autism spectrum disorder. *Radiology.* 2018;288(1):209–217.
170. Sporns O, Tononi G, Edelman GM. Connectivity and complexity: the relationship between neuroanatomy and brain dynamics. *Neural Netw.* 2000;13(8):909–922.
171. Goch CJ, et al. Quantification of changes in language-related brain areas in autism spectrum disorders using large-scale network analysis. *Int J Comput Assist Radiol Surg.* 2014;9(3):357–365.
172. Lin HY, et al. Development of frontoparietal connectivity predicts longitudinal symptom changes in young people with autism spectrum disorder. *Transl Psychiatry.* 2019;9(1).
173. Colizza V, et al. Detecting rich-club ordering in complex networks. *Nat Phys.* 2006;2(2):110–115.
174. Dennis EL, et al. Development of the "rich club" in brain connectivity networks from 438 adolescents & adults aged 12 to 30. In: *2013 IEEE 10th International Symposium on Biomedical Imaging.* IEEE; 2013.
175. McAuley JJ, da Fontoura Costa L, Caetano TS. Rich-club phenomenon across complex network hierarchies. *Appl Phys Lett.* 2007;91(8), 084103.

176. Van Den Heuvel MP, Sporns O. Rich-club organization of the human connectome. *J Neurosci.* 2011;31(44):15775–15786.
177. Ray S, et al. Structural and functional connectivity of the human brain in autism spectrum disorders and attention-deficit/hyperactivity disorder: a rich club-organization study. *Hum Brain Mapp.* 2014;35(12):6032–6048.
178. Watanabe T, Rees G. Age-associated changes in rich-club organisation in autistic and neurotypical human brains. *Sci Rep.* 2015;5:16152.
179. Wolff JJ, et al. Altered corpus callosum morphology associated with autism over the first 2 years of life. *Brain.* 2015;138(7):2046–2058.
180. Wei L, et al. Aberrant development of the asymmetry between hemispheric brain white matter networks in autism spectrum disorder. *Eur Neuropsychopharmacol.* 2018;28(1):48–62.
181. Conti E, et al. Lateralization of brain networks and clinical severity in toddlers with autism spectrum disorder: a HARDI diffusion MRI study. *Autism Res.* 2016;9(3):382–392.
182. Fründt O, et al. White matter microstructure of the human mirror neuron system is related to symptom severity in adults with autism. *J Autism Dev Disord.* 2018;48(2):417–429.
183. Nair A, et al. Impaired thalamocortical connectivity in autism spectrum disorder: a study of functional and anatomical connectivity. *Brain.* 2013;136(6):1942–1955.
184. Ameis SH, et al. A diffusion tensor imaging studyin children with ADHD, autism spectrum disorder, OCD, and matched controls: distinct and non-distinct white matter disruption and dimensional brain-behavior relationships. *Am J Psychiatr.* 2016;173(12):1213–1222.
185. Barnea-Goraly N, Lotspeich LJ, Reiss AL. Similar white matter aberrations in children with autism and their unaffected siblings: a diffusion tensor imaging study using tract-based spatial statistics. *Arch Gen Psychiatry.* 2010;67(10):1052–1060.
186. Carper RA, et al. Reduced hemispheric asymmetry of white matter microstructure in autism spectrum disorder. *J Am Acad Child Adolesc Psychiatry.* 2016;55(12):1073–1080.
187. Jou RJ, et al. Diffusion tensor imaging in autism spectrum disorders: preliminary evidence of abnormal neural connectivity. *Aust N Z J Psychiatry.* 2011;45(2):153–162.
188. Nagae L, et al. Elevated mean diffusivity in the left hemisphere superior longitudinal fasciculus in autism spectrum disorders increases with more profound language impairment. *Am J Neuroradiol.* 2012;33(9):1720–1725.
189. Naigles LR, et al. Neural correlates of language variability in preschool-aged boys with autism spectrum disorder. *Autism Res.* 2017;10(6):1107–1119.
190. Ni H-C, et al. Association of self-regulation with white matter correlates in boys with and without autism spectrum disorder. *Sci Rep.* 2020;10(1):1–12.
191. Sahyoun CP, Belliveau JW, Mody M. White matter integrity and pictorial reasoning in high-functioning children with autism. *Brain Cogn.* 2010;73(3):180–188.
192. Lin HY, et al. Neural substrates of behavioral variability in attention deficit hyperactivity disorder: based on ex-Gaussian reaction time distribution and diffusion spectrum imaging tractography. *Psychol Med.* 2014;44(8):1751–1764.
193. Courchesne E, Carper R, Akshoomoff N. Evidence of brain overgrowth in the first year of life in autism. *JAMA.* 2003;290(3):337–344.
194. Courchesne E, et al. Unusual brain growth patterns in early life in patients with autistic disorder: an MRI study. *Neurology.* 2001;57(2):245–254.
195. Courchesne E, et al. Mapping early brain development in autism. *Neuron.* 2007;56(2):399–413.
196. Herbert MR. Large brains in autism: the challenge of pervasive abnormality. *Neuroscientist.* 2005;11(5):417–440.
197. Lainhart JE, et al. Head circumference and height in autism: a study by the collaborative program of excellence in autism. *Am J Med Genet A.* 2006;140(21):2257–2274.
198. McAlonan GM, et al. Mapping the brain in autism. A voxel-based MRI study of volumetric differences and intercorrelations in autism. *Brain.* 2005;128(Pt 2):268–276.

199. Herbert MR, et al. Dissociations of cerebral cortex, subcortical and cerebral white matter volumes in autistic boys. *Brain.* 2003;126(Pt 5):1182–1192.
200. Sporns O, Zwi JD. The small world of the cerebral cortex. *Neuroinformatics.* 2004;2(2):145–162.
201. Wass S. Distortions and disconnections: disrupted brain connectivity in autism. *Brain Cogn.* 2011;75(1):18–28.
202. Lewis JD, Elman JL. Growth-related neural reorganization and the autism phenotype: a test of the hypothesis that altered brain growth leads to altered connectivity. *Dev Sci.* 2008;11(1):135–155.
203. Schmithorst VJ, et al. Correlation of white matter diffusivity and anisotropy with age during childhood and adolescence: a cross-sectional diffusion-tensor MR imaging study. *Radiology.* 2002;222(1):212–218.
204. Ben Bashat D, et al. Accelerated maturation of white matter in young children with autism: a high b value DWI study. *NeuroImage.* 2007;37(1):40–47.
205. Xiao Z, et al. Autism spectrum disorder as early neurodevelopmental disorder: evidence from the brain imaging abnormalities in 2-3 years old toddlers. *J Autism Dev Disord.* 2014;44(7):1633–1640.
206. McLaughlin K, et al. Longitudinal development of thalamic and internal capsule microstructure in autism spectrum disorder. *Autism Res.* 2018;11(3):450–462.
207. Groen WB, et al. Pervasive microstructural abnormalities in autism: a DTI study. *J Psychiatry Neurosci.* 2011;36(1):32.
208. Braden BB, et al. Executive function and functional and structural brain differences in middle-age adults with autism spectrum disorder. *Autism Res.* 2017;10(12):1945–1959.
209. Koolschijn PCMP, et al. Age-related differences in autism: the case of white matter microstructure. *Hum Brain Mapp.* 2017;38(1):82–96.
210. Duboc V, et al. Asymmetry of the brain: development and implications. *Annu Rev Genet.* 2015;49:647–672.
211. Springer SP, Deutsch G. *Left Brain, Right Brain: Perspectives From Cognitive Neuroscience.* 5th ed. New York, NY: W H Freeman/Times Books/Henry Holt & Co; 1998. xiii, 406-xiii, 406.
212. Prior MR, Bradshaw JL. Hemisphere functioning in autistic children. *Cortex.* 1979;15(1):73–81.
213. Kleinhans NM, et al. Atypical functional lateralization of language in autism spectrum disorders. *Brain Res.* 2008;1221:115–125.
214. Rentería ME. Cerebral asymmetry: a quantitative, multifactorial, and plastic brain phenotype. *Twin Res Hum Genet.* 2012;15(3):401–413.
215. Toga AW, Thompson PM. Mapping brain asymmetry. *Nat Rev Neurosci.* 2003;4(1):37–48.
216. Floris DL, et al. Atypical brain asymmetry in autism—a candidate for clinically meaningful stratification. *Biol Psychiatry Cogn Neurosci Neuroimaging.* 2021;8:802–812.
217. Postema MC, et al. Altered structural brain asymmetry in autism spectrum disorder in a study of 54 datasets. *Nat Commun.* 2019;10(1):1–12.
218. Knaus TA, et al. Language laterality in autism spectrum disorder and typical controls: a functional, volumetric, and diffusion tensor MRI study. *Brain Lang.* 2010;112(2):113–120.
219. Bletsch A, et al. Atypical measures of diffusion at the gray-white matter boundary in autism spectrum disorder in adulthood. *Hum Brain Mapp.* 2021;42(2):467–484.
220. D'Albis MA, et al. Superficial white matter integrity in autism spectrum disorders. *Biol Psychiatry.* 2017;81(10):S99–S100.
221. Hong S-J, et al. Atypical functional connectome hierarchy in autism. *Nat Commun.* 2019;10(1):1022.
222. Zikopoulos B, Barbas H. Changes in prefrontal axons may disrupt the network in autism. *J Neurosci.* 2010;30(44):14595–14609.
223. Zikopoulos B, García-Cabezas MÁ, Barbas H. Parallel trends in cortical gray and white matter architecture and connections in primates allow fine study of pathways in humans and reveal network disruptions in autism. *PLoS Biol.* 2018;16(2), e2004559.

224. Zikopoulos B, et al. Opposite development of short- and long-range anterior cingulate pathways in autism. *Acta Neuropathol.* 2018;136(5):759–778.
225. Avino TA, Hutsler JJ. Abnormal cell patterning at the cortical gray-white matter boundary in autism spectrum disorders. *Brain Res.* 2010;1360:138–146.
226. Nordahl CW, et al. Sex differences in the corpus callosum in preschool-aged children with autism spectrum disorder Dr Meng-Chuan Lai. *Mol Autism.* 2015;6(1).
227. Beacher FD, et al. Autism attenuates sex differences in brain structure: a combined voxel-based morphometry and diffusion tensor imaging study. *Am J Neuroradiol.* 2012;33(1):83–89.
228. Irimia A, et al. Support vector machines, multidimensional scaling and magnetic resonance imaging reveal structural brain abnormalities associated with the interaction between autism spectrum disorder and sex. *Front Comput Neurosci.* 2018;12.

CHAPTER

# 8

# Animal models of autism

*Elizabeth L. Berg and Jill L. Silverman*

**Department of Psychiatry and Behavioral Sciences, MIND Institute, University of California Davis School of Medicine, Sacramento, CA, United States**

## Introduction

Autism spectrum disorder is a complex, lifelong neurodevelopmental disorder that affects an estimated 1 in 54 children in the United States. While prevalence rates been rapidly increasing, up from an estimated 1 in 150 children in 2002,[1] there are not yet evidence-based treatments that target the core symptoms of autism. Crucial to the development of effective interventions are models of autism in which candidate treatments can be administered and the subsequent effects on autism-relevant outcomes can be assessed. Since autism is diagnosed using purely behavioral criteria (i.e., deficient social interaction and communication alongside restricted, repetitive patterns of behavior), the model systems used to develop therapies must be able to express behaviors that can be compared to the clinical criteria. Thereby, in vivo approaches using live animals that display observable behaviors offer the most appropriate model systems for autism. This chapter aims to introduce ways in which animal biology and behavior can be leveraged to study the etiology of autism and to test potential treatments.

## Characteristics of autism in humans

Since there are no reliable biomarkers of autism spectrum disorder, the clinical diagnosis of autism in humans is primarily based on evaluations of behavioral criteria. These criteria are outlined in the Diagnostic and Statistical Manual of Mental Disorders (DSM-V),[2] which was most recently updated in 2013.


https://doi.org/10.1016/B978-0-12-816393-1.00010-5

Compared to the criteria described in the previous DSM-IV, which was published in 1994, there were a few major changes made in the DSM-V:

**(1)** Four independent categories of autism, namely autistic disorder, Asperger syndrome, childhood disintegrative disorder, and pervasive developmental disorder-not otherwise specified (PDD-NOS), were combined into a single diagnosis labeled "autism spectrum disorder." This change reflects the current thinking that the high heterogeneity of autism, both in cause and presentation, is better represented by a spectrum rather than discrete categories and that the umbrella term of "autism spectrum disorder" can encapsulate a diversity of "autisms" similar to "cancer" encapsulating many different "cancers."[3]
**(2)** Instead of PDD-NOS, the diagnosis for an individual exhibiting social deficits but not restricted, repetitive behaviors was changed to "social communication disorder."
**(3)** The criteria of social impairment and language/communication impairment were combined into a single criterion.
**(4)** Sensory issues were added as a symptom under the restricted, repetitive behavior category. These include hypo- or hyperreactivity to sensory input or unusual responses to environmental stimuli.
**(5)** Assessments were added for the following: accompanying intellectual disability, accompanying language impairment, association with a known medical or genetic condition or environmental factor (e.g., anxiety, seizures, disrupted sleep), and association with another disorder (e.g., Fragile X or Rett syndrome).

Currently, in order to receive an autism diagnosis, an individual must:

**(1)** exhibit persistent deficits in social communication and interaction across multiple contexts, which may include:
  - **(a)** Aversion to maintaining eye contact and low proficiency with nonverbal gestures
  - **(b)** Low interest in peers and failure to initiate or respond to social interactions
  - **(c)** Deficits in social reciprocity
  - **(d)** Low proficiency in normal back-and-forth conversation (tendency to speak in monologues rather than interactively)
  - **(e)** Literal interpretation of abstract concepts and difficulty interpreting irony or sarcasm
  - **(f)** Difficulty appreciating emotions and reduced sharing of interests and/or emotions
  - **(g)** Difficulty adjusting behavior to suit different social contexts
  - **(h)** Difficulty making and/or maintaining friendships

**(2)** and engage in restricted, repetitive behaviors, interests, or activities, such as:
  **(a)** Stereotyped motor movements (e.g., hand flapping, rocking)
  **(b)** Repetitive use of objects or speech (e.g., arranging toys, echolalia)
  **(c)** Behavioral inflexibility, insistence on sameness, and rigid patterns of thinking
  **(d)** Difficulty tolerating new experiences or changes in routine
  **(e)** Hypersensitivity to or unusual interest in sensory stimuli (e.g., indifference to pain/temperature, adverse reaction to specific sounds or textures, fascination with lights, excessive smelling or touching of objects)
  **(f)** Intense, fixated interest on niche subjects.

## The causes of autism

There are considerable research efforts aimed at elucidating the causes of autism. To date, numerous genetic and environmental factors have been identified to contribute to an individual's risk of developing autism, with an estimated 81% of autism risk coming from genetic factors.[4] Thanks to early research on twins, the high heritability rate for autism has been well-established with monozygotic twins exhibiting 70%–90% concordance rates compared to less than 10% for dizygotic twins and siblings.[5–8] Subsequent studies aimed at identifying specific genes linked to autism led to the collection of over 1000 genes with at least one de novo likely-gene-disrupting mutation associating it with autism.[9,10] Advances in genetic technologies, such as whole genome/exome sequencing to detect variants across the entire genome, chromosomal microarrays to detect copy number variants (CNVs), and genome wide association studies (GWAS) to detect associations between genetic variants and autism,[11–17] helped narrow the list of genes down to hundreds. In most cases, the genes implicated in autism risk were identified as rare or de novo mutations that led to chromosomal abnormalities, CNVs, or single-gene disorders such as Fragile X, Rett, and Angelman syndromes.[7,12,18–21] Of the known genetic abnormalities linked to autism, at least 5% are caused by mutations in a single gene, and at least 10% are caused by CNVs resulting fromstructural changes in DNA such as duplications, deletions, inversions, and translocations.[12,17,22–26] In 2020, the largest exome sequencing study of autism to date, involving more than 35,000 samples, further refined the list of high confidence autism-associated genes to 102 and delineated these from the broader category of neurodevelopmental disorders.[27] The functional roles of these risk genes can be grouped into a handful of categories, suggesting that common mechanisms underlie the etiology of autism. These categories include synaptic functioning (e.g., *SCN2A*, *SYNGAP1*, *CACNA1C*, *SLC6A1*), synaptic structure (e.g., *SHANK3*, *NLGN*, *GRIN2B*), chromatin remodeling (e.g., *CHD8*, *ARID1B*, *MECP2*, *ADNP*, *POGZ*, *KMT5B*), transcriptional regulation (e.g., *FOXP1*, *FMR1*), and cell signaling (e.g., *CDKL5*, *TSC1*, *DYRK1A*, *PTEN*, *UBE3A*). The identification of these common biological mechanisms is highly encouraging for therapeutic development as each pathway provides a target to which genetic or pharmacological interventions can be directed.

The less than 100% concordance rate in identical twins, along with the recent rise in autism rates that cannot solely be attributed to genetic causes or diagnostic changes, has brought increased attention to environmental causes of autism, as well as gene-environment interactions such as epigenetics.[28–31] A 2013 study, for example, found that prenatal exposure to the anticonvulsant valproic acid led to an almost threefold greater risk of an autism diagnosis.[32] Additional epidemiological and clinical data helped strengthen this association as well as identify various environmental risk factors for autism, including but not limited to: exposure to chemicals and pollutants (e.g., pesticides, particulate matter, heavy metals, PCBs, flame retardants, phthalates), exposure to drugs and medications (e.g., valproic acid, thalidomide, misoprostol, SSRIs, antipyretics), infections (e.g., viruses, bacteria, fever, maternal immune activation), parental characteristics (e.g., age, diet, diabetes, interpregnancy interval, high blood pressure, anemia, melatonin, smoking, autoimmune disease), and pregnancy factors (e.g., preterm birth, low birth weight).[30,33–41] These factors may contribute to autism risk by disrupting neurodevelopment irrespective of genetic factors, but an individual's genetic background can also influence their responsivity to environmental stimuli and therefore susceptibility to pathology.[42,43] The interaction between genetic and environmental factors (G×E) can confer autism risk by causing de novo mutations in DNA, influencing patterns of gene expression via effects on epigenetic processes, and by having a combined effect that outweighs the individual effects.[33] This can occur when inherited genetic vulnerabilities, such as a mutation or CNV that affects neural functioning, is exacerbated by an experience or environmental exposure.

## Animal models of autism

The identification of various genetic and environmental risk factors for autism has allowed for the generation of animal models in which a genetic abnormality has been introduced and/or an environmental exposure has been carried out. Since the clinical diagnosis of autism in humans is based on observable behaviors, animal models capable of expressing analogous behaviors are essential to the study of autism. Animal models make it possible to manipulate individual biological factors, such as genes or immune responses, and then measure biological and behavioral outcomes throughout development, all within a controlled laboratory setting. The ability to investigate isolated causes of autism is especially important given the incredibly high heterogeneity in the biological etiology and symptom manifestation of the disorder. Experimentally evaluating risk factors that are identified via epidemiological or clinical research can help to establish causality and delineate the nature of the causal relationship. One compelling approach to test hypotheses about the numerous risk genes for autism is to generate analogous mutations in an animal and assess whether the animal displays phenotypes analogous to the symptoms of autism.[44–46] Animal models make it possible to identify biological metrics (e.g., neuroanatomy, epigenetics, microbiota, physiology) correlated with autism-like behavior, which can shed light on the etiology of autism as well as potential therapeutic targets. Although there are not yet reliable biological markers of autism available to date, a goal for the use of animal models is to identify novel translational biomarkers that can be applied across species for clinical diagnosis and/or treatment decisions in the future.

With the early identification of genetics as the major cause of autism, the initial animal models of autism were genetic models that exhibited autism-like behaviors (i.e., social deficits and repetitive behavior). These so-called "forward genetic models," which included the BTBR T + tf/J and BALB/c mouse models, were discovered as autism models based on their behavioral traits and subsequently had their underlying genetics investigated.[47,48] Mice have been advantageous for modeling autism due to their large behavioral repertoire, high degree of sociability, and high level of genetic conservation relative to humans. In following years, technological advances in manipulating the mouse genome were utilized to generate "first generation" preclinical genetic models carrying single gene mutations and CNVs implicated in autism. These "reverse genetic models," which modeled autism based on genetics and only subsequently had their behavior characterized, included mice with analogous disruptions to the causal genes of Fragile X (*Fmr1*) and Rett (*Mecp2*) syndromes, two of the leading genetic causes of autism,[49–53] as well as mice with mutations in synaptic and cell signaling genes (e.g., *Shank3, Nlgn3, Nlgn4, Pten*).[54–58]

The most commonly used mouse models of autism are those with either a gene of interest added to ("transgenic") or removed from ("knockout") the mouse genome. Rapid advances in mouse genetics have led to the ability to generate even more sophisticated models that allow for temporal-, spatial-, and cell-specific gene expression. These include the tetracycline-controlled transcriptional activation model of inducible gene expression in which double transgenic mice are generated to carry a tetracycline response element (*TRE*) upstream of the gene of interest and a tetracycline transactivator (*tTA*) gene downstream of a promoter of interest (e.g., *Camk2a* for forebrain expression).[59] Under basal conditions, the tTA protein binds to the *TRE* and leads to expression of the gene of interest. The presence of tetracycline or doxycycline, however, prevents tTA from binding *TRE* and thus the gene of interest is not expressed. Carefully timed systemic administration of tetracycline or doxycycline can therefore be used to investigate the role of a gene during specific developmental time windows and/or specific regions of the brain. Deliberate consideration of time is highly important in the study of neurodevelopmental disorders such as autism since causal factors act in utero, symptoms manifest early in life, and traits arise at different times throughout development. While the translational applications of such temporally and spatially specific genetic manipulations are still being investigated, these techniques lay the groundwork for therapeutic delivery through gene- and stem cell-based approaches, such as gene editing and gene replacement via viral vectors.[60] Humanized mouse models, or mice with the human sequence for a gene of interest added to their genome, are gaining popularity due to the enhanced translational power and ability to test the safety and efficacy of the same gene therapy that will be given to humans, rather than a mouse version of the treatment.

Although mice remain the most common species used for modeling autism, rats are becoming more widely available thanks to advances in gene-editing technologies such as CRISPR-Cas9, along with the 2004 publication of the rat genome.[61–63] Genetic rat models of autism now available include those with mutations in *Fmrp, Nlgn3, Mecp2, Nrxn1, Pten, Cntnap2, Met, mGluR5, Arid1b, Chd8, Dyrk1a, Fmr1, Grin2b, Scn2a, Shank2, Shank3, Pax6, Cacna1c,* and *Ube3a*.[64–74] Despite many commonalities between mice and rats, an estimated 12–24 million years of separate evolution has contributed to several notable differences in their biology and behavior. Of particular relevance to autism is the variety and complexity of the rat's social behavior and vocal communication system, as well as their enhanced cognitive capabilities and greater physiological similarity to humans.[75] Rats display social behaviors that are not observed in mice such as cooperative behaviors[76–78] and robust social play, which plays an important role in their social development similarly to humans.[79–81] Compared to mice, rats display a greater degree of motivation to engage with a social partner, thereby producing an elevated "social signal" that makes a social deficit easier to detect.[82,83] Rats also show greater sophistication in their vocal communication, using calls of different frequencies to bi-directionally transfer information regarding an animal's situation and affective state. One type of rat call is long low-frequency alarm calls, which rats use to warn others of potential dangers and which are not emitted by mice.[84,85] Therefore, although the genetic toolbox is still larger for mice and more financial resources and laboratory space are required for rats, the greater number of social and communication behaviors with complexities more similar to humans means that rats can provide additional insights on the social component of autism as compared to mice.[63,67,70,86–88]

While their social behavioral repertoire is more limited than mice and rats, nonrodent species such as the zebrafish provide numerous advantages for studying the genetic bases of autism. The zebrafish genome, which has been well-characterized, contains ortho- or homologous genes to over 70% of human genes.[89] Since they are relatively easy to house in large quantities, breed in large numbers, and develop rapidly, they are well-suited for high-throughput experiments involving transgene introduction or drug screening. Furthermore, the near transparency of zebrafish embryos offers the unique opportunity to visualize neurodevelopment and their aquatic environment is highly advantageous for the efficient delivery of drugs to multiple subjects at once.

Despite a limited availability of genetic technologies, other species with sophisticated social behavioral repertoires, such as voles[90] and nonhuman primates,[91–93] provide useful model systems for autism and particularly for investigating environmental risk factors.[94] Nonhuman primates, such as macaque monkeys, are far more similar to humans in their biology and behavior compared to rodents, only having been evolutionarily separated from humans by about 25 million years compared to 70 million years.[95,96] While nonhuman primate studies are significantly more expensive and time-intensive due to longer gestation times and fewer offspring compared to rodent research, nonhuman primates allow for the study of brain regions that are central to human social behavior and have been implicated in autism but are less developed in the rodent brain (e.g., the prefrontal cortex and fusiform gyrus).[97] The sensory dependency of nonhuman primates is also more analogous to humans, as they are heavily reliant on vision whereas rodents primarily rely on olfaction. Like humans, nonhuman primates live in complex, hierarchical social networks and transfer information with sophisticated communication systems involving vocalizations, facial expressions, gestures, and body positions. These social signals are learned over development such that young individuals must learn how to interpret, understand, and then use them in order to successfully navigate various social situations.[91]

The perfect animal model of autism does not exist, as each carries its own set of strengths and limitations, but a perfect model is not a necessary component of autism research. The unique advantages of different model species can each be leveraged to shed light on various components of autism etiology, manifestation, and treatment. Since the ultimate goal of preclinically modeling autism is to utilize animal models to elucidate underlying causes and effective therapies, the strength of a given model depends on (1) how closely its biological dysfunction (e.g., gene mutation or environmental exposure) resembles that which causes autism in humans ("construct validity"), (2) how closely it recapitulates the defining behavioral features exhibited by humans with autism ("face validity"), and (3) how well its responsiveness to treatments resembles the treatment response in humans with autism ("predictive validity").[97–99] Historically, in the assessment of autism models, emphasis was placed on face validity and the alignment between animal behavior and the behaviorally based diagnostic criteria. However, face validity is inherently limited by the disconnect between animal behavior and human behavior: autism-like behavior in animals can never fully capture the human phenotype and it can result from causes that are not related to autism specifically. For instance, there is a high degree of overlap between the symptomology of autism and that of other neurodevelopmental disorders. Therefore, without incorporating a biological mechanism to explain the behavioral phenotypes (i.e., construct validity), a model with only face validity to autism is indeed a model of disordered neurodevelopment more broadly.

As the biological bases for autism are becoming more fully elucidated, the strongest and most useful animal models of autism are those that maximize both construct and face validity and show reliability of phenotypes across time and laboratories. The etiology of the model should match the proposed etiology of the disorder, while the model's behavioral phenotypes should involve analogous neural circuitry and have translational relevance for the disorder. While some symptoms of autism, such as language impairments, may not be possible to model in an animal, a high face validity model is one that demonstrates social interaction impairments, communication deficits, restricted/repetitive behaviors, and comorbidities such as anxiety-like behavior, cognitive deficits, and seizure susceptibility. Phenotypes in each of these domains can be used as translational outcome measures in the discovery and assessment of novel interventions and therapies. Additionally, in the future, when a treatment demonstrates efficacy in humans with autism and is available to administer to animals, predictive validity should be the third criterion used to evaluate animal models.[100] The current prevalence of models with high construct and face validity, as well as the analogous outcomes found in rodents and humans following nonautism pharmacological treatments, is promising for the eventual discovery of models with all three validities.

## Examining autism symptoms in rodents

Given that the defining criteria for autism are social interaction and communication deficits along with restricted, repetitive patterns of behavior, how can these symptoms be studied in animals? Furthermore, how can we investigate the associated symptoms of autism such as intellectual disability, gross and fine motor abnormalities, altered responsiveness to sensory stimuli, anxiety, and comorbid neurological issues such as seizures and disrupted sleep? Since mice are the preeminent model species for autism and rats are on the rise, here we review the laboratory tests commonly used to detect autism-relevant phenotypes in mice and rats, along with essential control measures.

Thanks to decades of behavioral neuroscience research combining ethological information about natural rodent behaviors with guidance from autism clinicians, there currently exist a number of standardized assays for each clinical criterion of autism[3,45,99,101–110] (Table 1). These assays

TABLE 1 Examples of behavioral assays used to study rodent models of autism and their lab-to-clinic translational power.

| Behavioral domain | Assay | Strengths | Translational outcome(s) |
|---|---|---|---|
| Social interaction | Three-chambered social approach | Accounts for social motivation, social recognition memory, and/or preference for social novelty | |
| | Peer reciprocal social interactions | Detailed analysis of nuanced, discrete social behaviors. Expressive and receptive communication | ✓ |
| | Social conditioned place preference | Probes the rewarding aspects of social stimuli | |
| Social communication | Scent mark deposition/investigation | Expressive and receptive olfactory communication | |
| | Social transmission of food preference | Expressive and receptive olfactory and tactile communication | |
| | Olfactory habituation/dishabituation (OHDH) | Sensitivity to nonsocial and social odors. Can detect an olfactory deficit | |
| | Pup ultrasonic vocalizations (USV) | Early life functional readout | ✓ |
| | Juvenile and adult USV | USV can be linked to physical activity at the time of emission. Improved translation with rats | ✓ |
| | USV playback | Expressive and receptive auditory communication. Improved translation with rats | ✓ |

*Continued*

TABLE 1 Examples of behavioral assays used to study rodent models of autism and their lab-to-clinic translational power—cont'd

| Behavioral domain | Assay | Strengths | Translational outcome(s) |
|---|---|---|---|
| Restricted, repetitive behaviors | Repetitive behaviors and motor stereotypies | Easily assayed using an empty cage. Examples include grooming, flipping, and circling | ✓ |
| | Restricted interest and insistence on sameness | Observable during other behavioral assays | |
| | Perseverative behaviors and cognitive inflexibility | Observable during cognitive tests | ✓ |
| Comorbidities and associated symptoms | Cognitive abilities | Wide range of assays available. Touchscreen is highly translational | ✓ |
| | Anxiety-like behavior | Informative for interpreting other behavioral assays | |
| | Motor function | Informative for interpreting other behavioral assays. Gait is highly translational | ✓ |
| | Developmental delay | Early life functional readout | ✓ |
| | Reactivity to sensory stimuli | Informative for interpreting other behavioral assays | ✓ |
| | Seizure susceptibility | Can be observed spontaneously or induced. EEG detects subthreshold epileptiform activity. EEG is highly translational | ✓ |
| | Sleep abnormalities | Can be observed using EEG/EMG | ✓ |

have helped to identify autism-relevant behaviors in both genetic[111–114] (Table 2) and environmental rodent models of autism[115–119] (Table 3) and are designed to evaluate autism-relevant behavior in mice and rats based on species-typical behavior and the primary factors that regulate their behavior: olfactory, auditory, and tactile information. Both mice and rats are highly social species that quickly approach and affiliate with others, engage in communal nesting, investigate the pheromones emitted by conspecifics, and communicate through vocalizations.[120–123] The assays

**TABLE 2** Examples of behavioral phenotypes in genetic rodent models of autism.

| | | Reported domains affected | | |
|---|---|---|---|---|
| **Function** | **Gene** | **Core ASD** | **Comorbidities and associated symptoms** | **Example references** |
| Synaptic functioning | *SCN2A* | Social interaction<br>Repetitive behaviors | Cognition<br>Anxiety-like behavior<br>Motor<br>Seizures | 124,125 |
| | *SYNGAP1* | Social interaction | Cognition<br>Motor<br>Sensorimotor gating | 126–128 |
| | *CACNA1C* (Timothy Syndrome) | Social interaction<br>Reduced vocalizations<br>Repetitive behaviors | Cognition | 70,129,130 |
| Synaptic structure | *CNTNAP2* | Social interaction<br>Reduced vocalizations<br>Repetitive behaviors | Cognition<br>Motor<br>Sensory sensitivity<br>Behavioral flexibility<br>Seizures | 131,132 |
| | *SHANK2* | Social interaction<br>Communication<br>Repetitive behaviors | Cognition<br>Anxiety-like behavior<br>Motor | 133–136 |
| | *SHANK3* | Social interaction<br>Communication<br>Repetitive behaviors<br>Restricted interest | Cognition<br>Anxiety-like behavior<br>Motor<br>Sensory sensitivity | 54,56,130, 137–139 |
| | *NLGN3* | Social interaction<br>Communication | Cognition<br>Anxiety-like behavior<br>Motor<br>Sensory sensitivity<br>Development | 55,57, 140–142 |
| | *NLGN4* | Social interaction<br>Communication<br>Repetitive behavior<br>Restricted interest | Cognition<br>Motor | 58,143,144 |

*Continued*

**TABLE 2** Examples of behavioral phenotypes in genetic rodent models of autism—cont'd

| Function | Gene | Reported domains affected | | Example references |
|---|---|---|---|---|
| | | **Core ASD** | **Comorbidities and associated symptoms** | |
| Chromatin remodeling | *CHD8* | Social interaction<br>Communication<br>Repetitive behaviors | Cognition<br>Anxiety-like behavior<br>Motor | 145–148 |
| | *ARID1B* | Social interaction<br>Vocalizations<br>Repetitive behaviors | Cognition<br>Anxiety-like behavior<br>Motor<br>Development | 149–151 |
| | *POGZ* | Social interaction<br>Vocalizations | Cognition<br>Motor | 152,153 |
| Transcriptional regulation | *ADNP* | Social memory<br>Vocalizations | Cognition<br>Motor<br>Development<br>Sensory responsivity | 154–157 |
| | *TBR1* | Social interaction<br>Vocalizations | Cognition | 158 |
| Cell signaling | *DYRK1A* | Social interaction<br>Vocalizations<br>Repetitive behaviors | Cognition<br>Motor<br>Seizure susceptibility | 159 |
| | *PTEN* | Social interaction<br>Repetitive behavior<br>Restricted interest | Anxiety-like behavior<br>Sensory sensitivity<br>Sensorimotor gating<br>Seizures | 160–164 |
| | *TSC1/TSC2* (Tuberous sclerosis) | Social interaction<br>Vocalizations<br>Repetitive behaviors<br>Restricted interest | Seizures | 165–168 |
| | *UBE3A* (Angelman Syndrome) | Social interaction | Cognition<br>Motor<br>Seizures<br>Sleep | 86,169–172 |

TABLE 3 Examples of behavioral phenotypes in environmental models of autism.

| Environmental risk factor | Reported domains affected | | Example references |
|---|---|---|---|
| | Core ASD | Comorbidities and associated symptoms | |
| Valproic acid (VPA) | Social interaction<br>Repetitive behaviors | Cognition<br>Anxiety-like behavior<br>Motor<br>Pain sensitivity<br>Development<br>EEG activity | 115,173–176 |
| Maternal immune activation | Social interaction<br>Communication<br>Repetitive behaviors | Cognition<br>Motor | 34,177–180 |
| Pesticides | Social interaction<br>Communication<br>Restricted interest | Cognition<br>Anxiety-like behavior<br>Motor<br>Development | 72,181–185 |
| Air pollution | Social interaction<br>Repetitive behaviors | Cognition<br>Anxiety-like behavior | 72,118,181,182,186–188 |
| Polychlorinated biphenyls (PCBs) | Social interaction | Cognition<br>Motor<br>Anxiety-like behavior<br>Seizures | 117,189–192 |
| Paternal age | Social interaction<br>Communication<br>Repetitive behaviors | Anxiety-like behavior<br>Motor<br>Development | 119,193–195 |

standard to preclinical autism research are designed to take advantage of natural rodent behavior in a way that specifically maximizes its relevance to the types of social deficits and behaviors that are observed in humans with autism (e.g., playing alone instead of with others).[100]

## Social interaction assays

### Three-chambered social approach

To measure social motivation, subjects are placed in a central, empty chamber and allowed to freely explore two side chambers: one containing an unfamiliar conspecific inside an inverted wire cup and one chamber containing just a wire cup.[102,105] Subjects are essentially given the choice to spend time with the novel conspecific (social approach) or the novel object (wire cup). The wire cup containing the conspecific ensures that the animals can sniff each other, and all social behaviors are initiated by the subject, but they cannot engage in aggression. The empty wire cup in the other chamber serves as a control since the chamber containing the novel conspecific also contains a wire cup. Spending significantly more time with the conspecific compared to the empty cup constitutes typical rodent social behavior. Importantly, this task was not designed to quantify a subject's level of sociability, but rather to answer the yes/no question of whether a subject demonstrates typical sociability. A modified version of this assay using an unfamiliar conspecific and a familiar conspecific can also be used to measure social recognition and social novelty preference. Since mice and rats are naturally novelty-seeking, spending significantly more time with the novel conspecific than the familiar one constitutes typical social recognition and novelty preference.[45,102,105,196–198]

## Peer reciprocal social interactions

More nuanced and fine-grained analyses of social behavior can be obtained by allowing subjects to freely interact with one or more conspecifics and observing their reciprocal social interactions. When given this opportunity, the time that mice and rats spend sniffing, following, chasing, pushing past, crawling over, pushing under, and grooming their partner(s) can be quantified.[181,197,199–201] Nonsocial behaviors such as exploring, digging, eating, and self-grooming can also be scored and, for rats, rough-and-tumble play fighting can also be observed. Rat play is comparable to that of cats and dogs, consisting of fast-paced wrestling, pouncing, pinning, chasing, and boxing.[81,86] These parameters can be used to establish a subject's level of social motivation as well as the degree of social reciprocity between animals.

## Social conditioned place preference

To test the rewarding value of a social stimulus, subjects are provided with a social stimulus (e.g., a conspecific or social scent) while in a chamber containing unique environmental stimuli, such as markings on the walls or a textured floor.[202–204] They are also exposed to a second chamber with unique environmental cues but no social stimulus, which trains the subject to associate each chamber with either a social stimulus or with social isolation. Subjects are then reintroduced to the arena and allowed to explore both chambers, during which spending significantly more time in the chamber associated with the social stimulus indicates that the subject found the social context rewarding.

## Prosocial behavior

Rodent models may be inherently limited in their ability to recapitulate empathy or theory of mind deficits; however, a few notable studies show promise in this regard. In mice, the response to a painful stimulus was greater when the subject was able to observe a conspecific which also received the painful stimulus and the responses of two mice tested together were similar despite having received stimuli of different intensities.[205] Female mice also showed approach toward another mouse in pain, spending more time in proximity to a familiar conspecific in pain compared to an unfamiliar conspecific in pain or a familiar conspecific not in pain.[205] Studies of observational fear learning found that mice able to observe a conspecific experiencing a painful stimulus displayed fear responses despite no exposure to a painful stimulus themselves[206] and that rats able to observe a conspecific exhibiting a tone-elicited fear response subsequently showed a tone-elicited fear response despite no exposure to a painful stimulus themselves.[207,208] There is also a range of evidence showing cooperation and reciprocity in rats, possibly reflecting empathy.[76–78,209–212] Upon encountering a conspecific trapped inside a restrainer, subject rats will learn to quickly open a door to release the conspecific, and they allow the conspecific access to chocolate that could have been consumed before releasing the conspecific.[213,214] Rats also learned to help a conspecific in distress (stuck in a pool) by opening a door that enabled the distressed rat to escape the pool. Prior experience being stuck in the pool led rats to open the door faster.[215] Rats taught to play hide-and-seek with researchers displayed some behaviors suggestive of theory of mind capabilities, such as going to hide in a location previously inspected by the researcher, hiding in an opaque rather than transparent box, and remaining silent while hiding.[216] Although not yet routinely employed in rodent models of autism, assays of prosocial behavior may become increasingly useful for evaluating empathy and theory of mind capacities when potential confounders such as cognitive abilities are carefully considered.

# Social communication assays

## Pheromones and scent marking

Mice and rats are olfactory creatures and predominantly communicate via pheromones emitted from anogenital glands and in urine. Compounds in rodent urine, of which there are hundreds and potentially thousands, help convey identifying information such as species, strain, sex, rank, and reproductive status of the donor animal. These pheromones play important roles in marking territory, mating, kin recognition, and aggression. Olfactory communication can therefore be assessed by measuring the time a subject spends investigating a conspecific's anogenital region, urinary scent marks left in a cage by a conspecific, a cotton swab soaked with urine, or urinary odors delivered via an olfactometer.[45,71,109,122,217] A subject's propensity to transmit olfactory information can be measured by the frequency with which they deposit urinary scent marks near those left by others.[71,218–220]

## Social transmission of food preference

This assay tests whether subjects obtain information about a novel food from a cagemate who recently consumed the food.[107,221] First, the subject's cagemate is allowed to consume a food item with a flavor that is unfamiliar to the subject and is then allowed to interact with the subject. This gives the subject the opportunity to become familiar with the flavor by sniffing the cagemate's face, whiskers, and breath. Since rodents typically prefer familiar over novel foods, the transmission of food-related information can be tested by giving the subject the opportunity to consume that food item or a new one and evaluating whether a preference is shown.[197,203]

## Olfactory habituation/dishabituation (OHDH)

This task evaluates a subject's sensitivity to olfactory information and tests for enhanced investigation of social odors (which contain pheromones) over nonsocial odors.[104] Subjects are exposed to a cotton swab containing a novel odor and then presented with the same odor multiple times. Repeated presentation of the same odor leads to habituation and the subject spends less time sniffing the cotton swab each time it is presented. Dishabituation then takes place via introduction to a new odor, which reinstates a high level of sniffing. Both social (e.g., urine) and nonsocial (e.g., vanilla) odors are presented with subjects typically showing a significantly enhanced investigation of the social odor compared to nonsocial scents. If subjects demonstrate an ability to discriminate between odors but do not show a preference for sniffing social odors, this may indicate a social communication deficit. However, if subjects do not show normal odor discrimination, this would suggest an olfactory deficit which may confound other tests of social behavior.

## Pup ultrasonic vocalizations (USV)

Like human infants, mouse and rat pups are born immature and are highly dependent on their mother for food, thermoregulation, and cleaning.[222] During the first 2 weeks of life, pups communicate with their mother through ultrasonic vocalizations (USV) in the range of 40 kHz, which elicit maternal retrieval, help to ensure that pups receive adequate maternal care, and can be compared to the cries of a human infant.[223–226] As pups reach 2 weeks old and gain the ability to see and hear, the number of USV emitted drops substantially. Therefore, pup communication can be assessed by briefly removing a pup from the nest and recording its vocalizations when isolated from the mother. This can be carried out on a single day of development (e.g., postnatal day 7) or repeatedly across development (e.g., postnatal day 4 through 14). In the absence of thermoregulatory deficits and global developmental delay that might affect a pup's ability to produce USV, deviation from the typical quantity or pattern of USV emission can provide evidence of an early life social communication abnormality.[227]

## Juvenile and adult USV

During interactions with a conspecific of the same-sex, juvenile mice and rats emit affiliative USV that can be recorded and analyzed using acoustic software.[225,228–232] For mice, a period of social isolation before the test is usually required to promote USV production.[3] Since advanced techniques are required to differentiate the USV emitted from each individual, subjects are often paired with a member of the same experimental group and the resulting USV are analyzed as a single set.[133,135,230,233,234] This identification issue, however, can be circumvented by eliciting USV with a social odor (i.e., urine), a social context (i.e., a previously played-in arena), or prerecorded USV.[227,235,236] In rats, the identity issue can also be avoided by eliciting USV from a single subject using the experimenter's hand to mimic social play.[86,237–241]

Territorial USV can also be collected by introducing a same-sex intruder into the home environment of the subject. In mice, the resident mouse is reliably the source of emitted USV,[228,242–244] while in rats, the intruder who gets attacked produces the majority of the USV, which likely serve as alarm calls or signals of negative affect.[229] Subjects can also be given time to interact with a conspecific of the opposite sex, which is often carried out for male subjects since males emit high numbers of courtship USV when exposed to a female in estrus or to urine from an estrus female without the need for pretest isolation.[234,245–248] With different levels of complexity and underlying neurobiological substrates, rodent USV are not quite analogous to human language, however they are important signals that reflect a subject's responsivity to social stimuli, and they do provide useful behavioral read-outs. Considerable work is ongoing to better understand the communicative function of USV produced by mice and rats during specific types of social situations.

## USV playback

Both expressive and receptive communication can be assayed in rodents by quantifying the behavioral response to hearing the USV of a conspecific.[88,108,169,233,249–251] An ultrasonic speaker is used to play prerecorded USV to a single subject while both their movement in relation to the speaker (approach or avoidance) and any USV they emit in response are measured. Presentation of a time- and amplitude-matched nonsocial acoustic control stimulus, such as a scrambled USV or white noise, is important for correctly interpreting the subject's response to the USV. The control stimulus helps to show that the subject's response to the USV is due to the social salience of the USV and not simply the presentation of a novel sound, and it helps confirm that the subject's hearing abilities are intact.

Although possible to carry out in both mice and rats, this task is not commonly carried out in mouse models of autism, likely due to the rapid hearing loss that commonly afflicts inbred laboratory mice, including the highly popular C57BL/6J strain.[252–256] In rats, however, the USV playback assay is highly versatile due to the sophistication of the rat vocal communication system. Unlike mice, it is well-established that rats use vocalizations of different frequencies to transfer different types of information. High frequency USV (~ 50 kHz) are emitted by both mice and rats in positive contexts such as social interaction and are used to promote social affiliation, but only rats also emit low frequency USV (~ 22 kHz) in negative contexts and use them to warn others of potential danger.[84,106,257] These distinct call types make it possible to study a subject rat's behavioral reaction to both prosocial and alarm calls, in addition to characterizing the different types of USV emitted in response.

# Assays of restricted, repetitive behaviors

## Repetitive and stereotyped behaviors

Repetitive behaviors in rodents often manifest via normal activities, such as self-grooming, that last for an unusually long amount of time (e.g., 2 min rather than 10 s).[45,73,116,131,138,197,258] These are usually observed in an empty test cage and can be compared to repetitive behaviors in autism, such as playing the same game over and over. In addition to self-grooming, excessive digging can also be scored in the marble burying assay in which subjects are presented with a set of glass marbles on top of bedding material.[45,258] The number of marbles that a subject buries during the test session can be used as a measure of repetitive digging behavior. It is important to note that this test can be confounded by a motor phenotype (hypo- or hyperlocomotion) as well as anxiety-like behavior so additional assays in these domains should be carried out alongside the marble burying test. While marble burying is readily observed in mice, rats do not show the same degree of neophobia in response to the marbles as mice and they do not reliably engage in marble burying. Rather, a variety of responses to the marbles have been observed, including licking the marbles and picking them up.

Stereotypies are fixed predictable movements, seemingly with no purpose or goal, that are performed repeatedly in the same form. Motor stereotypies observed in autism include hand flapping, body rocking, and toe walking. In rodents, motor stereotypies take the form of species-typical behaviors such as jumping, circling, and backflipping that are performed at a much greater frequency than normal.[58,198,259,260] These are typically measured by observing the subject alone in an empty test cage for a defined period of time.

## Restricted interests and insistence on sameness

Restricted interests can be tested by exposing subjects to a novel environment containing several different stimuli, such as novel objects or holes in the walls or floor.[259,261,262] Since typical rodent exploration consists of investigating all novel stimuli, continued interaction with only one of the objects or holes may represent restricted interests. An example of this is a reduced number of spontaneous alternations in a Y-maze, which occurs when a subject does not explore all three arms in a typical fashion and instead revisits previously explored arms. If subjects are confirmed to have intact working memory, meaning that they are capable of identifying recently explored arms, then elevated re-visits can suggest restricted interest and insistence on sameness. Additionally, a lack of digging in the marble burying assay may also reflect reduced interests and disrupted performance in an operant task following the presentation of a novel stimulus may indicate an upset to a change.[45,263]

## Perseverative behaviors and cognitive inflexibility

Perseveration, or the continuation of a particular response despite the cessation of a stimulus, is most often measured in rodents with reversal learning tasks. The subject is first trained using a food reward to establish a new habit, which could be entering a particular arm of a T-maze, swimming to a particular area in a Morris water maze, or nose poking a particular hole inside an operant chamber.[196,264–266] Once the subject has learned the rule governing the reward, the rule is changed such that the reward is delivered upon entering a different area of the maze or nose poking a different hole. Perseverative, cognitively inflexible behavior can be observed when the subject continues to visit the previously reinforced location and fails to adapt to new conditions and learn the new rule governing the reward.

## Evaluating comorbidities and autism-associated symptoms

### Cognitive abilities

One of the most prevalent comorbidities in autism is intellectual disability, which is observed in about 70% of cases.[267,268] There are numerous laboratory tests used for evaluating both short-term and long-term learning and memory in rodents, including the previously mentioned Y-maze spontaneous alternation assay, novel object recognition (NOR), contextual and cued fear conditioned freezing, the Morris water maze spatial navigation task, and operant touchscreen learning assays.

The spontaneous alternation task tests working spatial memory by taking advantage of the natural novelty-seeking behavior of rodents. Subjects are allowed to freely explore a Y-maze, which consists of three identical arms. Cognitively intact rodents tend to alternate the arms that they explore and choose to visit a newer arm rather than a more recently visited arm. Therefore, a reduced rate of spontaneous arm alternation and elevated rate of arm revisits may indicate that a subject has impaired working memory for the recently visited arms. In the test of NOR, subjects are allowed to investigate and become familiar with two identical objects.[269] After a delay period, which can be adjusted to change the task's difficulty, subjects are re-introduced to one of the previously investigated objects and one novel object. Subjects with intact learning and memory abilities recognize the previously seen object and, due to their natural preference to explore novelty, spend significantly more time investigating the novel object compared to the familiar object.[270] This task can also be modified to test spatial recognition by changing one object's location within the arena, rather than changing an object's identity.

Fear conditioning paradigms are also frequently used to train rodents to associate an aversive foot shock with contextual cues (e.g., specific lighting, odor, floor texture) and/or an auditory cue (e.g., a loud tone).[271] After the subject has received a foot shock while being exposed to the cues, there is a delay period after which the subject is reintroduced to the cues without the foot shock. Since freezing is a natural fear response in rodents, it is used as a proxy metric for learning and memory. Memory of the aversive foot shock that was paired with the cues is reflected by the level of freezing behavior observed in response to the cues alone. In the Morris water maze task, a subject is placed inside a pool with a hidden escape platform.[272] Through repeated testing, the subject learns the location of the escape platform using spatial cues in the testing environment. The pace of learning, as well as the search strategy used to locate the platform, can be used to detect cognitive deficits. Instead of a pool, a large flat surface ("Barnes maze") with several holes but only one escape box can also be used. Long-term learning and memory are also commonly assayed using automated operant touchscreen chambers, which are highly efficient and translational tools for testing cognition as touchscreens are also used in clinical populations. In rodent touchscreen chambers, a food reward is delivered to the subject upon selection of a particular response on the touchscreen panel. The reinforced response may be to touch the image of a flower and not an airplane, or to touch the second hole from the left out of a set of five holes. Various metrics related to the rate of learning, such as the number of training sessions required or the number of incorrect responses made, can be used to characterize cognitive abilities.[72,273] Touchscreen chambers are highly customizable and can be tailored to test attention as well as various types of learning with varying degrees of difficulty.

## Anxiety-like behavior

As nocturnal, tunnel-dwelling animals, mice and rats prefer environments that are dark and enclosed. Anxiety-like behavior is therefore commonly assessed in rodents by presenting subjects with an approach-avoidance conflict in which the natural tendency to explore a novel environment is placed at odds with the natural preference for dark, sheltered environments.[59,99,274] The classic apparatus used for this purpose is the elevated plus maze (EPM), which consists of two open and two enclosed arms crossed in the shape of a plus sign that is elevated above the floor. When placed on this maze, subjects can choose to spend time in the darker, closed arms or explore the brighter, more exposed open arms. A light-dark box consisting of a dark, enclosed chamber attached to an open and brightly lit chamber can serve a similar purpose.[275–278] In both tests, increased anxiety-like behavior is represented by a subject spending unusually more time in the dark, closed arms or chamber.

## Motor function

Motor dysfunction and hyperactivity are autism-associated symptoms that are critical to evaluate in animal models since motor abnormalities can confound the interpretation of many other behavioral assays. Gross motor activity is easily assessed by allowing subjects the opportunity to explore a novel open field and quantifying their level of locomotion (e.g., distance moved) throughout the test session.[3,45] Motor abilities can also be assessed by testing whether a subject can cross an elevated beam, counting any foot slips, and timing how long it takes them to cross.[279,280] More fine motor skills such as specific parameters of gait can be measured through paw painting and manual footprint analyses, or automated tools such as the CatWalk XT footprint analysis system and the DigiGait automated treadmill system. Another highly utilized test of motor functioning is the accelerating rotarod task, in which subjects are placed on a horizontal rod that gradually accelerates over the course of several minutes. The amount of time a subject remains moving on the rod reflects their motor coordination and balance abilities, while improved performance across repeated test sessions indicates their motor learning capacity.[281]

## Developmental delay

The pace of maturation is assessed in mice and rats by studying the rate at which developmental milestones are achieved across the first 2–3 weeks of life.[282] In addition to physical characteristics, such as body mass, body length, head width, eye opening, pinnae detachment, and tooth emergence, various psychomotor reflexes are also tested.[140,283–286] These include the righting reflex measured by how quickly a pup can right itself from its back onto all four paws, cliff avoidance reflex measured by whether a pup can detect and avoid the edge of a cliff, grasping reflex measured by the forelimbs grasping onto a thin rod, rooting reflex measured by a turn of the head in response to whisker stimulation, and acoustic startle reflex measured by whether a pup turns its head in response to an auditory cue. Muscle tone can be tested by timing how long a pup can hang onto a rod or an inverted wire screen.

## Reactivity to sensory stimuli

Abnormal reactivity to sensory stimuli, which affects up to 90% of individuals with autism,[287,288] is tested in mice and rats using olfactory, acoustic, and tactile stimuli. In the previously described test of OHDH, in which a variety of odors are presented to each subject, hypo- or hyperreactivity to the stimuli is reflected in aberrant quantities of time spent sniffing the odors. Reactivity to acoustic stimuli is most often measured by how much a subject startles in response to a loud tone. The subject is placed inside a chamber with piezoelectric sensors that can detect the animal's level of movement. Tones of various intensities are presented while the automated system captures the subject's subsequent motor reactivity. An extended paradigm, called prepulse inhibition (PPI) of the startle response, is used to analyze sensorimotor gating, which is impaired in autism. In animals with intact sensorimotor gating, presentation of a weaker acoustic stimulus (prepulse) just before the intense startle stimulus (pulse) leads to a reduced startle response.[289,290] The startle response can also be quantified following a tactile stimulus, for which a sudden puff of air is often used.

Responsiveness to tactile stimuli is also frequently assayed with two tests common to pain research: the hot plate and tail flick tests.[291] For the hot plate test, a subject is placed onto a hot plate maintained at a constant temperature and the amount of time that passes until the animal exhibits a behavioral reaction (e.g., jumps, licks its paw) is measured. In the tail flick test, a heat source (e.g., water or light beam) is applied to the subject's tail and the amount of time that elapses before the animal moves their tail is recorded. An alternative method for testing mechanical reactivity is to place a subject onto a mesh surface and touch the bottom of their paw with a Von Frey monofilament. Each filament is designed to deliver a constant predetermined force for 2–5s before it bends, so filaments of differing forces are used until the subject shows a response (e.g., withdraws, licks, or shakes their paw).

## Seizures and sleep abnormalities

Sleep disturbances are highly prevalent in autism, occurring in as many as 80% of cases, while up to 30% of individuals with autism exhibit seizures and up to 60% display abnormal electroencephalograms (EEG).[292,293] Both seizures and sleep patterns can be precisely quantified with EEG techniques using electrodes placed within the skull to measure the brain's electrophysiological activity, along with simultaneous electromyography (EMG) to detect muscle movement.[170,294,295] Epileptiform activity, including subthreshold activity, can be quantified by the number of spikes that occur within a given timeframe and sleep/wake activity can be quantified by metrics such as the percent time spent in active wake, wake, slow-wave sleep, and deep paradoxical (REM-like) sleep. Active wake is characterized by low amplitude, high frequency EEG signal with accompanying EMG activity, while wake is differentiated from active awake by a lack of EMG activity. Slow-wave sleep has a high amplitude, low frequency EEG signal with no accompanying EMG activity and deep paradoxical sleep has low amplitude, low frequency EEG signal with no co-occurring EMG activity. The frequency of sleep spindles, which are bursts of activity characteristic of normal sleep and important for learning and memory, is another key metric as spindle density is often reduced in those with autism.

Sleep phenotypes can also be evaluated without the need for electrode implantation, including via home cage observation or automated monitoring of movement and respiration using piezoelectric sensors. For models that exhibit spontaneous seizures, home cage behavioral monitoring with videocameras may suffice for data collection; otherwise, seizures can be induced with a chemoconvulsant such as the $GABA_A$ receptor antagonist pentylenetetrazol or the glutamate receptor agonist kainic acid.[296,297] Both spontaneous and induced seizures can be scored behaviorally by the amount of time that elapses before a subject displays a myoclonic jerk, loss of righting reflex, generalized tonic-clonic seizure, and/or death. A greater frequency of seizures or faster onset and progression reflect enhanced seizure susceptibility, while fewer seizures and/or a longer time to onset indicates seizure resistance. EEG techniques are highly versatile as they can be coupled with behavioral assays to pair brain activity with behavioral outcomes (e.g., auditory evoked potentials) and are highly translational as the same EEG metrics can be compared across rodents to humans, allowing for the delineation of translational biomarkers.

## Methodological considerations

While many standardized tests of rodent behavior are available, social behavior and social communication are highly complex and should be interpreted with care. Assays designed to test social behavior do not solely involve social behavior, but also depend on sensory, motor, and cognitive abilities and can therefore be confounded by physical disabilities. It is important to be mindful that olfaction, not vision, is the predominant sensory modality in rodents and that social behavior is inextricably linked with olfaction and motor activity, therefore these should be assessed alongside social behavior. An impaired ability to smell can contribute to low social investigation times and be misinterpreted as reduced social behavior, so olfactory abilities should be tested by OHDH, timing how long it takes a subject to locate buried food, or another olfactory assay. Similarly, since low motor activity can lead to low social investigation times, a motor outcome such as distance moved or transitions between chambers should be quantified. Another potential confound of social assays that should be evaluated concomitantly is anxiety-like behavior, which has a suppressing effect on motor behavior.

In addition to addressing potential confounds, multiple corroborating tests should be used to support the discovery of social impairments and, furthermore, multiple domains of behavior (e.g., social, motor, cognitive, anxiety-like behavior) should be evaluated to demonstrate an unconfounded autism-like phenotype.[298] There is no single task that simply measures social behavior or social communication and the results from any single test may be artifactual. It therefore does not suffice to use a single test of behavior to demonstrate an autism-like phenotype, which is underscored by the diagnostic requirement that an individual must display persistent deficits in social interaction and communication across multiple contexts in order to be diagnosed with autism.

## Conclusions and future directions

Autism is a uniquely human disorder with rising prevalence rates, no established biomarkers, and an immense unmet need for effective treatments. Since the diagnostic criteria for autism are purely behavioral and genetics play the primary role in the disorder's etiology, live behaving animals with a high degree of genetic conservation relative to humans are central to the study of autism. While it may not be possible to study certain aspects of the human phenotype in animals, such as characteristics of language, numerous behavioral tests relevant to the diagnostic domains of autism provide researchers with powerful tools to investigate the genetic as well as environmental factors that contribute to autism risk and pathophysiology.

Thanks to the optimization of targeted genetic mutations in the mouse, hundreds of mouse models have been developed to help study the genetic bases of autism. Yet, despite decades of research with mouse models, there are still no treatments available to target the core symptoms of autism. The only effective interventions currently available are intensive behavioral therapies[299–301] and the only FDA-approved pharmacological treatments are risperidone and aripiprazole, which are both for the associated symptom of irritability and have been available since 2006 and 2009, respectively.[302,303]

The field, however, is moving in a promising direction toward novel therapies by putting greater emphasis on outcome measures with high lab-to-clinic translational value, such as touchscreen tasks, EEG, sleep, as well as neuroanatomical phenotypes obtained by magnetic resonance imaging.[304] These not only provide powerful translational metrics with a high degree of analogy to clinical outcomes, but physiological phenotypes ("biomarkers") can also be correlated with behavioral scores to inform and strengthen the interpretation of a given model, as well as provide linked outcome measures for assessing therapeutic efficacy.[305–307] As they become elucidated, biomarkers are bound to play an increasingly important role in evaluating treatment efficacy, as they are less susceptible to the robust placebo effect apparent in numerous clinical trials for neurodevelopmental disorders. The field has also been placing greater attention on enhancing rigor, reproducibility, and reliability by using high powered sample sizes, critically interpreting behavioral data, considering potential confounds, collecting crucial control measures, detailed reporting of methods, as well as closely collaborating with clinicians.[298,304,308] While behavioral neuroscientists can gain valuable insights into autism behaviors through observational assessments, trained clinicians can help to address more profound questions such as what the underlying motivations for various types of social interactions are, how phenotypes change across development, and which features show specificity versus commonality across different genetic syndromes.

New developments in behavioral neuroscience research elucidating the circuitry underlying specific rodent behaviors and improvements in the ability to manipulate circuits will also ensure that preclinical scientists have a clearer understanding of the circuitry that underlies their behaviors of interest and how analogous they are to the circuitry in humans. Moreover, with a handful of genetic rat models now available and more in development, the field is poised for tremendous advancements in modeling more complex social and communication phenotypes in genetic models of autism. A larger number and wider range of construct- and face-valid models to cover the autism spectrum and capture the disorder's high heterogeneity will help collect the information necessary to move the field toward the development of effective treatment strategies that prevent, ameliorate, or reverse the symptoms of autism.

Given the implication of synaptic genes, therapeutics that act on synaptic functioning are likely to be useful targets. Although gene and stem-cell therapies hold great promise for offering long-term disease-modifying treatments, the technologies are still undergoing significant development and substantial progress must be made with regards to optimization of delivery route, dose, and timing. In parallel to gene therapies, the ongoing investigation of pharmacological agents, which can be quickly discontinued if side effects present, will be central to treating populations for whom gene therapies are not well-suited, such as higher functioning individuals. Testing animal models with high construct and face validity to autism in well-validated behavioral assays targeting the core features of autism, as well as the associated symptoms and control measures, will be essential for evaluating whether candidate treatments can reduce the incidence or lessen the severity of autism spectrum disorder.

## References

1. Centers for Disease Control and Prevention. *Data & Statistics on Autism Spectrum Disorder*; 2020.
2. American Psychiatric Association. *Diagnostic and Statistical Manual of Mental Disorders*; 2013.
3. Kazdoba T, Leach P, Yang M, Silverman JL, Crawley JN. Translational mouse models of autism: advancing toward pharmacological therapeutics. *Curr Top Behav Neurosci.* 2012;28:1–52.
4. Bai D, et al. Association of genetic and environmental factors with autism in a 5-country cohort. *JAMA Psychiatry.* 2019;76:1035–1043.
5. Folstein S, Rutter M. Genetic influences and infantile autism. *Nature.* 1977;265:726–728.
6. Hallmayer J, et al. Genetic heritability and shared environmental factors among twin pairs with autism. *Arch Gen Psychiatry.* 2011;68:1095–1102.
7. Miles JH. Autism spectrum disorders—a genetics review. *Genet Med.* 2011;13:278–294.
8. Nordenbæk C, Jørgensen M, Kyvik KO, Bilenberg N. A Danish population-based twin study on autism spectrum disorders. *Eur Child Adolesc Psychiatry.* 2014;23:35–43.
9. Simons Foundation Autism Research Initiative. Gene scoring. In: *SFARI Gene.* SFARI; 2019. Available at: https://gene.sfari.org/database/gene-scoring/.
10. Abrahams BS, et al. SFARI gene 2.0: a community-driven knowledgebase for the autism spectrum disorders (ASDs). *Mol Autism.* 2013;4:1.
11. Glessner JT, et al. Autism genome-wide copy number variation reveals ubiquitin and neuronal genes. *Nature.* 2009;459:569–572.
12. Iossifov I, et al. The contribution of de novo coding mutations to autism spectrum disorder. *Nature.* 2014;515:216–221.
13. Pinto D, et al. Convergence of genes and cellular pathways dysregulated in autism spectrum disorders. *Am J Hum Genet.* 2014;94:677–694.
14. Sebat J, et al. Strong association of de novo copy number mutations with autism. *Science.* 2007;316:445–449.
15. Weiss LA, et al. A genome-wide linkage and association scan reveals novel loci for autism. *Nature.* 2009;461:802–808.
16. O'Roak BJ, State MW. Autism genetics: strategies, challenges, and opportunities. *Autism Res.* 2008;1:4–17.
17. De Rubeis S, et al. Synaptic, transcriptional and chromatin genes disrupted in autism. *Nature.* 2014;515:209–215.

18. Abrahams BS, Geschwind DH. Connecting genes to brain in the autism spectrum disorders. *Arch Neurol.* 2010;67:395–399.
19. Devlin B, Scherer SW. Genetic architecture in autism spectrum disorder. *Curr Opin Genet Dev.* 2012;22:229–237.
20. Murdoch JD, State MW. Recent developments in the genetics of autism spectrum disorders. *Curr Opin Genet Dev.* 2013;23:310–315.
21. Turkmen AS, Lin S. Detecting X-linked common and rare variant effects in family-based sequencing studies. *Genet Epidemiol.* 2021;45:36–45.
22. Lim ET, et al. Rare complete knockouts in humans: population distribution and significant role in autism Spectrum disorders. *Neuron.* 2013;77:235–242.
23. Marshall CR, et al. Structural variation of chromosomes in autism spectrum disorder. *Am J Hum Genet.* 2008;82:477–488.
24. Rosenfeld JA, et al. Copy number variations associated with autism spectrum disorders contribute to a spectrum of neurodevelopmental disorders. *Genet Med.* 2010;12:694–702.
25. Matsunami N, et al. Identification of rare recurrent copy number variants in high-risk autism families and their prevalence in a large ASD population. *PLoS One.* 2013;8:1–14.
26. Poultney CS, et al. Identification of small exonic CNV from whole-exome sequence data and application to autism spectrum disorder. *Am J Hum Genet.* 2013;93:607–619.
27. Satterstrom FK, et al. Large-scale exome sequencing study implicates both developmental and functional changes in the neurobiology of autism. *Cell.* 2020;180:568–584.e23.
28. Abrahams BS, Geschwind DH. Advances in autism genetics: on the threshold of a new neurobiology. *Nat Rev Genet.* 2008;9:341–355.
29. Ashwood P, Wills S, Van De Water J. The immune response in autism: a new frontier for autism. *J Leukoc Biol.* 2006;80:1–15.
30. Chaste P, Leboyer M. Autism risk factors: genes, environment, and gene-environment interactions. *Dialogues Clin Neurosci.* 2012;14:281–292.
31. Hertz-Picciotto I, et al. The CHARGE study: an epidemiologic investigation of genetic and environmental factors contributing to autism. *Environ Health Perspect.* 2006;114:1119–1125.
32. Christensen J, et al. Prenatal valproate exposure and risk of autism spectrum disorders and childhood autism. *JAMA.* 2013;309:1696–1703.
33. Hertz-picciotto I, Schmidt RJ, Krakowiak P. Understanding environmental contributions to autism: causal concepts and the state of science. *Austim Res.* 2018;554–586. https://doi.org/10.1002/aur.1938.
34. Smith SEP, Li J, Garbett K, Mirnics K, Patterson PH. Maternal immune activation alters fetal brain development through interleukin-6. *J Neurosci.* 2007;27:10695–10702. https://doi.org/10.1523/JNEUROSCI.2178-07.2007.
35. Bruce MR, et al. Sexually dimorphic neuroanatomical differences relate to ASD-relevant behavioral outcomes in a maternal autoantibody mouse model. *Mol Psychiatry.* 2021;1–8. https://doi.org/10.1038/s41380-021-01215-w.
36. Ramirez-Celis A, et al. Risk assessment analysis for maternal autoantibody-related autism (MAR-ASD): a subtype of autism. *Mol Psychiatry.* 2021;26:1551–1560.
37. Modabbernia A, Velthorst E, Reichenberg A. Environmental risk factors for autism: an evidence-based review of systematic reviews and meta-analyses. *Mol Autism.* 2017;8:1–16.
38. Bölte S, Girdler S, Marschik PB. The contribution of environmental exposure to the etiology of autism spectrum disorder. *Cell Mol Life Sci.* 2018. https://doi.org/10.1007/s00018-018-2988-4.
39. Ashwood P, et al. Elevated plasma cytokines in autism spectrum disorders provide evidence of immune dysfunction and are associated with impaired behavioral outcome. *Brain Behav Immun.* 2011;25:40–45.
40. Volk HE, et al. Maternal immune response and air pollution exposure during pregnancy: insights from the early markers for autism (EMA) study. *J Neurodev Disord.* 2020;12:1–12.

41. Volk HE, Lurmann F, Penfold B, Hertz-Picciotto I, McConnell R. Traffic-related air pollution, particulate matter, and autism. *Arch Gen Psychiatry.* 2013;70:71–77.
42. Caspi A, Moffitt TE. Gene—environment interactions in psychiatry: joining forces with neuroscience. *Nat Rev Neurosci.* 2006;7:583–590.
43. Duncan L, Pollastri A, Smoller J. Why many geneticists and psychological scientists have discrepant views about gene–environment interaction (GxE) research. *Am Psychol.* 2014;69:249–268.
44. Crawley JN. Mouse behavioral assays relevant to the symptoms of autism. *Brain Pathol.* 2007;17:448–459.
45. Silverman JL, Yang M, Lord C, Crawley JN. Behavioural phenotyping assays for mouse models of autism. *Nat Rev Neurosci.* 2010;11.
46. Crawley JN. Testing hypotheses about autism. *Science.* 2007;318:56–57.
47. Moy SS, Nadler JJ. Advances in behavioral genetics: mouse models of autism. *Mol Psychiatry.* 2008;13:4–26.
48. Brodkin ES. BALB/c mice: low sociability and other phenotypes that may be relevant to autism. *Behav Brain Res.* 2007;176:53–65.
49. Farzin F, et al. Autism spectrum disorders and attention-deficit/hyperactivity disorder in boys with the fragile X premutation. *J Dev Behav Pediatr.* 2006;27:137–144.
50. Wang LW, Berry-Kravis E, Hagerman RJ. Fragile X: leading the way for targeted treatments in autism. *Neurotherapeutics.* 2010;7:264–274.
51. Hagerman R, Hoem G, Hagerman P. Fragile X and autism: intertwined at the molecular level leading to targeted treatments. *Mol Autism.* 2010;1:1–14.
52. Guy J, Hendrich B, Holmes M, Martin JE, Bird A. A mouse Mecp2-null mutation causes neurological symptoms that mimic rett syndrome. *Nat Genet.* 2001;27:322–326.
53. Chen RZ, Akbarian S, Tudor M, Jaenisch R. Deficiency of methyl-CpG binding protein-2 in CNS neurons results in a Rett-like phenotype in mice. *Nat Genet.* 2001;27:327–331.
54. Bozdagi O, Sakurai T, Papapetrou D, et al. Haploinsufficiency of the autism-associated Shank3 gene leads to deficits in synaptic function, social interaction, and social communication. *Mol Autism.* 2010;1:1–15. https://doi.org/10.1186/2040-2392-1-15.
55. Tabuchi K, Blundell J, Etherton MR, et al. A neuroligin-3 mutation implicated in autism increases inhibitory synaptic transmission in mice. *Science.* 2007;318:71–76. https://doi.org/10.1126/science.1146221.
56. Yang M, Bozdagi O, Scattoni ML, et al. Reduced excitatory neurotransmission and mild autism-relevant phenotypes in adolescent shank3 null mutant mice. *J Neurosci.* 2012;32:6525–6541. https://doi.org/10.1523/JNEUROSCI.6107-11.2012.
57. Radyushkin K, Hammerschmidt K, Boretius S, et al. Neuroligin-3-deficient mice: model of a monogenic heritable form of autism with an olfactory deficit. *Genes Brain Behav.* 2009;8:416–425. https://doi.org/10.1111/j.1601-183X.2009.00487.x.
58. El-Kordi A, Winkler D, Hammerschmidt K, et al. Development of an autism severity score for mice using Nlgn4 null mutants as a construct-valid model of heritable monogenic autism. *Behav Brain Res.* 2013;251:41–49. https://doi.org/10.1016/j.bbr.2012.11.016.
59. Copping NA, et al. Neuronal overexpression of Ube3a isoform 2 causes behavioral impairments and neuroanatomical pathology relevant to 15q11.2-q13.3 duplication syndrome. *Hum Mol Genet.* 2017;26:3995–4010.
60. Copping NA, McTighe SM, Fink KD, Silverman JL. Emerging gene and small molecule therapies for the neurodevelopmental disorder Angelman syndrome. *Neurotherapeutics.* 2021. https://doi.org/10.1007/s13311-021-01082-x.
61. Geurts AM, et al. Knockout rats via embryo microinjection of zinc-finger nucleases. *Science.* 2009;325:433.
62. Shao Y, et al. CRISPR/Cas-mediated genome editing in the rat via direct injection of one-cell embryos. *Nat Protoc.* 2014;9:2493–2512.

63. Hamilton SM, et al. Fmr1 and Nlgn3 knockout rats: novel tools for investigating autism spectrum disorders. *Behav Neurosci.* 2014;128:103–109.
64. Engineer CT, et al. Degraded speech sound processing in a rat model of fragile X syndrome. *Brain Res.* 2014;1564:72–84.
65. Engineer CT, et al. Degraded neural and behavioral processing of speech sounds in a rat model of Rett syndrome. *Neurobiol Dis.* 2015;83:26–34.
66. Hughes V. *Researchers Unveil Seven New Rat Models of Autism.* Spectrum; 2011.
67. Berg EL, et al. Developmental social communication deficits in the Shank3 rat model of phelan-mcdermid syndrome and autism spectrum disorder. *Autism Res.* 2018;11:587–601.
68. Modi ME, et al. Hyperactivity and hypermotivation associated with increased striatal mglur1 signaling in a Shank2 rat model of autism. *Front Mol Neurosci.* 2018;11:1–17.
69. Umeda T, et al. Evaluation of pax6 mutant rat as a model for autism. *PLoS One.* 2010;5:1–10.
70. Redecker TM, Kisko TM, Schwarting RKW, Wöhr M. Effects of Cacna1c haploinsufficiency on social interaction behavior and 50-kHz ultrasonic vocalizations in adult female rats. *Behav Brain Res.* 2019;367:35–52. https://doi.org/10.1016/j.bbr.2019.03.032.
71. Wöhr M, Scattoni ML. Behavioural methods used in rodent models of autism spectrum disorders: current standards and new developments. *Behav Brain Res.* 2013;251:5–17.
72. Berg EL, et al. Translational outcomes in a full gene deletion of ubiquitin protein ligase E3A rat model of Angelman syndrome. *Transl Psychiatry.* 2020;10:1–16. 2020 101.
73. Hamilton SM, et al. Multiple autism-like behaviors in a novel transgenic mouse model. *Behav Brain Res.* 2011;218:29–41.
74. Simons Foundation Autism Research Initiative. *SFARI Rat Models;* 2021. Available at: https://www.sfari.org/resource/rat-models/.
75. Ellenbroek B, Youn J. Rodent models in neuroscience research: is it a rat race? *DMM Dis Model Mech.* 2016;9:1079–1087.
76. Gerber N, Schweinfurth MK, Taborsky M. The smell of cooperation: rats increase helpful behaviour when receiving odour cues of a conspecific performing a cooperative task: the smell of cooperation. *Proc R Soc B Biol Sci.* 2020;287:1–9.
77. Schneeberger K, Dietz M, Taborsky M. Reciprocal cooperation between unrelated rats depends on cost to donor and benefit to recipient. *BMC Evol Biol.* 2012;12:1–7.
78. Wood RI, Kim JY, Li GR. Cooperation in rats playing the iterated Prisoner's dilemma game. *Anim Behav.* 2016;114:27–35.
79. Gordon NS, Kollack-Walker S, Akil H, Panksepp J. Expression of c-fos gene activation during rough and tumble play in juvenile rats. *Brain Res Bull.* 2002;57:651–659.
80. Panksepp J, Gordon N, Burgdorf J. Empathy and the action-perception resonances of basic socio-emotional systems of the brain. *Behav Brain Sci.* 2002;25:43–44.
81. Panksepp J. The ontogeny of play in rats. *Dev Psychobiol.* 1981;14:327–332.
82. Netser S, et al. Distinct dynamics of social motivation drive differential social behavior in laboratory rat and mouse strains. *Nat Commun.* 2020;11.
83. Reppucci CJ, Brown LA, Chambers AQ, Veenema AH. Wistar rats and C57BL/6 mice differ in their motivation to seek social interaction versus food in the social versus food preference test. *Physiol Behav.* 2020;227, 113162.
84. Blanchard DC, Agullana R, Squirrels G. Twenty-two kHz alarm cries to presentation of a predator, by laboratory rats living in visible burrow systems. *Physiol Behav.* 1991;50:967–972.
85. Sadananda M, Wöhr M, Schwarting RKW. Playback of 22-kHz and 50-kHz ultrasonic vocalizations induces differential c-fos expression in rat brain. *Neurosci Lett.* 2008;435:17–23.
86. Berg EL, et al. Excessive laughter-like vocalizations, microcephaly, and translational outcomes in the Ube3a deletion rat model of Angelman syndrome. *J Neurosci.* 2021;41(42):8801–8814.

87. Till SM, et al. Conserved hippocampal cellular pathophysiology but distinct behavioural deficits in a new rat model of FXS. *Hum Mol Genet.* 2015;24:5977–5984.
88. Wöhr M, Seffer D, Schwarting RKW. Studying socio-affective communication in rats through playback of ultrasonic vocalizations. *Curr Protoc Neurosci.* 2016;2016:8.35.1–8.35.17.
89. Stewart AM, Braubach O, Spitsbergen J, Gerlai R, Kalueff AV. Zebrafish models for translational neuroscience research: from tank to bedside. *Trends Neurosci.* 2014;37:264–278.
90. Bales KL, et al. Long-term exposure to intranasal oxytocin in a mouse autism model. *Transl Psychiatry.* 2014;4:1–10.
91. Bauman MD, Schumann CM. Advances in nonhuman primate models of autism: integrating neuroscience and behavior. *Exp Neurol.* 2018;299:252–265.
92. Bauman MD, et al. Activation of the maternal immune system during pregnancy alters behavioral development of rhesus monkey offspring. *Biol Psychiatry.* 2014;75:332–341.
93. Jennings CG, et al. Opportunities and challenges in modeling human brain disorders in transgenic primates. *Nat Neurosci.* 2016;19:1123–1130.
94. Curtis B, et al. Examination of the safety of pediatric vaccine schedules in a non-human primate model: assessments of neurodevelopment, learning, and social behavior. *Environ Health Perspect.* 2015;123:579–589.
95. Gibbs RA, et al. Genome sequence of the Brown Norway rat yields insights into mammalian evolution. *Nature.* 2004;428:493–521.
96. Kumar S, Hedges SB. A molecular timescale for vertebrate development. *Nature.* 1998;392:917–920.
97. Bauman MD, Amaral DG. Nonhuman primate models for autism spectrum disorders. In: *The Neuroscience of Autism Spectrum Disorders.* Elsevier; 2013. https://doi.org/10.1016/B978-0-12-391924-3.00027-2.
98. Chadman KK, Yang M, Crawley JN. Criteria for validating mouse models of psychiatric diseases. *Am J Med Genet B Neuropsychiatr Genet.* 2009;150:1–11.
99. Crawley JN. Designing mouse behavioral tasks relevant to autistic-like behaviors. *Ment Retard Dev Disabil Res Rev.* 2004;10:248–258.
100. Crawley JN. Translational animal models of autism and neurodevelopmental disorders. *Dialogues Clin Neurosci.* 2012;14:293–305.
101. Pasciuto E, et al. Autism Spectrum disorders: translating human deficits into mouse behavior. *Neurobiol Learn Mem.* 2015;124:71–87.
102. Nadler JJ, et al. Automated apparatus for quantitation of social approach behaviors in mice. *Genes Brain Behav.* 2004;3:303–314.
103. Chang YC, Cole TB, Costa LG. Behavioral phenotyping for autism spectrum disorders in mice. *Curr Protoc Toxicol.* 2017;2017:1–21.
104. Yang M, Crawley JN. Simple behavioral assessment of mouse olfaction. *Curr Protoc Neurosci.* 2009;1–12. https://doi.org/10.1002/0471142301.ns0824s48.
105. Yang M, Silverman JL, Crawley JN. Automated three-chambered social approach task for mice. *Curr Protoc Neurosci.* 2011;1–16. https://doi.org/10.1002/0471142301.ns0826s56.
106. Portfors CV. Types and functions of ultrasonic vocalizations in laboratory rats and mice. *J Am Assoc Lab Anim Sci.* 2007;46:28–34.
107. Wrenn CC. Social transmission of food preference in mice. *Curr Protoc Neurosci.* 2004;1–7 [chapter 8].
108. Seffer D, Schwarting RKW, Wöhr M. Pro-social ultrasonic communication in rats: insights from playback studies. *J Neurosci Methods.* 2014;234:73–81.
109. Arakawa H, Blanchard DC, Arakawa K, Dunlap C, Blanchard RJ. Scent marking behavior as an odorant communication in mice. *Neurosci Biobehav Rev.* 2008;32:1236–1248.
110. Servadio M, Vanderschuren LJMJ, Trezza V. Modeling autism-relevant behavioral phenotypes in rats and mice: do 'autistic' rodents exist? *Behav Pharmacol.* 2015;26:522–540.

111. Ey E, Leblond CS, Bourgeron T. Behavioral profiles of mouse models for autism spectrum disorders. *Autism Res.* 2011;4:5–16.
112. Ergaz Z, Weinstein-Fudim L, Ornoy A. Genetic and non-genetic animal models for autism spectrum disorders (ASD). *Reprod Toxicol.* 2016;64:116–140.
113. Bey A, Jiang YH. Current protocols in pharmacology: overview of mouse models of autism spectrum disorders. *Curr Protoc Pharmacol.* 2014;4.
114. Kazdoba TM, Leach PT, Crawley JN. Behavioral phenotypes of genetic mouse models of autism. *Genes Brain Behav.* 2016;15:7–26.
115. Wagner GC, Reuhl KR, Cheh M, McRae P, Halladay AK. A new neurobehavioral model of autism in mice: pre- and postnatal exposure to sodium valproate. *J Autism Dev Disord.* 2006;36:779–793. https://doi.org/10.1007/s10803-006-0117-y.
116. Schwartzer JJ, et al. Maternal immune activation and strain specific interactions in the development of autism-like behaviors in mice. *Transl Psychiatry.* 2013;3:e240–e249.
117. Poon E, Bandara SB, Allen JB, Sadowski RN, Schantz SL. Developmental PCB exposure increases susceptibility to audiogenic seizures in adulthood. *Neurotoxicology.* 2015;46:117–124. https://doi.org/10.1016/j.neuro.2014.12.007.
118. Allen JL, Oberdorster G, Morris-Schaffer K, et al. Developmental neurotoxicity of inhaled ambient ultrafine particle air pollution: parallels with neuropathological and behavioral features of autism and other neurodevelopmental disorders. *Neurotoxicology.* 2017;59:140–154. https://doi.org/10.1016/j.neuro.2015.12.014.
119. Krug A, Wöhr M, Seffer D, et al. Advanced paternal age as a risk factor for neurodevelopmental disorders: a translational study. *Mol Autism.* 2020;11:1–19. https://doi.org/10.1186/s13229-020-00345-2.
120. Terranova ML, Laviola G, Alleva E. Ontogeny of amicable social behavior in the mouse: gender differences and ongoing isolation outcomes. *Dev Psychobiol.* 1993;26:467–481.
121. Terranova ML, Laviola G. Scoring of social interactions and play in mice during adolescence. *Curr Protoc Toxicol.* 2005;26:1–11.
122. Arakawa H, Arakawa K, Blanchard DC, Blanchard RJ. A new test paradigm for social recognition evidenced by urinary scent marking behavior in C57BL/6J mice. *Behav Brain Res.* 2008;190:97–104.
123. Portfors CV, Perkel DJ. The role of ultrasonic vocalizations in mouse communication. *Curr Opin Neurobiol.* 2014;28:115–120.
124. Eaton M, Zhang J, Ma Z, et al. Generation and basic characterization of a gene-trap knockout mouse model of Scn2a with a substantial reduction of voltage-gated sodium channel Nav1.2 expression. *Genes Brain Behav.* 2021;20:1–15. https://doi.org/10.1111/gbb.12725.
125. Tatsukawa T, Raveau M, Ogiwara I, et al. Scn2a haploinsufficient mice display a spectrum of phenotypes affecting anxiety, sociability, memory flexibility and ampakine CX516 rescues their hyperactivity. *Mol Autism.* 2019;10:1–15. https://doi.org/10.1186/s13229-019-0265-5.
126. Clement JP, Aceti M, Creson TK, et al. Pathogenic SYNGAP1 mutations impair cognitive development by disrupting maturation of dendritic spine synapses. *Cell.* 2012;151:709–723. https://doi.org/10.1016/j.cell.2012.08.045.
127. Creson TK, Rojas C, Hwaun E, et al. Re-expression of SynGAP protein in adulthood improves translatable measures of brain function and behavior. *Elife.* 2019;8:1–19. https://doi.org/10.7554/eLife.46752.
128. Nakajima R, Takao K, Hattori S, et al. Comprehensive behavioral analysis of heterozygous Syngap1 knockout mice. *Neuropsychopharmacol Rep.* 2019;39:223–237. https://doi.org/10.1002/npr2.12073.
129. Bader PL, Faizi M, Kim LH, et al. Mouse model of Timothy syndrome recapitulates triad of autistic traits. *Proc Natl Acad Sci U S A.* 2011;108:15432–15437. https://doi.org/10.1073/pnas.1112667108.

130. Kabitzke PA, Brunner D, He D, et al. Comprehensive analysis of two Shank3 and the Cacna1c mouse models of autism spectrum disorder. *Genes Brain Behav.* 2018;17:4–22. https://doi.org/10.1111/gbb.12405.
131. Peñagarikano O, Abrahams BS, Herman EI, et al. Absence of CNTNAP2 leads to epilepsy, neuronal migration abnormalities, and core autism-related deficits. *Cell.* 2011;147:235–246. https://doi.org/10.1016/j.cell.2011.08.040.
132. Peñagarikano O, Lázaro MT, Lu X, et al. Exogenous and evoked oxytocin restores social behavior in the Cntnap2 mouse model of autism. *Sci Transl Med.* 2015;7:1–26. https://doi.org/10.1126/scitranslmed.3010257.Exogenous.
133. Ey E, Torquet N, Le Sourd AM, et al. The autism ProSAP1/Shank2 mouse model displays quantitative and structural abnormalities in ultrasonic vocalisations. *Behav Brain Res.* 2013;256:677–689. https://doi.org/10.1016/j.bbr.2013.08.031.
134. Ey E, Torquet N, de Chaumont F, et al. Shank2 mutant mice display hyperactivity insensitive to methylphenidate and reduced flexibility in social motivation, but normal social recognition. *Front Mol Neurosci.* 2018;11:1–9. https://doi.org/10.3389/fnmol.2018.00365.
135. Schmeisser MJ, Ey E, Wegener S, et al. Autistic-like behaviours and hyperactivity in mice lacking ProSAP1/Shank2. *Nature.* 2012;486:256–260. https://doi.org/10.1038/nature11015.
136. Won H, Lee HR, Gee HY, et al. Autistic-like social behaviour in Shank2-mutant mice improved by restoring NMDA receptor function. *Nature.* 2012;486:261–265. https://doi.org/10.1038/nature11208.
137. Mei Y, Monteiro P, Zhou Y, et al. Adult restoration of Shank3 expression rescues selective autistic-like phenotypes. *Nature.* 2016;530:481–484. https://doi.org/10.1038/nature16971.
138. Peça J, Feliciano C, Ting JT, et al. Shank3 mutant mice display autistic-like behaviours and striatal dysfunction. *Nature.* 2011;472:437–442. https://doi.org/10.1038/nature09965.
139. Speed HE, Kouser M, Xuan Z, et al. Autism-associated insertion mutation (InsG) of shank3 exon 21 causes impaired synaptic transmission and behavioral deficits. *J Neurosci.* 2015;35:9648–9665. https://doi.org/10.1523/JNEUROSCI.3125-14.2015.
140. Chadman KK, Gong S, Scattoni ML, et al. Minimal aberrant behavioral phenotypes of neuroligin-3 R451C knockin mice. *Autism Res.* 2008;1:147–158. https://doi.org/10.1002/aur.22.
141. Jaramillo TC, Escamilla CO, Liu S, Peca L, Birnbaum SG, Powell CM. Genetic background effects in Neuroligin-3 mutant mice: minimal behavioral abnormalities on C57 background. *Autism Res.* 2018;11:234–244. https://doi.org/10.1002/aur.1857.
142. Jaramillo TC, Liu S, Pettersen A, Birnbaum SG, Powell CM. Autism-related neuroligin-3 mutation alters social behavior and spatial learning. *Autism Res.* 2014;7:264–272. https://doi.org/10.1002/aur.1362.
143. Jamain S, Radyushkin K, Hammerschmidt K, et al. Reduced social interaction and ultrasonic communication in a mouse model of monogenic heritable autism. *Proc Natl Acad Sci U S A.* 2008;105:1710–1715. https://doi.org/10.1073/pnas.0711555105.
144. Ju A, Hammerschmidt K, Tantra M, Krueger D, Brose N, Ehrenreich H. Juvenile manifestation of ultrasound communication deficits in the neuroligin-4 null mutant mouse model of autism. *Behav Brain Res.* 2014;270:159–164. https://doi.org/10.1016/j.bbr.2014.05.019.
145. Gompers AL, Su-Feher L, Ellegood J, et al. Germline Chd8 haploinsufficiency alters brain development in mouse. *Nat Neurosci.* 2017;20:1062–1073. https://doi.org/10.1038/nn.4592.
146. Katayama Y, Nishiyama M, Shoji H, et al. CHD8 haploinsufficiency results in autistic-like phenotypes in mice. *Nature.* 2016;537:675–679. https://doi.org/10.1038/nature19357.

147. Platt RJ, Zhou Y, Slaymaker IM, et al. Chd8 mutation leads to autistic-like behaviors and impaired striatal circuits. *Cell Rep.* 2017;19:335–350. https://doi.org/10.1016/j.celrep.2017.03.052.
148. Suetterlin P, Hurley S, Mohan C, et al. Altered neocortical gene expression, brain overgrowth and functional over-connectivity in chd8 haploinsufficient mice. *Cereb Cortex.* 2018;28:2192–2206. https://doi.org/10.1093/cercor/bhy058.
149. Celen C, Chuang JC, Luo X, et al. Arid1b haploinsufficient mice reveal neuropsychiatric phenotypes and reversible causes of growth impairment. *Elife.* 2017;6:1–22. https://doi.org/10.7554/eLife.25730.
150. Ellegood J, Petkova SP, Kinman A, et al. Neuroanatomy and behavior in mice with a haploinsufficiency of AT-rich interactive domain 1B (ARID1B) throughout development. *Mol Autism.* 2021;12:1–24. https://doi.org/10.1186/s13229-021-00432-y.
151. Jung EM, Moffat JJ, Liu J, Dravid SM, Gurumurthy CB, Kim WY. Arid1b haploinsufficiency disrupts cortical interneuron development and mouse behavior. *Nat Neurosci.* 2017;20:1694–1707. https://doi.org/10.1038/s41593-017-0013-0.
152. Matsumura K, Seiriki K, Okada S, et al. Pathogenic POGZ mutation causes impaired cortical development and reversible autism-like phenotypes. *Nat Commun.* 2020;11:1–16. https://doi.org/10.1038/s41467-020-14697-z.
153. Suliman-Lavie R, Title B, Cohen Y, et al. Pogz deficiency leads to transcription dysregulation and impaired cerebellar activity underlying autism-like behavior in mice. *Nat Commun.* 2020;11:1–15. https://doi.org/10.1038/s41467-020-19577-0.
154. Hacohen-Kleiman G, Sragovich S, Karmon G, et al. Activity-dependent neuroprotective protein deficiency models synaptic and developmental phenotypes of autism-like syndrome. *J Clin Invest.* 2018;128:4956–4969. https://doi.org/10.1172/JCI98199.
155. Malishkevich A, Amram N, Hacohen-Kleiman G, Magen I, Giladi E, Gozes I. Activity-dependent neuroprotective protein (ADNP) exhibits striking sexual dichotomy impacting on autistic and Alzheimer's pathologies. *Transl Psychiatry.* 2015;5:1–9. https://doi.org/10.1038/tp.2014.138.
156. Vandeweyer G, Helsmoortel C, VanDijck A, et al. The transcriptional regulator ADNP links the BAF (SWI/SNF) complexes with autism. *Am J Med Genet C Semin Med Genet.* 2014;166:315–326. https://doi.org/10.1002/ajmg.c.31413.
157. Vulih-Shultzman I, Pinhasov A, Mandel S, et al. Activity-dependent neuroprotective protein snippet NAP reduces tau hyperphosphorylation and enhances learning in a novel transgenic mouse model. *J Pharmacol Exp Ther.* 2007;323:438–449. https://doi.org/10.1124/jpet.107.129551.
158. Huang TN, Chuang HC, Chou WH, et al. Tbr1 haploinsufficiency impairs amygdalar axonal projections and results in cognitive abnormality. *Nat Neurosci.* 2014;17:240–247. https://doi.org/10.1038/nn.3626.
159. Levy J, LaFlemme C, Tsaprailis G, Crynen G, Page DT. Dyrk1a mutations cause undergrowth of cortical pyramidal neurons via dysregulated growth factor signaling. *Biol Psychiatry.* 2021;90:295–306.
160. Clipperton-Allen AE, Page DT. Decreased aggression and increased repetitive behavior in Pten haploinsufficient mice. *Genes Brain Behav.* 2015;14:145–157. https://doi.org/10.1111/gbb.12192.
161. Clipperton-Allen AE, Page DT. Pten haploinsufficient mice show broad brain overgrowth but selective impairments in autism-relevant behavioral tests. *Hum Mol Genet.* 2014;23:3490–3505. https://doi.org/10.1093/hmg/ddu057.
162. Kwon CH, Luikart BW, Powell CM, et al. Pten regulates neuronal arborization and social interaction in mice. *Neuron.* 2006;50:377–388. https://doi.org/10.1016/j.neuron.2006.03.023.
163. Lugo JN, Smith GD, Arbuckle EP, et al. Deletion of PTEN produces autism-like behavioral deficits and alterations in synaptic proteins. *Front Mol Neurosci.* 2014;7:1–13. https://doi.org/10.3389/fnmol.2014.00027.

164. Zhou J, Blundell J, Ogawa S, et al. Pharmacological inhibition of mTORCl suppresses anatomical, cellular, and behavioral abnormalities in neural-specific PTEN knock-out mice. *J Neurosci.* 2009;29:1773–1783. https://doi.org/10.1523/JNEUROSCI.5685-08.2009.
165. Saré RM, Lemons A, Figueroa C, Song A, Levine M, Smith CB. Sex-selective effects on behavior in a mouse model of tuberous sclerosis complex. *eNeuro.* 2020;7:1–9. https://doi.org/10.1523/ENEURO.0379-19.2020.
166. Tang G, Gudsnuk K, Kuo SH, et al. Loss of mTOR-dependent macroautophagy causes autistic-like synaptic pruning deficits. *Neuron.* 2014;83:1131–1143. https://doi.org/10.1016/j.neuron.2014.07.040.
167. Tsai PT, Hull C, Chu Y, et al. Autistic-like behaviour and cerebellar dysfunction in Purkinje cell Tsc1 mutant mice. *Nature.* 2012;488:647–651. https://doi.org/10.1038/nature11310.
168. Young DM, Schenk AK, Yang SB, Jan YN, Jan LY. Altered ultrasonic vocalizations in a tuberous sclerosis mouse model of autism. *Proc Natl Acad Sci U S A.* 2010;107:11074–11079. https://doi.org/10.1073/pnas.1005620107.
169. Berg EL, et al. Insulin-like growth factor-2 does not improve behavioral deficits in mouse and rat models of Angelman syndrome. *Mol Autism.* 2021;12:59.
170. Copping NA, Silverman JL. Abnormal electrophysiological phenotypes and sleep deficits in a mouse model of Angelman syndrome. *Mol Autism.* 2021;12:1–14. https://doi.org/10.1186/s13229-021-00416-y.
171. Jiang YH, Armstrong D, Albrecht U, et al. Mutation of the Angelman ubiquitin ligase in mice causes increased cytoplasmic p53 and deficits of contextual learning and long-term potentiation. *Neuron.* 1998;21:799–811. https://doi.org/10.1016/S0896-6273(00)80596-6.
172. Sonzogni M, Wallaard I, Santos SS, et al. A behavioral test battery for mouse models of Angelman syndrome: a powerful tool for testing drugs and novel Ube3a mutants. *Mol Autism.* 2018;9:1–19. https://doi.org/10.1186/s13229-018-0231-7.
173. Bambini-Junior V, Rodrigues L, Behr GA, Moreira JCF, Riesgo R, Gottfried C. Animal model of autism induced by prenatal exposure to valproate: behavioral changes and liver parameters. *Brain Res.* 2011;1408:8–16. https://doi.org/10.1016/j.brainres.2011.06.015.
174. Gandal MJ, Edgar JC, Ehrlichman RS, Mehta M, Roberts TPL, Siegel SJ. Validating γ oscillations and delayed auditory responses as translational biomarkers of autism. *Biol Psychiatry.* 2010;68:1100–1106. https://doi.org/10.1016/j.biopsych.2010.09.031.
175. Markram K, Rinaldi T, La Mendola D, Sandi C, Markram H. Abnormal fear conditioning and amygdala processing in an animal model of autism. *Neuropsychopharmacology.* 2008;33:901–912. https://doi.org/10.1038/sj.npp.1301453.
176. Schneider T, Przewłocki R. Behavioral alterations in rats prenatally to valproic acid: animal model of autism. *Neuropsychopharmacology.* 2005;30:80–89. https://doi.org/10.1038/sj.npp.1300518.
177. Careaga M, Murai T, Bauman MD. Maternal immune activation and autism spectrum disorder: from rodents to nonhuman and human primates. *Biol Psychiatry.* 2016;81:391–401.
178. Garay PA, Hsiao EY, Patterson PH, McAllister AK. Maternal immune activation causes age- and region-specific changes in brain cytokines in offspring throughout development. *Brain Behav Immun.* 2013;31:54–68. https://doi.org/10.1016/j.bbi.2012.07.008.
179. Hsiao EY, McBride SW, Chow J, Mazmanian SK, Patterson PH. Modeling an autism risk factor in mice leads to permanent immune dysregulation. *Proc Natl Acad Sci U S A.* 2012;109:12776–12781. https://doi.org/10.1073/pnas.1202556109.
180. Hsiao EY, McBride SW, Hsien S, et al. Microbiota modulate behavioral and physiological abnormalities associated with neurodevelopmental disorders. *Cell.* 2013;155:1451–1463. https://doi.org/10.1016/j.cell.2013.11.024.

181. Berg EL, Pedersen LR, Pride MC, et al. Developmental exposure to near roadway pollution produces behavioral phenotypes relevant to neurodevelopmental disorders in juvenile rats. *Transl Psychiatry.* 2020;10:1–16. https://doi.org/10.1038/s41398-020-00978-0.
182. Berg EL, Ching TM, Bruun DA, et al. Translational outcomes relevant to neurodevelopmental disorders following early life exposure of rats to chlorpyrifos. *J Neurodev Disord.* 2020;12:40. https://doi.org/10.1186/s11689-020-09342-1.
183. De Felice A, Scattoni ML, Ricceri L, Calamandrei G. Prenatal exposure to a common organophosphate insecticide delays motor development in a mouse model of idiopathic autism. *PLoS One.* 2015;10:1–19. https://doi.org/10.1371/journal.pone.0121663.
184. Lan A, Kalimian M, Amram B, Kofman O. Prenatal chlorpyrifos leads to autism-like deficits in C57Bl6/J mice. *Environ Health A Glob Access Sci Source.* 2017;16:1–10. https://doi.org/10.1186/s12940-017-0251-3.
185. Pu Y, Yang J, Chang L, et al. Maternal glyphosate exposure causes autism-like behaviors in offspring through increased expression of soluble epoxide hydrolase. *Proc Natl Acad Sci U S A.* 2021;117:11753–11759. https://doi.org/10.1073/pnas.2100100118.
186. Chang YC, Cole TB, Costa LG. Prenatal and early-life diesel exhaust exposure causes autism-like behavioral changes in mice. *Part Fibre Toxicol.* 2018;15:1–14. https://doi.org/10.1186/s12989-018-0254-4.
187. Church JS, Tijerina PB, Emerson FJ, et al. Perinatal exposure to concentrated ambient particulates results in autism-like behavioral deficits in adult mice. *Neurotoxicology.* 2018;65:231–240. https://doi.org/10.1016/j.neuro.2017.10.007.
188. Li K, Li L, Cui B, et al. Early postnatal exposure to airborne fine particulate matter induces autism-like phenotypes in male rats. *Toxicol Sci.* 2017;162:189–199. https://doi.org/10.1093/toxsci/kfx240.
189. Bell MR, Thompson LM, Rodriguez K, Gore AC. Two-hit exposure to polychlorinated biphenyls at gestational and juvenile life stages: 1. Sexually dimorphic effects on social and anxiety-like behaviors. *Horm Behav.* 2016;78:168–177. https://doi.org/10.1016/j.yhbeh.2015.11.007.
190. Gillette R, Reilly MP, Topper VY, Thompson LM, Crews D, Gore AC. Anxiety-like behaviors in adulthood are altered in male but not female rats exposed to low dosages of polychlorinated biphenyls in utero. *Horm Behav.* 2017;87:8–15. https://doi.org/10.1016/j.yhbeh.2016.10.011.
191. Jolous-Jamshidi B, Cromwell HC, McFarland AM, Meserve LA. Perinatal exposure to polychlorinated biphenyls alters social behaviors in rats. *Toxicol Lett.* 2010;199:136–143. https://doi.org/10.1016/j.toxlet.2010.08.015.
192. Tian YH, Hwan Kim S, Lee SY, Jang CG. Lactational and postnatal exposure to polychlorinated biphenyls induces sex-specific anxiolytic behavior and cognitive deficit in mice offspring. *Synapse.* 2011;65:1032–1041. https://doi.org/10.1002/syn.20934.
193. Foldi CJ, Eyles DW, McGrath JJ, Burne THJ. Increasing paternal age alters anxiety-related behaviour in adult mice. *Genes Brain Behav.* 2019;18:1–11. https://doi.org/10.1111/gbb.12522.
194. Foldi CJ, Eyles DW, McGrath JJ, Burne THJ. Advanced paternal age is associated with alterations in discrete behavioural domains and cortical neuroanatomy of C57BL/6J mice. *Eur J Neurosci.* 2010;31:556–564. https://doi.org/10.1111/j.1460-9568.2010.07074.x.
195. Smith RG, Kember RL, Mill J, et al. Advancing paternal age is associated with deficits in social and exploratory behaviors in the offspring: A mouse model. *PLoS One.* 2009;4:4–8. https://doi.org/10.1371/journal.pone.0008456.
196. Moy SS, et al. Mouse behavioral tasks relevant to autism: phenotypes of 10 inbred strains. *Behav Brain Res.* 2007;176:4–20.
197. McFarlane HG, et al. Autism-like behavioral phenotypes in BTBR T+tf/J mice. *Genes Brain Behav.* 2008;7:152–163.

198. Silverman JL, et al. Negative allosteric modulation of the mGluR5 receptor reduces repetitive behaviors and rescues social deficits in mouse models of autism. *Sci Transl Med.* 2012;4.
199. Kaidanovich-Beilin O, Lipina T, Vukobradovic I, Roder J, Woodgett JR. Assessment of social interaction behaviors. *J Vis Exp.* 2010;0:1–6.
200. Bolivar VJ, Walters SR, Phoenix JL. Assessing autism-like behavior in mice: variations in social interactions among inbred strains. *Behav Brain Res.* 2007;176:21–26.
201. Panksepp J. Play behavior. *Encycl Behav Neurosci.* 2010;87–92. https://doi.org/10.1016/B978-0-08-045396-5.00204-9.
202. Panksepp JB, Lahvis GP. Rodent empathy and affective neuroscience. *Neurosci Biobehav Rev.* 2011;35:1864–1875.
203. Ryan BC, Young NB, Crawley JN, Bodfish JW, Moy SS. Social deficits, stereotypy and early emergence of repetitive behavior in the C58/J inbred mouse strain. *Behav Brain Res.* 2010;208:178–188.
204. Peartree NA, et al. Limited physical contact through a mesh barrier is sufficient for social reward-conditioned place preference in adolescent male rats. *Physiol Behav.* 2012;105:749–756.
205. Langford DJ, et al. Social modulation of pain as evidence for empathy in mice. *Science.* 2006;312:1967–1970.
206. Chen QL, Panksepp JB, Lahvis GP. Empathy is moderated by genetic background in mice. *PLoS One.* 2009;4:1–14.
207. Jones CE, Agee L, Monfils MH. Fear conditioning by proxy: social transmission of fear between interacting conspecifics. *Curr Protoc Neurosci.* 2018;83, e43.
208. Jones CE, Monfils MH. The social transmission of associative fear in rodents-individual differences in fear conditioning by proxy. In: *Neuronal Correlates of Empathy: From Rodent to Human.* Elsevier Inc; 2018. https://doi.org/10.1016/B978-0-12-805397-3.00008-5.
209. Rutte C, Taborsky M. Generalized reciprocity in rats. *PLoS Biol.* 2007;5:1421–1425.
210. Viana DS, Gordo I, Sucena É, Moita MAP. Cognitive and motivational requirements for the emergence of cooperation in a rat social game. *PLoS One.* 2010;5:1–9.
211. Schweinfurth MK, Taborsky M. Reciprocal trading of different commodities in Norway rats. *Curr Biol.* 2018;28:594–599.e3.
212. Kettler N, Schweinfurth MK, Taborsky M. Rats show direct reciprocity when interacting with multiple partners. *Sci Rep.* 2021;11:1–8.
213. Ben-Ami Bartal I, Rodgers DA, Bernardez Sarria MSO, Decety J, Mason P. Pro-social behavior in rats is modulated by social experience. *Elife.* 2014;3, e01385.
214. Ben-Ami Bartal I, Decety J, Mason P. Helping a cagemate in need: empathy and pro-social behavior in rats. *Science.* 2013;334:1427–1430.
215. Sato N, Tan L, Tate K, Okada M. Rats demonstrate helping behavior toward a soaked conspecific. *Anim Cogn.* 2015;18:1039–1047.
216. Reinhold AS, Sanguinetti-Scheck JI, Hartmann K, Brecht M. Behavioral and neural correlates of hide-and-seek in rats. *Science.* 2019;365:1180–1183.
217. Wersinger SR, et al. Vasopressin 1a receptor knockout mice have a subtle olfactory deficit but normal aggression. *Genes Brain Behav.* 2007;6:540–551.
218. Wöhr M, Roullet FI, Crawley JN. Reduced scent marking and ultrasonic vocalizations in the BTBR T+tf/J mouse model of autism. *Genes Brain Behav.* 2011;10:35–43.
219. Roullet FI, Wöhr M, Crawley JN. Female urine-induced male mice ultrasonic vocalizations, but not scent-marking, is modulated by social experience. *Behav Brain Res.* 2011;216:19–28.
220. Wöhr M, Roullet FI, Hung AY, Sheng M, Crawley JN. Communication impairments in mice lacking shank1: reduced levels of ultrasonic vocalizations and scent marking behavior. *PLoS One.* 2011;6.
221. Wrenn CC, Harris AP, Saavedra MC, Crawley JN. Social transmission of food preference in mice: methodology and application to galanin-overexpressing transgenic mice. *Behav Neurosci.* 2003;117:21–31.

222. Hofer MA, Shair HN, Brunelli SA. Ultrasonic vocalizations in rat and mouse pups. *Curr Protoc Neurosci.* 2001;17:1–16.
223. Ehret G. Infant rodent ultrasounds—a gate to the understanding of sound communication. *Behav Genet.* 2005;35:19–29.
224. D'Amato FR, Scalera E, Sarli C, Moles A. Pups call, mothers rush: does maternal responsiveness affect the amount of ultrasonic vocalizations in mouse pups? *Behav Genet.* 2005;35:103–112.
225. Fischer J, Hammerschmidt K. Ultrasonic vocalizations in mouse models for speech and socio-cognitive disorders: insights into the evolution of vocal communication. *Genes Brain Behav.* 2011;10:17–27.
226. Okabe S, et al. The effects of social experience and gonadal hormones on retrieving behavior of mice and their responses to pup ultrasonic vocalizations. *Zoolog Sci.* 2010;27:790–795.
227. Scattoni ML, Michetti C, Ricceri L. Rodent vocalization studies in animal models of the autism spectrum disorder. In: *Handbook of Behavioral Neuroscience.* vol. 25. Elsevier B.V; 2018.
228. Maggio JC, Maggio JH, Whitney G. Experience-based vocalization of male mice to female chemosignals. *Physiol Behav.* 1983;31:269–272.
229. Burgdorf J, et al. Ultrasonic vocalizations of rats (*Rattus norvegicus*) during mating, play, and aggression: behavioral concomitants, relationship to reward, and self-administration of playback. *J Comp Psychol.* 2008;122:357–367.
230. Scattoni ML, Ricceri L, Crawley JN. Unusual repertoire of vocalizations in adult BTBR T+tf/J mice during three types of social encounters. *Genes Brain Behav.* 2011;10:44–56.
231. Panksepp JB, et al. Affiliative behavior, ultrasonic communication and social reward are influenced by genetic variation in adolescent mice. *PLoS One.* 2007;2.
232. Pellis SM, Burke CJ, Kisko TM, Euston DR. 50-kHz vocalizations, play and the development of social competence. In: *Handbook of Behavioral Neuroscience.* vol. 25. Elsevier B.V; 2018.
233. Kisko TM, et al. Sex-dependent effects of Cacna1c haploinsufficiency on juvenile social play behavior and pro-social 50-kHz ultrasonic communication in rats. *Genes Brain Behav.* 2020;19:1–17.
234. Wang H, Liang S, Burgdorf J, Wess J, Yeomans J. Ultrasonic vocalizations induced by sex and amphetamine in M2, M4, M5 muscarinic and D2 dopamine receptor knockout mice. *PLoS One.* 2008;3:30–33.
235. Knutson B, Burgdorf J, Panksepp J. Anticipation of play elicits high-frequency ultrasonic vocalizations in young rats. *J Comp Psychol.* 1998;112:65–73.
236. Willey AR, Spear LP. Development of anticipatory 50kHz USV production to a social stimuli in adolescent and adult male Sprague-Dawley rats. *Behav Brain Res.* 2012;226:613–618.
237. LaFollette MR, O'Haire ME, Cloutier S, Gaskill BN. Practical rat tickling: determining an efficient and effective dosage of heterospecific play. *Appl Anim Behav Sci.* 2018;208:82–91.
238. Cloutier S, LaFollette MR, Gaskill BN, Panksepp J, Newberry RC. Tickling, a technique for inducing positive affect when handling rats. *J Vis Exp.* 2018;1–10. https://doi.org/10.3791/57190.
239. Burgdorf J, Panksepp J. Tickling induces reward in adolescent rats. *Physiol Behav.* 2001;72:167–173.
240. Schwarting RKW, Jegan N, Wöhr M. Situational factors, conditions and individual variables which can determine ultrasonic vocalizations in male adult Wistar rats. *Behav Brain Res.* 2007;182:208–222.
241. Wöhr M, et al. New insights into the relationship of neurogenesis and affect: tickling induces hippocampal cell proliferation in rats emitting appetitive 50-khz ultrasonic vocalizations. *Neuroscience.* 2009;163:1024–1030.

242. Ey E, et al. Absence of deficits in social behaviors and ultrasonic vocalizations in later generations of mice lacking neuroligin4. *Genes Brain Behav.* 2012;11:928–941.
243. Hammerschmidt K, Radyushkin K, Ehrenreich H, Fischer J. The structure and usage of female and male mouse ultrasonic vocalizations reveal only minor differences. *PLoS One.* 2012;7:1–7.
244. Gourbal BEF, Barthelemy M, Petit G, Gabrion C. Spectrographic analysis of the ultrasonic vocalisations of adult male and female BALB/c mice. *Naturwissenschaften.* 2004;91:381–385.
245. Whitney G. Vocalization of mice influenced by a single gene in a heterogeneous population. *Behav Genet.* 1973;3:57–64.
246. White NR, Prasad M, Barfield RJ, Nyby JG. 40- and 70-kHz vocalizations of mice (*Mus musculus*) during copulation. *Physiol Behav.* 1998;63:467–473.
247. Sugimoto H, et al. A role for strain differences in waveforms of ultrasonic vocalizations during male-female interaction. *PLoS One.* 2011;6.
248. Warburton VL, Sales GD, Milligan SR. The emission and elicitation of mouse ultrasonic vocalizations: the effects of age, sex and gonadal status. *Physiol Behav.* 1989;45:41–47.
249. Hammerschmidt K, Radyushkin K, Ehrenreich H, Fischer J. Female mice respond to male ultrasonic 'songs' with approach behaviour. *Biol Lett.* 2009;5:589–592.
250. Chabout J, Jones-Macopson J, Jarvis ED. Eliciting and analyzing male mouse ultrasonic vocalization (USV) songs. *J Vis Exp.* 2017;2017:1–13.
251. Shepard KN, Liu RC. Experience restores innate female preference for male ultrasonic vocalizations. *Genes Brain Behav.* 2011;10:28–34.
252. Kas MJ, et al. Assessing behavioural and cognitive domains of autism spectrum disorders in rodents: current status and future perspectives. *Psychopharmacology (Berl).* 2014;231:1125–1146.
253. Erway LC, Shiau YW, Davis RR, Krieg EF. Genetics of age-related hearing loss in mice. III. Susceptibility of inbred and F1 hybrid strains to noise-induced hearing loss. *Hear Res.* 1996;93:181–187.
254. Henry KR, Chole RA. Genotypic differences in behavioral, physiological and anatomical expressions of age-related hearing loss in the laboratory mouse: original papers travaux originaux. *Int J Audiol.* 1980;19:369–383.
255. Johnson KR, Erway LC, Cook SA, Willott JF, Zheng QY. A major gene affecting age-related hearing loss in C57BL/6J mice. *Hear Res.* 1997;114:83–92.
256. Zheng QY, Johnson KR, Erway LC. Assessment of hearing in 80 inbred strains of mice by ABR threshold analyses. *Hear Res.* 1999;130:94–107.
257. Brudzynski SM. Communication of adult rats by ultrasonic vocalization: biological, sociobiological, and neuroscience approaches. *ILAR J.* 2009;50:43–50.
258. Thomas A, et al. Marble burying reflects a repetitive and perseverative behavior more than novelty-induced anxiety. *Psychopharmacology (Berl).* 2009;204:361–373.
259. Moy SS, et al. Development of a mouse test for repetitive, restricted behaviors: relevance to autism. *Behav Brain Res.* 2008;188:178–194.
260. Lewis MH, Tanimura Y, Lee LW, Bodfish JW. Animal models of restricted repetitive behavior in autism. *Behav Brain Res.* 2007;176:66–74.
261. Moy SS, et al. Repetitive behavior profile and supersensitivity to amphetamine in the C58/J mouse model of autism. *Behav Brain Res.* 2014;259:200–214.
262. Roullet FI, Crawley JN. Mouse models of autism: testing hypotheses about molecular mechanisms. In: Hagan J, ed. *Current Topics in Behavioral Neurosciences: Molecular and Functional Models in Neuropsychiatry.* Springer; 2011:187–212.
263. Moon J, et al. Attention, arousal regulation, and inhibitory control in FMR1 knockout mice: a mouse model of fragile X syndrome. *Behav Neurosci.* 2006;120:1367–1379.
264. Guariglia SR, Chadman KK. Water T-maze: a useful assay for determination of repetitive behaviors in mice. *J Neurosci Methods.* 2013;220:24–29.

265. Nakatani J, et al. Abnormal behavior in a chromosome- engineered mouse model for human 15q11-13 duplication seen in autism. *Cell.* 2009;137:1235–1246.
266. Hoeffer CA, et al. Removal of FKBP12 enhances mTOR-raptor interactions, LTP, memory, and perseverative/repetitive behavior. *Neuron.* 2008;60:832–845.
267. Fombonne E, et al. Psychiatric and medical profiles of autistic adults in the SPARK cohort. *J Autism Dev Disord.* 2020;50:3679–3698.
268. La Malfa G, Lassi S, Bertelli M, Salvini R, Placidi GF. Autism and intellectual disability: a study of prevalence on a sample of the Italian population. *J Intellect Disabil Res.* 2004;48:262–267.
269. Vogel-Ciernia A, Wood MA. Examining object location and object recognition memory in mice. *Curr Protoc Neurosci.* 2014;2014:8.31.1–8.31.17.
270. Adhikari A, et al. Cognitive deficits in the Snord116 deletion mouse model for Prader-Willi syndrome. *Neurobiol Learn Mem.* 2019;165, 106874.
271. Wehner JM, Radcliffe RA. Cued and contextual fear conditioning in mice. *Curr Protoc Neurosci.* 2004;1–14 [chapter 8].
272. Wenk GL. Assessment of spatial memory using the radial arm maze and Morris water maze. *Curr Protoc Neurosci.* 2004;26:1–12.
273. Copping NA, et al. Touchscreen learning deficits and normal social approach behavior in the Shank3B model of Phelan-McDermid Syndrome and autism. *Neuroscience.* 2017;345:155–165.
274. File SE, Lippa AS, Beer B, Lippa MT. Animal tests of anxiety. *Curr Protoc Neurosci.* 2004;26:1–22.
275. Crawley JN. Exploratory behavior models of anxiety in mice. *Neurosci Biobehav Rev.* 1985;9:37–44.
276. Takao K, Miyakawa T. Light/dark transition test for mice. *J Vis Exp.* 2006;1–3. https://doi.org/10.3791/104.
277. Bourin M, Hascoët M. The mouse light/dark box test. *Eur J Pharmacol.* 2003;463:55–65.
278. Misslin R, Belzung C, Vogel E. Behavioural validation of a light/dark choice procedure for testing anti-anxiety agents. *Behav Processes.* 1989;18:119–132.
279. Adhikari A, et al. Functional rescue in an Angelman syndrome model following treatment with lentivector transduced hematopoietic stem cells. *Hum Mol Genet.* 2021;ddab104:1–59.
280. Luong TN, Carlisle HJ, Southwell A, Patterson PH. Assessment of motor balance and coordination in mice using the balance beam. *J Vis Exp.* 2011;5–7. https://doi.org/10.3791/2376.
281. Carter RJ, Morton J, Dunnett SB. Motor coordination and balance in rodents. *Curr Protoc Neurosci.* 2001;15:1–14.
282. Heyser CJ. Assessment of developmental milestones in rodents. *Curr Protoc Neurosci.* 2003;25:1–15.
283. Scattoni ML, Gandhy SU, Ricceri L, Crawley JN. Unusual repertoire of vocalizations in the BTBR T+tf/J mouse model of autism. *PLoS One.* 2008;3:48–52.
284. Wöhr M, et al. Developmental delays and reduced pup ultrasonic vocalizations but normal sociability in mice lacking the postsynaptic cell adhesion protein neuroligin2. *Behav Brain Res.* 2013;251:50–64.
285. Hill JM, Lim MA, Stone MM. Developmental milestones in the newborn mouse. *Neuromethods.* Vol. 39. Humana Press; 2008:131–149.
286. Fox WM. Reflex-ontogeny and behavioural development of the mouse. *Anim Behav.* 1965;13.
287. Tavassoli T, Miller LJ, Schoen SA, Nielsen DM, Baron-Cohen S. Sensory over-responsivity in adults with autism spectrum conditions. *Autism.* 2014;18:428–432.
288. Tomchek SD, Dunn W. Sensory processing in children with and without autism: a comparative study using the short sensory profile. *Am J Occup Ther.* 2007;61:190–200.

289. Geyer MA, Swerdlow NR. Measurement of startle response, prepulse inhibition, and habituation. *Curr Protoc Neurosci.* 1998;3:1–15.
290. Geyer MA, Dulawa SC. Assessment of murine startle reactivity, prepulse inhibition, and habituation. *Curr Protoc Neurosci.* 2003;24:1–15.
291. Bannon AW, Malmberg AB. Models of nociception: hot-plate, tail-flick, and formalin tests in rodents. *Curr Protoc Neurosci.* 2007;1–16 [chapter 8].
292. Al-Beltagi M. Autism medical comorbidities. *World J Clin Pediatr.* 2021;10:15–28.
293. Jeste SS. The neurology of autism spectrum disorders. *Curr Opin Neurol.* 2011;24:132–139.
294. Haigh JL, et al. Deletion of a non-canonical regulatory sequence causes loss of Scn1a expression and epileptic phenotypes in mice. *Genome Med.* 2021;13:1–22.
295. Born HA, et al. Early developmental eeg and seizure phenotypes in a full gene deletion of ubiquitin protein ligase e3a rat model of angelman syndrome. *eNeuro.* 2021;8.
296. Dhir A. Pentylenetetrazol (PTZ) kindling model of epilepsy. *Curr Protoc Neurosci.* 2012;1:1–12.
297. Copping NA, Adhikari A, Petkova SP, Silverman JL. Genetic backgrounds have unique seizure response profiles and behavioral outcomes following convulsant administration. *Epilepsy Behav.* 2019;101:1–27.
298. Sukoff Rizzo SJ, Silverman JL. Methodological considerations for optimizing and validating behavioral assays. *Curr Protoc Mouse Biol.* 2016;6:364–379.
299. Dawson G, Burner K. Behavioral interventions in children and adolescents with autism spectrum disorder: a review of recent findings. *Curr Opin Pediatr.* 2011;23:616–620.
300. Xu G, et al. Prevalence and treatment patterns of autism spectrum disorder in the United States, 2016. *JAMA Pediatr.* 2019;173:153–159.
301. Reichow B, Hume K, Barton EE, Boyd BA. Early intensive behavioral intervention (EIBI) for young children with autism spectrum disorders (ASD). *Cochrane Database Syst Rev.* 2018;1–50. https://doi.org/10.1002/14651858.CD009260.pub3.
302. Scahill L, Koenig K, Carroll DH, Pachler M. Risperidone approved for the treatment of serious behavioral problems in children with autism. *Psychopharmacology (Berl).* 2007;20:188–190.
303. Wink LK, Erickson CA, McDougle CJ. Pharmacologic treatment of behavioral symptoms associated with autism and other pervasive developmental disorders. *Curr Treat Options Neurol.* 2010;12:529–538.
304. Silverman JL, Nithianantharajah J, Der-Avakian A, Young J, Sukoff Rizzo SJ. Lost in translation: at the crossroads of face validity and translational utility of behavioral assays in animal models for the development of therapeutics. *Neurosci Biobehav Rev.* 2020;116:452–453.
305. Ellegood J, et al. Clustering autism: using neuroanatomical differences in 26 mouse models to gain insight into the heterogeneity. *Mol Psychiatry.* 2015;20:118–125.
306. Silverman JL, Ellegood J. Behavioral and neuroanatomical approaches in models of neurodevelopmental disorders: opportunities for translation. *Curr Opin Neurol.* 2018;31:126–133.
307. Ellegood J, Crawley JN. Behavioral and neuroanatomical phenotypes in mouse models of autism. *Neurotherapeutics.* 2015;12:521–533.
308. Kentner AC, et al. Maternal immune activation: reporting guidelines to improve the rigor, reproducibility, and transparency of the model. *Neuropsychopharmacology.* 2019;44:245–258.

CHAPTER

# 9

# Genetic etiologies of autism: Unpacking pathogenic mechanisms and characteristics

*Caitlin M. Hudac*[a,b], *Nicole R. Friedman*[a], *and Tychele N. Turner*[c]

**[a]Center for Youth Development and Intervention and Department of Psychology, University of Alabama, Tuscaloosa, AL, United States, [b]Department of Psychology, University of South Carolina, Columbia, SC, United States, [c]Department of Genetics, Washington University School of Medicine, St. Louis, MO, United States**

## Abbreviations

| | |
|---|---|
| CNV | copy number variation |
| FMRP | fragile X mental retardation protein |
| GWAS | genome wide association study |
| PRS | polygenic risk score |
| RTT | Rett syndrome |
| SNV | single nucleotide variation |
| STR | short tandem repeats |
| WES | whole-exome sequencing |
| WGS | whole-genome sequencing |

## Introduction

Autism spectrum disorder (ASD) is a complex neurodevelopmental disorder with heterogeneity (i.e., diverse variety of presentation) across levels of the genotype and phenotype.[1] This is particularly challenging when seeking to discover underlying biological causes, such as genetic etiologies, in order to improve the ability to identify young infants and



*The Neuroscience of Autism*
https://doi.org/10.1016/B978-0-12-816393-1.00001-4

children with increased likelihood of receiving an ASD diagnosis by clarifying biological mechanisms. Initial karyotyping efforts of ASD began over 50 years ago, in which a rudimentary "snap-shot" of the structural features was not sufficient to identify specific chromosomal abnormalities.[2] As early as 1977, twin and family studies confirmed the heritability of ASD between 38% and 90%,[3–5] such that if one monozygotic ("identical") twin is autistic, the other twin is 0.83 likely to also receive an ASD diagnosis.[6] Upwards of 30% of autistic individuals carry a de novo copy number or single nucleotide variant associated with ASD.[7] Building on decades of ASD genetic discoveries looking at shared genetic variance in populations with ASD, there are currently ~100 genes and genomic regions implicated with high-confidence ASD associations.[8–10] This work is critical for understanding the key genes and molecular pathways involved in ASD. Identification of genome-wide significant genes has allowed for the development of a "genetics-first" approach. In this strategy, populations are ascertained based upon shared genetic variants in order to characterize the clinical, medical, behavioral, and neural phenotypes in individuals.[11,12] In other words, the genetics-first approach builds upon identified genetic variations (i.e., genes related to ASD above and beyond statistical chance) by characterizing specific phenotypic presentations, or potential subgroups of ASD. Here, we provide examples of identified genetic variations associated with ASD and work describing the associated phenotype as it pertains to ASD and other clinical, medical, and behavioral neurodevelopmental disorders.

## ASD genetics primer

As the inherited "blueprint" containing code for proteins and other molecules, our genome consisting of our full set of coding genes and noncoding sections of deoxyribonucleic acid (DNA) builds and maintains our body's structure and function. All human cells ostensibly carry the same genome and each gene codes for a specific protein with a particular function, though genetic expression does vary based upon characteristics including cell type, developmental stage, age, and sex.[13] Genetic alterations or mutations are necessary within a species to promote phenotypic variation[14] and these variations are commonly distributed across locations in the genome.

The goal of a genetics-first approach is to link genetic etiology to resultant biological mechanisms and capture shared phenotypic traits, including behavior and clinical features (see Fig. 1). Discovery in the genomics of ASD are driven by genomic technological and statistical advances (Table 1), generating the identification of specific genes and mutations (Fig. 2). These include ASD-related genetic syndromes, rare copy

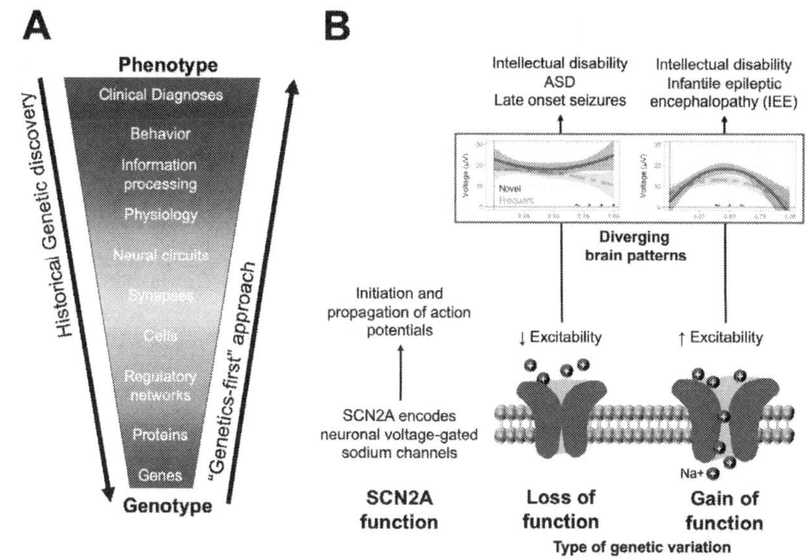


FIG. 1 (A) Framework for genetics-first approach. Building from the progress of historical genetic discovery, the genetics first approach explores how different levels of the phenotype are related to unique genetic variation. (B) Example of genetics-first approach: *SCN2A* likely gene disrupting mutations impact the role of SCN2A in sodium ion channel regulation, ultimately affecting initiation and propagation of action potentials and being associated with intellectual disability and global developmental delay diagnoses. When the variant causes a loss of SCN2A function, this decreases neuronal excitability, and we see this related to unique, ASD-like brain patterns, as well as clinical diagnoses of ASD and late onset seizures. In contrast, gain of SCN2A function is related to increased neuronal excitability, and phenotypes include brain patterns that are atypical yet different than ASD, and infantile epileptic encephalopathy.

**TABLE 1** Overview of the capabilities of different genetic techniques to capture different mutation types.

| Mutation type | Karyotype | SNP microarray | Whole-exome sequencing | Short-read whole-genome sequencing | Long-read whole-genome sequencing |
|---|---|---|---|---|---|
| | **Technology** | | | | |
| Single nucleotide variation (SNV) | - | **Partial** (specific sites) | **Partial** (protein-coding only) | **Partial** (regions w/high mappability) | + |
| Small insertion (<50 bp) | - | | | | + |
| Small deletion (<50 bp) | - | | | | + |
| Multi-nucleotide variation (MNV) | - | - | | | + |
| Short tandem repeats (STR) expansion | - | - | - | **Partial** | + |
| Duplication (>50 bp and <1000 bp) | - | - | - | - | + |
| Deletion (>50 bp and <1000 bp) | - | - | - | - | + |
| Duplication (>1000 bp) | **Partial** (Mbp in size) | **Partial** (>25K bp) | **Partial** (>3 exons) | + | + |
| Deletion (> 1000 bp) | | | | + | + |
| Inversion | | - | - | **Partial** | + |
| Translocation | + | - | - | **Partial** | **Partial** |

Positive evidence indicated by "+."

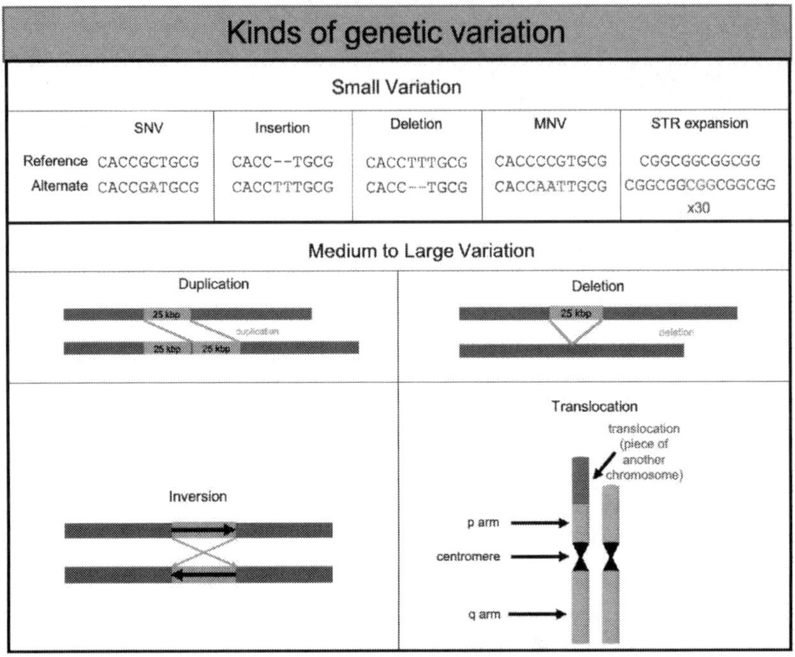


FIG. 2 Kinds of genetic variation. Genetic variation can include small variations of single nucleotide variations (SNV; i.e., one nucleotide changed), insertion or deletion variants (i.e., additional nucleotides inserted or deleted), multinucleotide variations (MNV; i.e., more than one nucleotide changed), and short-term repeat expansion (STR; as in fragile X). Medium to large variation can occur wherein large sections (≥ 25 kilobase pairs) are duplicated or repeated, deleted, or inverted. Translocation can also occur wherein a chromosomal section is transferred to another chromosome.

number variants (CNVs), de novo protein-coding variants (particularly likely gene-disrupting mutations), common variants, and polygenic risk. There is also active investigation into the role of rare inherited variation, as well as de novo and rare inherited noncoding variation. After identifying recurring pathogenic genetic variants in ASD, the genetics-first approach to research seeks to improve our understanding of the consequences of affecting the ability to produce proteins that support cellular function, creating cascading problems with development of protein-protein networks and cellular circuits, such as information processing between neurons. With these identified variants and knowledge about the molecular and cellular basis of ASD, it is important to capture aspects of the human phenotype, including physiology, information processing, behavior, and clinical diagnoses. For instance, genetic variants may subsequently impair brain processes and behaviors, often resulting in a constellation of symptoms and features that lead to a clinical diagnosis.

## ASD-related genetic syndromes

Early karyotyping and microarray work identified genetic syndromes that manifest ASD at higher than expected frequencies compared to the general population.[2,15] Different syndromes converge upon common biological backgrounds, which may provide insight into the shared mechanisms for their association with ASD. The syndromes briefly described here (and others) involve distinctive clinical and medical features, as well as overlap with ASD symptoms, with each syndrome thought initially to be linked to a common genetic variant. Yet, as is becoming evident from Down syndrome,[16] variation exists within syndromes due to multilevel multifactorial elements (e.g., epigenetics, developmental timing, other variants in the genome).

**Fragile X Syndrome** is the most common inherited cause of intellectual disability and ASD.[17] Current estimates suggest that ASD occurs in 21%–50% of males with fragile X syndrome,[18] with increased prevalence among individuals with greater degree of intellectual disability. Patients present with severe behavioral symptoms including hyperactivity, impulsivity, and anxiety, poor language development, and seizures. Fragile X syndrome is caused by a trinucleotide repeat expansion of three bases (CGG) that occurs in the fragile X mental retardation 1 gene (*FMR1*) at Xq27.3. A small expansion, or premutation, has 55–200 CGG repeats and is not usually associated with intellectual disability, unlike larger expansions (i.e., full mutation; > 200 CGG) that are associated with fragile X syndrome. When a full mutation is present, the gene becomes silenced and no protein (FMRP) is created. FMRP has a central role in gene expression and regulates the translation of hundreds of mRNAs,[7] which are involved in development and maintenance of neuronal synaptic connections. Additionally, fragile X syndrome was one of the first disorders shown to be caused by short tandem repeats (STR) that involve sequences of 1–20 base pairs repeated consecutively. Recent research suggests de novo STR mutations are similar in magnitude to de novo point mutations per child and are observed as genome-wide excess in probands compared with non-ASD siblings. Overall, STRs may account for approximately 4% of simplex ASD cases, which is comparable in magnitude to noncoding point mutations.[19]

**Rett Syndrome (RTT)** is a severe disorder that contributes significantly to severe intellectual disability in females.[20] Estimate rates of ASD range from 25% to 40%[18] and RTT is additionally characterized by normal early development followed by a loss of purposeful hand skills between 6 months and 2.5 years, characteristic movements, social withdrawal, and communication dysfunction. RTT is caused by mutations in the gene encoding methyl-CpG binding protein 2 (MeCP2), a transcriptional repressor involved in chromatin remodeling and the modulation of RNA splicing. MECP2 dysfunction results in a variety of neuropsychiatric abnormalities, where both loss of function and gain in MECP2 dosage lead to similar phenotypes.

**Dup15q Syndrome** is caused by mutations in 15q11–13 that are associated with copy number duplication. Estimate rates of ASD in Dup15 q range from 20% to 40%. Dup15q mutations lead to one of two resulting syndromes, based upon absence of maternal vs paternal gene expression. **Prader-Willi Syndrome** occurs as the result of absence of expression of paternal genes. This lack of expression occurs by three primary mechanisms: (1) deletion of a 5–6 Megabase pair region from paternally contributed chromosome 15 (65%–75%), (2) maternal uniparental disomy (20%–30%), (3) a rare defect in the genomic region that controls the imprinting process (1%–3%). Prader-Willi syndrome is a complex multisystem disorder that includes hypothalamic dysfunction that is responsible for hormonal dysfunctions and absence of sense of satiety.[21,22] Prader-Willi syndrome children develop hyperphagia (i.e., abnormally strong sensation of hunger) during infancy that can lead to obesity. In addition, behavioral problems that interfere with quality of life intensify during adolescence and adulthood. **Angelman Syndrome** results from the absence of expression of maternal genes. More specifically, Angelman syndrome results from the loss of function of the *UBE3A* gene, which in the brain is expressed from the maternal chromosome only. Angelman syndrome is characterized by severe learning disabilities with a majority of Angelman syndrome patients not developing speech, as well as ataxia, seizure disorder, subtle dysmorphic facial features, and a happy, sociable disposition.[23]

## Copy number variations (CNVs)

CNVs include deletions and duplications which are losses and gains of DNA, respectively, often encompassing a section of DNA > 1 kb. Although CNVs themselves are common (i.e., with no apparent influence on phenotype), early work from large genotyped cohorts identified several ASD-associated CNVs considered rare (i.e., not appearing in the general population) and recurrent (i.e., re-appearing in ASD populations) CNVs, defined based upon their location. For instance, Prader-Willi syndrome and Angelman syndrome are derived from 15q11–13 duplications[24] and appear on the chromosome 15 with breakpoints (i.e., position where allelic shifts are present) at chromosome bands 11 through 13. The amount of DNA either deleted or duplicated is known to be associated with autistic symptom severity with certain "hotspots" proposed as unique in ASD,[25] though there is evidence suggesting a broad overlap with ASD and other neurodevelopmental disorders.[26,27]

For several high-impact CNVs, opposing or "mirror" phenotypes are observed between deletion and duplication variants, including 16p11.2

and 22q11.2 CNV.[11] As one such CNV well-studied from both the genomic and clinical perspective, ~ 1% of individuals with ASD exhibit 16p11.2 CNVs[28] within a genomic region encompassing 28 genes.[29] Evidence from dose-dependent animal models[30] provide support for the opposing 16p11.2 phenotypes observed in humans. For example, relative to non-CNV controls, deletion carriers exhibit large head circumference (macrocephaly), increased brain volume, and obesity, whereas duplication carriers exhibit reduced head circumference (microcephaly), decreased brain volume, and lower to normal body mass index.[31,32] Additional opposing phenotypes are observed in functional brain responses, including visual evoked potentials[33] and responses to biological/social motion.[34] However, a graded dose-dependence model may be imprecise. In a rare case with a 16p11.2 triplication (4 copies instead of 2 copies; inherited as an expansion from a maternal duplication carrier), although some behavioral features resembled duplication carriers, a majority of the clinical and medical phenotype aligned with the 16p11.2 deletion phenotype.[35] This indicates a more complex phenomenon, wherein certain genes within the CNV may be more sensitive to the level of increased (or decreased) dosage or that certain regions of the chromosomal rearrangements may be more likely to mimic the effect of a deletion of the same region.

## De novo protein-coding likely gene-disrupting mutations

Whole-exome sequencing (WES) is a technology where only the protein-coding regions of the genome are sequenced in an individual, and this focus on the protein-coding regions aides in the assessment of rare variants with large-effect size in a practical manner.[36] In the use of WES in ASD, an early choice was made to not just sequence the children (often called "proband") but to also sequence their parents in a trio-based approach. By sequencing the parents, researchers could look at de novo variants that are variants present in children but not their parents.[37] Early genetic studies[38] focused on simplex families (i.e., only one affected child/proband and no other affected family members), such that using this trio-based approach, variants identified were both de novo and likely gene-disrupting, including the genes *CHD8* and *SCN2A*.[39,40] These early discoveries indicated WES in larger sample sizes would likely yield somewhere between 500 and 1000 genes involved in ASD. In fact, recent work identified 102 genes with enrichment for de novo likely gene-disrupting variants from 11,986 individuals with ASD.[10] Over time, it has also been clear that combining individuals with neurodevelopmental disorders more broadly would yield additional enriched genes. Researchers combined WES data from 31,058 trios to find 285 genes with an enrichment of de novo likely gene-disrupting variants[41] that contribute overall in ~ 21% of all individuals with simplex ASD.[7] Considering the relevance and importance of de novo likely gene-disrupting variants, we encourage the utility of combining data across studies, for instance through common website resources,[42] in order improve genomic discoveries.

## Common variation and polygenic risk

In addition to rare variations, common variants contribute to ASD and have been studied by two main approaches: genome-wide association studies (GWAS) and polygenic risk scores (PRS). Early GWAS identified few significant variants; however, many of these were not replicated in follow-up efforts. In one of these early studies, there were 1031 multiplex ASD families assessed with a total of 1553 individuals with ASD.[43] More recent studies increased that sample size 12-fold, subsequently detecting 5 replicated GWAS signals.[44] A second strategy has been to look at overall common variant signal in the form of PRS, which entails computing the genetic susceptibility of disease by evaluating possible cumulative burden from (potentially) common variants. For instance, an excess of polygenic risk was transmitted to individuals with ASD, but not unaffected siblings.[45] Altogether, narrow-sense heritability rates of ASD are ~ 53%, accounting for phenotypic variance attributed to cumulative or additive effects of genes.[46] Modern approaches seek to garner knowledge of common variants via GWAS and PRS in tandem with known rare variants to better assess familial associations (e.g., parent-proband relationships) related to ASD genetics.

## Linking ASD genetics to phenotypes

An important goal of studying the genetics of ASD is to link biological mechanisms (i.e., genetic etiology and its consequences) to aspects of the clinical, medical, behavioral, and neural phenotype, often described as "deep phenotyping." This is a particularly promising avenue for developing precision medicine in ASD,[47] wherein constellations of the phenotype for a particular "subgroup" of ASD may have clinical relevance. For instance, individuals with de novo variants in *CHD8* exhibit common features including facial dysmorphisms, gastrointestinal dysfunction, sleep disturbance, and macrocephaly,[48] whereas a different set of features is observed in individuals with de novo variants in *DYRK1A*, including different facial dysmorphisms, intellectual disability, speech delay, and microcephaly.[49] Continued efforts to link between biological mechanisms and aspects of the phenotype in these potentially unique (or systematically overlapping) subgroups will inform clinical assessments, particularly given that rare variants are anticipated in 20%–40% of clinical populations.[7]

The identification of many genes involved in ASD has provided key insights into the molecular biology of ASD. By assessment of protein-protein interactions and coexpression, researchers found that genes involved in ASD are broadly involved in chromatin, gene regulation, and synaptic biology.[50–53] As an example, the underlying functional cellular mechanism of *SCN2A* is well characterized (Fig. 1B): *SCN2A* encodes $Na_V1.2$ sodium channels that are primarily expressed within the axon and are responsible for the generation and propagation of action potentials.[54] There is evidence that altered levels of $Na_V1.2$ function are particularly consequential during early brain development-effects of $Na_V1.2$ disruption in mouse models extend into childhood and beyond in the form of increased seizure susceptibility and elevated anxiety.[55] Lab-based research illuminated the specificity between the *SCN2A* variant and its effect on $Na_V1.2$ function,[56,57] such that *loss* of SCN2A function results in an ASD phenotype (ASD phenotype), while *gain* of SCN2A function results in infantile seizures and/or epileptic encephalopathy (IEE phenotype). Pyramidal neuronal modeling of the two types of variants suggests opposing developmental patterns of neuronal excitability, such that reductions persist in the mature brain following gain but not loss of SCN2A function. This suggests that the ASD phenotype includes substantial downstream reductions (e.g., excitatory/inhibitory circuit balance) beyond reduction of neuronal excitability during early development.

Deep phenotyping is essential to better understand commonalties associated with particular genetic variation, such that unique profiles or subgroups of ASD may be identified. From the perspective of *SCN2A*, clinical and medical features make standardized behavioral testing difficult, including severe intellectual disabilities (96%), hypotonia (83%), and motor issues (85%) common to individuals with both loss and gain of *SCN2A* function.[58] However, modern techniques such as human electroencephalography provide an opportunity to assess cognitive systems in minimally verbal or nonverbal children. Our own efforts identified potential neural correlates in support of distinct functional profiles, including patterns of auditory attention and general resting state aligned with ASD in loss-of-function carriers, and atypical yet diverging from ASD in gain-of-function carriers.[59,60]

However, the rarity of specific genetic events is a considerable obstacle in phenotypic subtyping of mutations. A promising avenue of research evaluates possible shared biological mechanisms and pathway shared by multiple ASD-associated risk genes, seeking to examine the consequences of the disrupted genetic function. For instance, genes serving as an FMRP target gene (e.g., *GRIN2B*, *SCN2A*) are associated with lower cognitive scores, consistent with the role of FMRP in neuroplasticity.[7] Another example involves genes that have a dominant role during early embryonic development (e.g., *DYRK1A, ADNP, POGZ*), which are associated with disrupted neuronal signaling pathways[61] that may explain the ASD phenotype including atypical social brain processes.[62]

Given the high confidence of CHD8, recent efforts have focused on potential shared pathways specific to genes targeted or otherwise regulated by *CHD8*. As a chromatin modifier, *CHD8* has a role in dynamically modifying the structure of chromatin (i.e., the material that uses proteins called histones to package DNA) to regulate gene expression. More specifically, CHD8 is a transcriptional regulator implicated in the suppression of the Wnt-β-catenein signaling pathway through histone H1 recruitment.[63] Cross-species models of the human midfetal brain, neural stem cells, and embryonic mouse cortex indicate that *CHD8* targets other ASD-associated genes, including *ADNP, ARID1B,* and *DYRK1A*.[64] Children with *CHD8* and *CHD8*-targeted LGDs exhibit shared phenotypes, including strengths in adaptive communication and functional language, social challenges and low social motivation, and large head circumference,[65] providing evidence linking the phenotype to molecular functions.

Further consideration is necessary regarding ASD genetic etiologies associated with co-occurring clinical diagnoses.[66] We caution expectations of discovering "ASD (only) genes," given the extensive overlap between the genes identified as significant in individuals with ASD, intellectual disability, developmental delay, epilepsy, and schizophrenia.[67,68] An approach seeking to identify "ASD (only) genes" is likely to generate a simple classification that does not truly account for background variation or stochasticity seen in developmental processes. Instead, a genetics-first approach to ASD (and other neurodevelopmental disorders) focuses on the biological function of the gene, often implicating a role in brain development. It is likely the case that perturbations of these genes by variants of different effect sizes and location yield differing neural and subsequent clinical phenotypes at the level of the individual (e.g., SCN2A diverging phenotypes based upon functional impact, see Fig. 1B).

## The future of genetic discovery

Future advances in genetic discovery in ASD will move forward through both technology and a focus on novel areas of biological interpretation. For instance, as we gain technological innovations and biological knowledge, it will be increasingly critical to consider sex as a factor in ASD genomics. Over 80% of individuals with ASD are male, yet autistic females demonstrate enrichment in genetic variants of high effect (e.g., de novo LGD and large CNVs). This supports a biologically derived female-protective effect wherein autistic females may have more severe genomic etiologies.[69] However, autistic females are also enriched for other diagnoses of intellectual disability and/or developmental delay,[70] which may suggest a potential ascertainment bias (i.e., reason for receiving genetic testing). Efforts to exponentially increase genetic testing in ASD (The SPARK[71]) will improve the capacity to consider these critical individual differences, including the sex bias.

Thus far, a majority of genomic analyses focus on surveying predefined regions of the genome. This limits the ability to detect de novo and rare variation in the 98.5% of the genome that is noncoding and to detect small to medium size structural variation across the genome. Recently, short-read whole-genome sequencing has enabled a look at the variation across the full genome in thousands of individuals with ASD. Approximately 3.5% of the noncoding genome is highly conserved and is likely of functional importance.[72,73] Noncoding DNA involved in the regulation of genes include promoters, enhancers, silencers, untranslated regions, topologically associating domain boundaries, noncoding RNAs, and miRNA binding sites ([74]). Initial work examining upwards of 2500 families with ASD has highlighted an excess of de novo variation in promoters and enhancers.[75–78] The future in this area will involve identifying noncoding regions reaching genome-wide significance. As of yet, no one has assessed enough samples to reach this hallmark but it is predicted to be seen in ~ 8000 families.[69] Early work utilizing whole-exome and whole-genome sequencing identified an excess of rare inherited coding variation and in particular shown an excess of variation in highly constrained genes in the genome.[79] On the noncoding side, an excess of paternally inherited variants are enriched in ASD.[80] Whole-genome sequencing is allowing for the comprehensive assessment of both coding and noncoding as well as rare and common variants. Once full variant detection is enabled for each individual, the opportunity to assess different combinations of variants in individuals (known as oligogenicity) will be possible. Early glimpses into this area identified individuals with excess of multiple variant types.[77,81]

Long-read sequencing is a major genomic technological advance that will innovate the field of ASD genomics. In particular, the newest of these technologies (Pacific Biosciences HiFi sequencing) are able to generate highly accurate long reads (~ 20,000 basepairs). These reads are ~ 130 × longer than the current state-of-the-art and are enabling the detection of variation intractable with previous technologies, full phasing or assignment of variants to the chromosome on which they reside and in orientation with other variants, and the ability to build de novo assemblies whereby full reconstruction of a patient genome is possible from only the read data itself. Recently, this technology identified previously undetected critical and likely pathogenic structural variants in individuals with neurodevelopmental disorders.[82] As costs drop, this technology will likely be the greatest revolution to full resolution of genomic variation in ASD.

The final aspect of advances in ASD genomics involves connecting identified ASD genes with the underlying biology. Many genes are now known and they fit within defined biological categories (e.g., gene regulation, chromatin, synapse). It is important to define these biological functions, because if they were otherwise random genes, it would be hard to understand their connection to ASD and ASD macro-level phenotypes. Now that we know the first set of ~ 100 genes and as we continue to identify the remaining 400–900 genes, we can begin to put them together in gene regulatory networks. For instance, our work describing the *CHD8* clinical, medical, and behavioral phenotypes within the gene itself, as well as the downstream targets of CHD8.[65] Orthogonal genomic technologies such as single-cell sequencing, high-throughput proteomics, and spatial temporal resolution of genes and their function will be critical parallel works to support definitions of gene regulatory networks in ASD.

## Conclusions

As a highly heritable neurodevelopmental disorder, it is vital to consider genetic etiologies of ASD and understand the implication(s) for precision medicine. As genetic methodologies rapidly progressed over the past half-century, specific genetic contributions of ASD became more evident, including chromosomal re-arrangements (e.g., 16p11.2 CNVs, 15q11–13 duplications) de novo protein coding mutations, and aspects of common variation. Together with modern genetic approaches assessing polygenic risk and the emerging relevance of noncoding regions, continued work connecting these fundamental genetic foundations to distinct neural, cognitive, and behavioral phenotypes will aide in identification of potential subgroups of ASD. This information will be instrumental in evaluating the functional and structural mechanisms of ASD, as explored by other chapters in this book.

## References

1. Lord C, Brugha TS, Charman T, et al. Autism spectrum disorder. *Nat Rev Dis Primers.* 2020;6(1):5. https://doi.org/10.1038/s41572-019-0138-4.
2. Judd LL, Mandell AJ. Chromosome studies in early infantile autism. *Arch Gen Psychiatry.* 1968;18(4):450–457. https://doi.org/10.1001/archpsyc.1968.01740040066008.
3. Folstein S, Rutter M. Infantile autism: a genetic study of 21 twin pairs. *J Child Psychol Psychiatry.* 1977;18(4). https://doi.org/10.1111/j.1469-7610.1977.tb00443.x.

4. Hallmayer J, Cleveland S, Torres A, et al. Genetic heritability and shared environmental factors among twin pairs with autism. *Arch Gen Psychiatry.* 2011;68(11):1095–1102. https://doi.org/10.1001/archgenpsychiatry.2011.76.
5. Tick B, Bolton P, Happé F, Rutter M, Rijsdijk F. Heritability of autism spectrum disorders: a meta-analysis of twin studies. *J Child Psychol Psychiatry.* 2016;57(5):585–595. https://doi.org/10.1111/jcpp.12499.
6. Sandin S, Lichtenstein P, Kuja-Halkola R, Hultman C, Larsson H, Reichenberg A. The heritability of autism spectrum disorder. *JAMA.* 2017;318(12):1182–1184. https://doi.org/10.1001/jama.2017.12141.
7. Iossifov I, O'Roak BJ, Sanders SJ, et al. The contribution of de novo coding mutations to autism spectrum disorder. *Nature.* 2014;515(7526):216–221. https://doi.org/10.1038/nature13908.
8. O'Roak BJ, Stessman HA, Boyle EA, et al. Recurrent de novo mutations implicate novel genes underlying simplex autism risk. *Nat Commun.* 2014;5(1):5595. https://doi.org/10.1038/ncomms6595.
9. Sanders SJ, He X, Willsey AJ, et al. Insights into autism spectrum disorder genomic architecture and biology from 71 risk loci. *Neuron.* 2015;87(6):1215–1233. https://doi.org/10.1016/j.neuron.2015.09.016.
10. Satterstrom FK, Kosmicki JA, Wang J, et al. Large-scale exome sequencing study implicates both developmental and functional changes in the neurobiology of autism. *Cell.* 2020;180(3):568–584.e23. https://doi.org/10.1016/j.cell.2019.12.036.
11. Chawner SJRA, Doherty JL, Anney RJL, et al. A genetics-first approach to dissecting the heterogeneity of autism: phenotypic comparison of autism risk copy number variants. *Am J Psychiatry.* 2021;178(1):77–86. https://doi.org/10.1176/appi.ajp.2020.20010015.
12. Stessman HA, Bernier R, Eichler EE. A genotype-first approach to defining the subtypes of a complex disease. *Cell.* 2014;156(5):872–877. https://doi.org/10.1016/j.cell.2014.02.002.
13. Murrell A, Rakyan VK, Beck S. From genome to epigenome. *Hum Mol Genet.* 2005;14(suppl_1):R3–R10. https://doi.org/10.1093/hmg/ddi110.
14. Skinner MK. Environmental epigenetics and a unified theory of the molecular aspects of evolution: a neo-Lamarckian concept that facilitates neo-Darwinian evolution. *Genome Biol Evol.* 2015;7(5):1296–1302. https://doi.org/10.1093/gbe/evv073.
15. Moss J, Howlin P. Autism spectrum disorders in genetic syndromes: implications for diagnosis, intervention and understanding the wider autism spectrum disorder population. *J Intellect Disabil Res.* 2009;53(10):852–873. https://doi.org/10.1111/j.1365-2788.2009.01197.x.
16. Thomas MSC, Alfageme OO, D'Souza H, et al. A multi-level developmental approach to exploring individual differences in down syndrome: genes, brain, behaviour, and environment. *Res Dev Disabil.* 2020;104. https://doi.org/10.1016/j.ridd.2020.103638, 103638.
17. Hagerman RJ, Berry-Kravis E, Hazlett HC, et al. Fragile X syndrome. *Nat Rev Dis Primers.* 2017;3(1):17065. https://doi.org/10.1038/nrdp.2017.65.
18. Ornoy A, Fudim LW, Ergaz Z. Genetic syndromes, maternal diseases and antenatal factors associated with autism spectrum disorders (ASD). *Front Neurosci.* 2016;10:316. https://doi.org/10.3389/fnins.2016.00316.
19. Mitra I, Huang B, Mousavi N, et al. Patterns of de novo tandem repeat mutations and their role in autism. *Nature.* 2021;589(7841):246–250. https://doi.org/10.1038/s41586-020-03078-7.
20. Chahrour M, Zoghbi HY. The story of rett syndrome: from clinic to neurobiology. *Neuron.* 2007;56(3):422–437. https://doi.org/10.1016/j.neuron.2007.10.001.
21. Buiting K. Prader–Willi syndrome and Angelman syndrome. *Am J Med Genet C Semin Med Genet.* 2010;154C(3):365–376. https://doi.org/10.1002/ajmg.c.30273.
22. Elena G, Bruna C, Benedetta M, Stefania DC, Giuseppe C. Prader-Willi syndrome: clinical aspects. *J Obes.* 2012;2012. https://doi.org/10.1155/2012/473941, 473941.

23. Clayton-Smith J, Laan L. Angelman syndrome: a review of the clinical and genetic aspects. *J Med Genet.* 2003;40(2):87. https://doi.org/10.1136/jmg.40.2.87.
24. Cook EH, Lindgren V, Leventhal BL, et al. Autism or atypical autism in maternally but not paternally derived proximal 15q duplication. *Am J Hum Genet.* 1997;60(4):928–934.
25. Girirajan S, Dennis MY, Baker C, et al. Refinement and discovery of new hotspots of copy-number variation associated with autism spectrum disorder. *Am J Hum Genet.* 2013;92(2):221–237. https://doi.org/10.1016/j.ajhg.2012.12.016.
26. Coe BP, Witherspoon K, Rosenfeld JA, et al. Refining analyses of copy number variation identifies specific genes associated with developmental delay. *Nat Genet.* 2014;46(10):1063–1071. https://doi.org/10.1038/ng.3092.
27. Cooper GM, Coe BP, Girirajan S, et al. A copy number variation morbidity map of developmental delay. *Nat Genet.* 2011;43(9):838–846. https://doi.org/10.1038/ng.909.
28. Weiss LA, Shen Y, Korn JM, et al. Association between microdeletion and microduplication at 16p11.2 and autism. *N Engl J Med.* 2008;358(7):667–675. https://doi.org/10.1056/nejmoa075974.
29. Chung WK, Roberts TP, Sherr EH, Snyder LG, Spiro JE. 16p11.2 deletion syndrome. *Curr Opin Genet Dev.* 2021;68:49–56. https://doi.org/10.1016/j.gde.2021.01.011.
30. Horev G, Ellegood J, Lerch JP, et al. Dosage-dependent phenotypes in models of 16p11.2 lesions found in autism. *Proc Natl Acad Sci.* 2011;108(41):17076–17081. https://doi.org/10.1073/pnas.1114042108.
31. Jacquemont S, Reymond A, Zufferey F, et al. Mirror extreme BMI phenotypes associated with gene dosage at the chromosome 16p11.2 locus. *Nature.* 2011;478(7367):97–102. https://doi.org/10.1038/nature10406.
32. Qureshi AY, Mueller S, Snyder AZ, et al. Opposing brain differences in 16p11.2 deletion and duplication carriers. *J Neurosci.* 2014;34(34):11199–11211. https://doi.org/10.1523/jneurosci.1366-14.2014.
33. LeBlanc JJ, Nelson CA. Deletion and duplication of 16p11.2 are associated with opposing effects on visual evoked potential amplitude. *Mol Autism.* 2016;7(1):30. https://doi.org/10.1186/s13229-016-0095-7.
34. Hudac CM, Kresse A, Aaronson B, DesChamps TD, Webb SJ, Bernier RA. Modulation of mu attenuation to social stimuli in children and adults with 16p11.2 deletions and duplications. *J Neurodev Disord.* 2015;7(1):25. https://doi.org/10.1186/s11689-015-9118-5.
35. Wallace AS, Hudac CM, Steinman KJ, et al. Longitudinal report of child with de novo 16p11.2 triplication. *Clin Case Rep.* 2018;6(1):147–154. https://doi.org/10.1002/ccr3.1236.
36. Ng SB, Turner EH, Robertson PD, et al. Targeted capture and massively parallel sequencing of 12 human exomes. *Nature.* 2009;461(7261):272–276. https://doi.org/10.1038/nature08250.
37. O'Roak BJ, Deriziotis P, Lee C, et al. Exome sequencing in sporadic autism spectrum disorders identifies severe de novo mutations. *Nat Genet.* 2011;43(6):585–589. https://doi.org/10.1038/ng.835.
38. Fischbach GD, Lord C. The Simons simplex collection: a resource for identification of autism genetic risk factors. *Neuron.* 2010;68(2):192–195. https://doi.org/10.1016/j.neuron.2010.10.006.
39. O'Roak BJ, Vives L, Girirajan S, et al. Sporadic autism exomes reveal a highly interconnected protein network of de novo mutations. *Nature.* 2013;485(7397):246–250. https://doi.org/10.1038/nature10989.
40. Sanders SJ, Murtha MT, Gupta AR, et al. De novo mutations revealed by whole-exome sequencing are strongly associated with autism. *Nature.* 2012;485(7397):237–241. https://doi.org/10.1038/nature10945.
41. Kaplanis J, Samocha KE, Wiel L, et al. Evidence for 28 genetic disorders discovered by combining healthcare and research data. *Nature.* 2020;586(7831):757–762. https://doi.org/10.1038/s41586-020-2832-5.

42. Turner TN, Yi Q, Krumm N, et al. denovo-db: a compendium of human de novo variants. *Nucleic Acids Res.* 2017;45(D1):D804–D811. https://doi.org/10.1093/nar/gkw865.
43. Weiss LA, Arking DE, Daly MJ, et al. A genome-wide linkage and association scan reveals novel loci for autism. *Nature.* 2009;461(7265):802–808. https://doi.org/10.1038/nature08490.
44. Grove J, Ripke S, Als TD, et al. Identification of common genetic risk variants for autism spectrum disorder. *Nat Genet.* 2019;51(3):431–444. https://doi.org/10.1038/s41588-019-0344-8.
45. Weiner DJ, Wigdor EM, Ripke S, et al. Polygenic transmission disequilibrium confirms that common and rare variation act additively to create risk for autism spectrum disorders. *Nat Genet.* 2017;49(7):978–985. https://doi.org/10.1038/ng.3863.
46. Gaugler T, Klei L, Sanders SJ, et al. Most genetic risk for autism resides with common variation. *Nat Genet.* 2014;46(8):881–885. https://doi.org/10.1038/ng.3039.
47. Geschwind DH, State MW. Gene hunting in autism spectrum disorder: on the path to precision medicine. *Lancet Glob Health.* 2015;14(11):1. https://doi.org/10.1016/s1474-4422(15)00044-7.
48. Bernier R, Golzio C, Xiong B, et al. Disruptive CHD8 mutations define a subtype of autism early in development. *Cell.* 2014;158(2):263–276. https://doi.org/10.1016/j.cell.2014.06.017.
49. Earl RK, Turner TN, Mefford HC, et al. Clinical phenotype of ASD-associated DYRK1A haploinsufficiency. *Mol Autism.* 2017;8(1). https://doi.org/10.1186/s13229-017-0173-5.
50. Hormozdiari F, Penn O, Borenstein E, Eichler EE. The discovery of integrated gene networks for autism and related disorders. *Genome Res.* 2015;25(1):142–154. https://doi.org/10.1101/gr.178855.114.
51. Iakoucheva LM, Muotri AR, Sebat J. Getting to the cores of autism. *Cell.* 2019;178(6):1287–1298. https://doi.org/10.1016/j.cell.2019.07.037.
52. Parikshak NN, Luo R, Zhang A, et al. Integrative functional genomic analyses implicate specific molecular pathways and circuits in autism. *Cell.* 2013;155(5):1008–1021. https://doi.org/10.1016/j.cell.2013.10.031.
53. Voineagu I. Gene expression studies in autism: moving from the genome to the transcriptome and beyond. *Neurobiol Dis.* 2011;45(1):69–75. https://doi.org/10.1016/j.nbd.2011.07.017.
54. Li T, Tian C, Scalmani P, et al. Action potential initiation in neocortical inhibitory interneurons. *PLoS Biol.* 2014;12(9). https://doi.org/10.1371/journal.pbio.1001944.
55. Gazina EV, Leaw BTW, Richards KL, et al. "Neonatal" Nav1.2 reduces neuronal excitability and affects seizure susceptibility and behaviour. *Hum Mol Genet.* 2015;24(5):1457–1468. https://doi.org/10.1093/hmg/ddu562.
56. Ben-Shalom R, Keeshen CM, Berrios KN, An JY, Sanders SJ, Bender KJ. Opposing effects on NaV1.2 function underlie differences between SCN2A variants observed in individuals with autism spectrum disorder or infantile seizures. *Biol Psychiatry.* 2017;82(3):1–9. https://doi.org/10.1016/j.biopsych.2017.01.009.
57. Spratt PWE, Ben-Shalom R, Keeshen CM, et al. The autism-associated gene Scn2a contributes to dendritic excitability and synaptic function in the prefrontal cortex. *Neuron.* 2019;103(4):673–685.e5. https://doi.org/10.1016/j.neuron.2019.05.037.
58. Sanders SJ, Campbell AJ, Cottrell JR, et al. Progress in understanding and treating SCN2A-mediated disorders. *Trends Neurosci.* 2018;41(7):1–15. https://doi.org/10.1016/j.tins.2018.03.011.
59. Hall LT, Sargent CL, Ganz WR, et al. EEG resting state spectral differences between SCN2A, idiopathic ASD, and typically-developing controls. In: *Presented at the International Society for Autism Research (INSAR) annual meeting*; 2021, May.
60. Hudac CM, Cairney B, DesChamps TD, et al. Brain correlates of the SCN2A phenotype. In: *Presented at the American Academy of Child and Adolescent Psychiatry annual meeting*; 2018, October.

61. Kumar S, Reynolds K, Ji Y, Gu R, Rai S, Zhou CJ. Impaired neurodevelopmental pathways in autism spectrum disorder: a review of signaling mechanisms and crosstalk. *J Neurodev Disord.* 2019;11(1):10. https://doi.org/10.1186/s11689-019-9268-y.
62. Hudac CM, Stessman HAF, DesChamps TD, et al. Exploring the heterogeneity of neural social indices for genetically distinct etiologies of autism. *J Neurodev Disord.* 2017;9(1):24. https://doi.org/10.1186/s11689-017-9199-4.
63. Nishiyama M, Oshikawa K, Tsukada Y, et al. CHD8 suppresses p53-mediated apoptosis through histone H1 recruitment during early embryogenesis. *Nat Cell Biol.* 2009;11(2):172–182. https://doi.org/10.1038/ncb1831.
64. Cotney J, Muhle RA, Sanders SJ, et al. The autism-associated chromatin modifier CHD8 regulates other autism risk genes during human neurodevelopment. *Nat Commun.* 2015;6(1):1–11. https://doi.org/10.1038/ncomms7404.
65. Beighley JS, Hudac CM, Arnett AB, et al. Clinical phenotypes of carriers of mutations in CHD8 or its conserved target genes. *Biol Psychiatry.* 2019. https://doi.org/10.1016/j.biopsych.2019.07.020.
66. Kurtz-Nelson EC, Beighley JS, Hudac CM, et al. Co-occurring medical conditions among individuals with ASD-associated disruptive mutations. *Child Health Care.* 2020;1–24. https://doi.org/10.1080/02739615.2020.1741361.
67. McCarthy SE, Gillis J, Kramer M, et al. De novo mutations in schizophrenia implicate chromatin remodeling and support a genetic overlap with autism and intellectual disability. *Mol Psychiatry.* 2014;19(6):652–658. https://doi.org/10.1038/mp.2014.29.
68. Owen MJ, O'Donovan MC. Schizophrenia and the neurodevelopmental continuum:evidence from genomics. *World Psychiatry.* 2017;16(3):227–235. https://doi.org/10.1002/wps.20440.
69. Werling DM, Brand H, An J-Y, et al. An analytical framework for whole-genome sequence association studies and its implications for autism spectrum disorder. *Nat Genet.* 2018;50(5):727–736. https://doi.org/10.1038/s41588-018-0107-y.
70. Turner TN, Wilfert AB, Bakken TE, et al. Sex-based analysis of De novo variants in neurodevelopmental disorders. *Am J Hum Genet.* 2019;105(6):1274–1285. https://doi.org/10.1016/j.ajhg.2019.11.003.
71. Consortium TS, Feliciano P, Daniels AM, et al. SPARK: A US cohort of 50,000 families to accelerate autism research. *Neuron.* 2018;97(3):488–493. https://doi.org/10.1016/j.neuron.2018.01.015.
72. Bejerano G, Haussler D, Blanchette M. Into the heart of darkness: large-scale clustering of human non-coding DNA. *Bioinformatics.* 2004;20(suppl_1):i40–i48. https://doi.org/10.1093/bioinformatics/bth946.
73. Lander ES, Linton LM, Birren B, et al. Initial sequencing and analysis of the human genome. *Nature.* 2001;409(6822):860–921. https://doi.org/10.1038/35057062.
74. Turner TN, Eichler EE. The role of De novo noncoding regulatory mutations in neurodevelopmental disorders. *Trends Neurosci.* 2019;42(2):115–127. https://doi.org/10.1016/j.tins.2018.11.002.
75. An J-Y, Lin K, Zhu L, et al. Genome-wide de novo risk score implicates promoter variation in autism spectrum disorder. *Science.* 2018;362(6420). https://doi.org/10.1126/science.aat6576, eaat6576.
76. Markenscoff-Papadimitriou E, Whalen S, Przytycki P, et al. A chromatin accessibility atlas of the developing human telencephalon. *Cell.* 2020;182(3):754–769.e18. https://doi.org/10.1016/j.cell.2020.06.002.
77. Turner TN, Coe BP, Dickel DE, et al. Genomic patterns of De novo mutation in simplex autism. *Cell.* 2017;171(3):710–722.e12. https://doi.org/10.1016/j.cell.2017.08.047.
78. Zhou J, Park CY, Theesfeld CL, et al. Whole-genome deep-learning analysis identifies contribution of noncoding mutations to autism risk. *Nat Genet.* 2019;51(6):973–980. https://doi.org/10.1038/s41588-019-0420-0.

79. Krumm N, Turner TN, Baker C, et al. Excess of rare, inherited truncating mutations in autism. *Nat Genet.* 2015;47(6):582–588. https://doi.org/10.1038/ng.3303.
80. Brandler WM, Antaki D, Gujral M, et al. Paternally inherited cis-regulatory structural variants are associated with autism. *Science.* 2018;360(6386):327–331. https://doi.org/10.1126/science.aan2261.
81. Guo H, Duyzend MH, Coe BP, et al. Genome sequencing identifies multiple deleterious variants in autism patients with more severe phenotypes. *Genet Med.* 2019;21(7):1611–1620. https://doi.org/10.1038/s41436-018-0380-2.
82. Hiatt SM, Lawlor JMJ, Handley LH, et al. Long-read genome sequencing for the molecular diagnosis of neurodevelopmental disorders. *Hum Genet Genomics Adv.* 2021;2(2). https://doi.org/10.1016/j.xhgg.2021.100023, 100023.

CHAPTER

# 10

# Cellular and molecular neurobiology of autism spectrum disorder

*Gareth Chapman, Irene Antony, Mishka Narasimhan, Renata Shen, Rachel Elman, and Kristen L. Kroll*

**Department of Developmental Biology, Washington University School of Medicine, Saint Louis, MO, United States**

## Introduction

Autism spectrum disorder (ASD) is a genetically complex disorder with significant effects on the lives of affected individuals and their families; however, its etiology remains poorly understood. Recent improvements in techniques for using human pluripotent stem cells (hPSCs) to model aspects of human brain development have spurred significant advancement in our understanding of the cellular pathology associated with ASD. While genetic abnormalities that contribute substantially to ASD etiology were previously in studied in animal models, differences between humans and other animals, both in the genome sequence and in key aspects of human fetal brain development, necessitate human models.[1] However, the inaccessibility of the human fetal brain and inability to experimentally manipulate human brain-derived materials represent major challenges for studying the basis of ASD and other neurodevelopmental disorders. Over the past decade, hPSC models have begun to fill this gap, enabling derivation of human neurons and glia bearing ASD genetic liability. These models have been used to dissect contributors to disease and to test potential molecular and pharmacologic interventions to reverse ASD-associated cellular and molecular phenotypes. Here, we present genetic



https://doi.org/10.1016/B978-0-12-816393-1.00007-5

liabilities associated with ASD and major approaches used to model these in human pluripotent stem cell models of neurodevelopment. We then describe ASD-associated cellular and molecular phenotypes frequently observed in these hPSC models, including proliferative, metabolic, and synaptic phenotypes, imbalances in neuronal excitation versus inhibition, and alterations in glial development and function. Collectively, these studies provide insights into how alteration of neurodevelopmental programs may contribute to ASD, while also providing platforms for testing approaches for phenotype reversal, which could enable the development of interventions for individuals with ASD.

## Genetic liability for ASD

Genetic liability for ASD falls into three general categories. The first involves copy number variants (CNVs) that duplicate or delete genomic intervals often encompassing multiple genes and other noncoding elements.[2] While these mutations are generally very rare, they significantly increase the risk for ASD and other neurodevelopmental disorders. By contrast, liability also stems from single nucleotide polymorphisms (SNPs). These single base changes in the genetic code have been linked to an increased risk of developing ASD through recent large scale genome and exome sequencing of human populations.[3] Unlike CNVs, most SNPs are unlikely to confer major increases in risk; instead, they function additively or synergistically, with the presence of many liability-associated SNPs affecting an individual's overall risk of developing ASD (often referred to as a polygenic risk score). Despite their frequently low penetrance, modeling of genetic risk for ASD can be done by manipulating the expression and/or sequence of genes associated with these SNPs. Finally, cellular models can also be created from idiopathic ASD cases.[4] In these cases, while it is presumed that there is a genetic component to the development of the disorder, this remains unknown or undiscovered.

## Human pluripotent stem cell models of ASD

There are two major ways in which human pluripotent stem cell models (hPSCs, encompassing both embryonic and induced pluripotent stem cells (hESCs/iPSCs)) can be generated, based upon the nature of the genetic aberration being studied (Fig. 1). The first and perhaps simplest approach is to create induced pluripotent stem cell (iPSC) models by reprogramming somatic cells from an individual or individuals carrying the genetic anomaly of interest.[5] This is a popular approach for studying CNV-based risk for autism,[2] as CNVs are large and difficult to model using other methods.

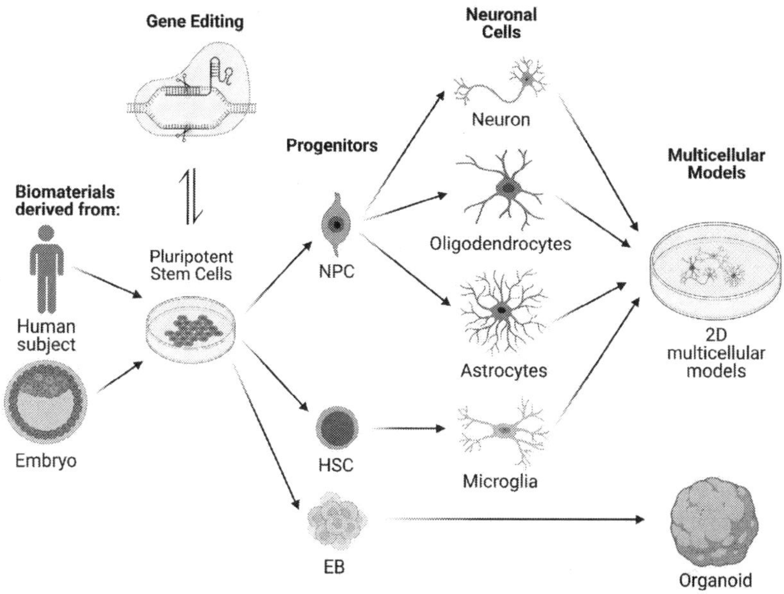


**FIG. 1** Approaches for the generation of human pluripotent stem cell models and their differentiation into neurons and glia. Pluripotent stem cells can be derived either by reprogramming of human somatic cells to generate induced pluripotent stem cells or obtained directly from embryos (embryonic stem cells). The genome of these pluripotent stem cells can be edited using techniques such as CRISPR/Cas9 gene editing to introduce a mutation of interest. The pluripotent stem cells can then be differentiated into the required progenitor population. Neural progenitor cells (NPCs) can be used to produce neurons, oligodendrocytes, and astrocytes. Microglia are instead produced from hematopoietic stem cells (HSC). Finally, organoids can be generated from embryoid bodies (EBs), which are collections of undifferentiated stem cells.

This is also the only viable method for studying idiopathic ASD as, without a known genetic cause, these cases cannot be modeled using other methods. However, the use of iPSC models presents its own challenges. A major challenge is to develop valid controls with which to match iPSC models from subjects with ASD, as human patients are genetically heterogeneous and carry many additional genetic variants that may contribute to ASD, beyond the gene or genes under study. In some cases, it is possible to correct the mutation of interest to create an isogenic pair of hPSC lines[6] with and without a given mutation. However, depending on the size and complexity of the genetic aberration being studied, this is not always possible. Therefore, in many cases, it is necessary to use large numbers of control iPSC lines to account for contributors to cellular phenotypes that relate to differences in the genetic background between individuals. Other technical challenges that must be addressed for iPSC modeling involve assuring that these lines maintain pluripotency, as well as the high cost and labor associated with their generation and maintenance.

A second commonly used approach involves creating models by using gene editing techniques such as CRISPR/Cas9 editing.[7] This allows the introduction of ASD-associated mutations, ranging from single nucleotide changes to gene ablations, into a known cell type (often an iPSC or ESC). This approach offers the advantage that the genetic changes under study are precisely defined and an isogenic control line is available. However, production of the required mutation can be technically challenging and concerns remain regarding the potential to introduce unwanted mutations when using CRISPR/Cas9 and other gene editing systems.[8] This methodology is particularly popular for studying ASD risk that is associated with a single mutation or gene (the origin of which could be derived from SNP or CNV data). Techniques based on CRISPR/Cas9 have also been developed for modulating the expression of genes without altering the genome sequence.[9] In summary, while challenges remain, advancements in the manipulation and use of hPSC models have enabled the development of nuanced cellular models of complex genetic abnormalities, which can then be used to model cellular and molecular alterations of neurodevelopment or function associated with ASD.

## Deriving neurons from iPSCs to model ASD

Having developed an hPSC model with the desired characteristics for modeling ASD, the next goal is to generate disease-relevant cell type(s) for study. There are two general approaches to generate neuronal cell types of interest from pluripotent stem cells: developmental patterning and direct reprogramming. The goal of developmental patterning is to recapitulate aspects of early human neuronal development by activating or repressing key signaling pathways to recapitulate a developmental trajectory in vitro that resembles events that occur during fetal brain development in vivo.[10] On the other hand, direct reprogramming skips multiple stages of development, using the overexpression of key transcription factors to directly convert pluripotent stem cells into the desired cell type.[11] While both methodologies can be used to produce a similar end product, developmental patterning approaches have proved more popular for cellular modeling of ASD, as they more faithfully recapitulate the early stages of neuronal development that are often disrupted to contribute to ASD.[12]

The development of the cerebral cortex has been a particular focus for cellular models of ASD. The human cerebral cortex is the outermost layer of the brain and functions as the processing center of the central nervous system. The core of the cerebral cortex is a layered structure of excitatory glutamatergic neurons formed from the base (or ventricular zone), which forms in the dorsal telencephalon of the developing brain (Fig. 2). Cortical patterning occurs in an inside-out direction, with the earliest born neurons occupying deep, while later born neurons occupy more superficial layers of the cortex. As it develops, the cortex is infiltrated by inhibitory GABAergic cortical neurons; a majority of these are generated in a subcortical, ventral telencephalic progenitor territory called the medial ganglionic eminence (MGE) and then migrate tangentially to establish connections with excitatory neurons in the different layers of the developing cortex. Cortical excitatory and inhibitory neurons represent a major focus of ASD modeling studies because altered development of either or both of these neuronal cell types, or imbalances in their activities, appear to contribute substantially to ASD etiology.[13,14] Therefore, major efforts have been made to develop effective protocols to differentiate hPSCs into these cortical neuron cell types in vitro.

Early protocols for generating neurons from iPSCs exploited the general principle that pluripotent cells can undergo default specification into

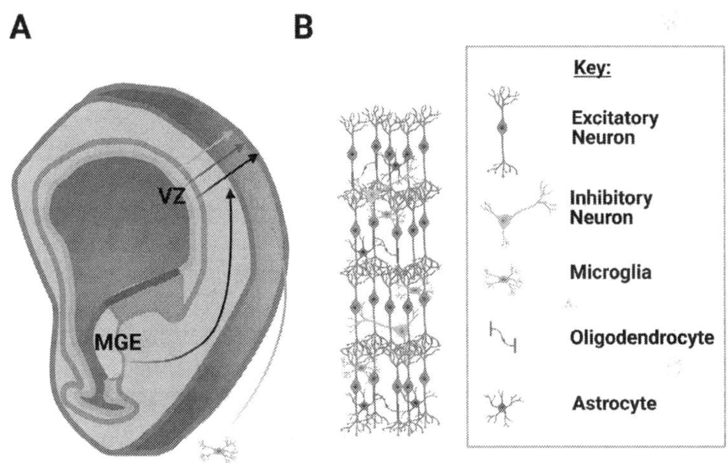


FIG. 2 Cortical development and organization. (A) Schematized view of a coronal section through the human telencephalon at 15 postconception weeks. The cerebral cortex is a complex and highly organized structure comprised of 5 cell types. The structure is derived from layers of excitatory neurons that form in the ventricular zone (VZ, green) and radially migrate outward (green arrow). Inhibitory neurons are generated in a subcortical progenitor territory called the medial ganglionic eminence (MGE, blue, with the adjoining lateral ganglionic eminence shown in purple). MGE-derived inhibitory neurons migrate tangentially into the developing cortex (blue arrow). Astrocytes are later produced by the same neuronal progenitors that produced the excitatory neurons (brown arrow). Oligodendrocytes are originally generated in the MGE and infiltrate the cortex; however, most of these cells are replaced by oligodendrocytes that develop in the VZ by birth (black arrows). Finally, microglia infiltrate the brain through the developing circulatory system (yellow arrow). (B) The five neuronal and glial cell types present and their general arrangement to form cortical layers.

neuroectoderm when media that retains pluripotency is removed, and these cells then form neuronal precursors with minimal interference.[15] However, while this protocol could generate neurons and glia, it allowed very little control over the specific cell types produced, resulting in high variability. More advanced protocols instead used signaling cues to specify a particular type of neuronal precursor, which could then differentiate into a particular type of neuron. The use of inhibitors of SMAD transcription factors that mediate responses to bone morphogenetic protein (BMP) and Activin/Nodal-type TGF-beta signaling (so-called dual SMAD inhibition) to induce neuroectoderm provided a critical stepping stone for developing more robust protocols to generate particular types of neuronal cells.[10] Dual SMAD inhibition drives loss of pluripotency and specification of neural progenitor cells (NPCs) with a forebrain regional identity. During brain development, cortical neurons migrate to form different cortical layers, with earlier born neurons occupying deep and later born neurons occupying upper, more superficial layers. This in vitro scheme models some of these events, producing primarily deep layer excitatory glutamatergic neurons, but also having the potential to generate upper layer glutamatergic neurons and small numbers of GABAergic interneurons. Importantly, these protocols also recapitulate some aspects of the time course of early human cortical development, with specification of neural progenitors followed by differentiation into immature neurons, which mature into electrophysiologically active functional neurons.

Further protocols have been developed for deriving cortical glutamatergic neurons, with a focus on decreasing the time required, as dual SMAD inhibition-based protocols can take 40–50 days to generate neurons and a further 40–50 days for development of fully functional neuronal networks.[16] These efforts focused on using mitotic inhibitors to synchronize neuronal differentiation, while simultaneously preventing continued neuronal precursor proliferation.[17,18] While this approach does depart from the aim of recapitulating neuronal development in vivo, it produces a more homogeneous product that may allow more subtle phenotypes relevant to neurodevelopmental and psychiatric disorders to be detected. Recent work has used these concepts in combination with developmental patterning approaches to substantially shorten protocols for the generation of cortical excitatory neurons.[19] Alternatively, the most rapid approach for producing cortical excitatory neurons remains direct reprogramming by overexpressing the transcription factor neurogenin-2 (NGN2). While this method bypasses key stages of neuronal development, it can efficiently convert pluripotent stem cells into functional neurons in ~ 2–4 weeks.[11] Neurons produced using this methodology are glutamatergic cortical excitatory neurons. However, while the population of neurons generated using this method are highly similar to one another, they do not recapitulate the diversity of glutamatergic neurons present in the human cerebral cortex and may not as closely resemble a genuine cell type found in vivo.

Compared to generating excitatory glutamatergic neurons, more complex protocols are required to generate relatively pure populations of inhibitory GABAergic interneurons. The critical modifications involve inducing neural progenitors that have a ventral rather than dorsal forebrain identity, by activating sonic hedgehog (SHH) signaling and reducing WNT signaling.[20] While these modifications can robustly produce GABAergic interneurons, it is still challenging to generate certain subtypes of GABAergic interneurons, such as those expressing Parvalbumin. Therefore, the development of protocols for generating particular GABAergic interneuron subtypes remains a key area of research, with developments in this area allowing this complex family of neurons to be utilized for further interrogation of phenotypes. Direct reprogramming approaches have also been developed for the production of GABAergic neurons: while multiple combinations of transcription factors can successfully produce GABAergic interneurons, systematic examination has shown that the combination of achaete-scute family BHLH transcription factor 1 (ASCL1), distal-less homeobox 2 (DLX2), and myelin transcription factor 1 like (MYT1L) was most effective in generating functional GABAergic interneurons.[21] However, similar to the concerns related to direct reprogramming of excitatory glutamatergic neurons, there are concerns over the ability of this methodology to recapitulate the extant diversity, particularly considering the high diversity of interneuron subtypes present in the brain in vivo.

## Deriving astrocytes and oligodendrocytes from iPSC models

While most prior work has focused on modeling neuronal dysfunction associated with neurodevelopmental disorders, more recently, deficits in glia have also been assessed. Glial cells, including astrocytes, oligodendrocytes, and microglia, support neuronal function. While their activity was previously considered less central to neurodevelopmental disorders, more recent work has shown that their activities are critical to proper nervous system function, while disruption of glial development or function can contribute to ASD.[22,23] Astrocytes are the most common cell type found in the central nervous system (CNS) and are as diverse a cell population as neurons. Astrocytes are responsible for a variety of functions including trophic support, neuronal synapse formation, mediation of inflammation, and facilitating axonal guidance, among many others.

The simplest way to produce astrocytes from hPSCs is to differentiate them into NPCs and then supplement the media with serum (e.g. fetal bovine serum; FBS) while removing all other signaling modifiers.[24] To aid in the production of functionally mature astrocytes, supplements that support astrocyte differentiation and function can be added.[25] More recent publications have also begun to examine the complexity of astrocyte biology by producing white matter-like (fibrous) and gray matter-like (protoplasmic) astrocytes.[26] Classical astrocyte production is thought to produce gray matter-like astrocytes, whereas using ciliary neurotrophic factor (CNTF) instead of FBS to induce astrocytic differentiation has been shown to produce a gray matter-like population. Further research in this area may further delineate astrocytic subtypes, reminiscent of similar efforts that have been made to derive neuronal derivatives in the GABAergic interneuron family. Direct reprogramming approaches to produce astrocytes have also been developed, with the most effective protocol focused on SRY-box transcription factor 9 (SOX9) and nuclear factor I B-type (NFIB) overexpression.[27] However, given the comparative ease with which astrocytes can be produced, the developmental patterning approach remains a more accessible option.

While generating neurons and astrocytes from human PSCs was relatively simple, the induction of oligodendrocytes has proven significantly more challenging. While oligodendrocytes do not have the subtype variability seen in neurons and astrocytes, they develop through multiple developmental stages [SRY-box transcription factor 10 (SOX10) and oligodendrocyte transcription factor 2 (OLIG2) expressing (+) progenitors, oligodendrocyte marker O4 + migratory progenitors, and myelin basic protein (MBP) + functional cells]. Recapitulating this developmental program is critical to generating functional oligodendrocytes. Oligodendrocytes are required to myelinate neurons, encircling them with a complex structure called a myelin sheath, which allows faster signal conduction of signals and protects neurons. Early protocols were developed that used hESCs to generate glial cells by the addition of brain-derived neurotrophic factor (BDNF), epidermal growth factor (EGF), retinoic acid, and triiodothyronine (T3). While these cells did go through SOX10 + and O4 + oligodendrocyte progenitor stages and could myelinate neurons when transplanted into myelin deficient mice, they did not produce myelin in monoculture.[28]

Developmental patterning-based approaches to generate oligodendrocytes by mimicking early human neural development involved generating neural precursors with a ventral forebrain identity, to mirror early waves of oligodendrocyte production. Protocols for deriving MGE-like progenitors provided a starting point for these protocols, which used dual SMAD inhibition plus an SHH agonist and a low dose of retinoic acid to derive ventral forebrain like progenitors.[29] This approach produced large numbers of OLIG2 expressing cells, which could then be induced to form O4 + oligodendrocyte progenitor cells (OPCs) with the addition of growth factors and supplements including platelet derived growth factor (PDGF), hepatocyte growth factor (HGF), T3, and cyclic AMP (cAMP). While this protocol robustly generated oligodendrocytes from an array of iPSC lines, it was very long, requiring at least 95 days to produce myelinating oligodendrocytes. In subsequent work, minor modifications were made to this protocol by treating progenitors for a more limited time with specific growth factors (PDGF, HGF, insulin-like growth factor 1 (IGF-1) and neurotrophin 3 (NT3)), reducing the time taken to generate MBP + cells to 75 days.[30]

Given the high utility of producing oligodendrocytes from pluripotent stem cells, there are comparatively few protocols for generating oligodendrocytes by direct reprogramming. One such published protocol enables conversion of fibroblasts to oligodendrocytes; however, the efficiency of OPC production, as measured by O4 positivity, was relatively low (15%–30%).[31] Two additional published protocols[32,33] use a combination of developmental patterning and direct reprogramming to achieve conversion of iPSCs into oligodendrocytes. Human iPSCs are first differentiated into neuronal precursors employing protocols developed using developmental patterning approaches; however, when complex media conditions would otherwise have been used to enrich for oligodendrocyte precursors, overexpression of key transcription factors (OLIG2, SOX10, and NK6 homeobox 2 (NKX6–2)) is instead used to convert the NPCs into functional oligodendrocytes. While this technique does produce oligodendrocytes significantly faster than the conventional developmental patterning approaches, the efficiency remains low, with only ~ 50%–60% of cells transduced with the transcription factor overexpression constructs expressing the oligodendrocyte marker O4, while only one fifth of these cells subsequently express MBP (a key marker of functional oligodendrocytes).[32,33]

## Deriving microglia from iPSC models

As described above for other glial cell types, original protocols for generating microglia from pluripotent stem cells focused on deriving microglia from a neuroectodermal lineage. However, investigations into the developmental origins of microglia provided clear evidence that microglia instead originate from mesodermally derived primitive yolk sac progenitors.[34] Therefore, more recent protocols have focused on deriving microglia from hematopoietic precursors. Most current protocols[35–37] follow three stages, successively inducing hematopoietic stem cells (using growth factors such as stem cell factor (SCF) and vascular endothelial growth factor (VEGF)), microglia progenitors (using cytokines such as macrophage colony-stimulating factor (M-CSF)) and mature microglia (using cytokines such as interleukin-34 (IL-34)). Unlike other neuronal cell types, direct reprogramming approaches have not yet been developed for deriving into microglia from pluripotent stem cells.

## Using iPSCs to derive cerebral organoids

More recently, the advent of complex 3D cellular models otherwise known as organoids has begun to allow the examination of cellular phenotypes in a more complex and physiologically relevant system. The original protocol for organoid generation relied on a self-organizing system with minimal addition patterning cues[38]; therefore, the results were highly varied, including the production of nonneuronal tissues.[39] More recent advances in the field, using the knowledge gained from the generation of developmental patterning approaches for effectively deriving specific neuronal cell types, have led to more complex organoid protocols that more closely recapitulate the development of discrete areas of the developing brain.[40] Further research has also shown that organoids can be used to develop astrocytes, neurons and oligodendrocytes[41] and can also be supplemented with microglia generated from pluripotent stem cells.[42] Therefore, this system provides the closest facsimile to a developing human brain. However, while the intrinsic complexity of these models allows a greater understanding of the interplay between neuronal cell types, this can make understanding the precise nature of the deficit in question challenging. There also remain concerns about the reproducibility of organoid-based studies, due to the relative lack of control over the developing system. To examine the interaction between multiple neuronal cell types of interest without incurring some of the limitations of highly complex organoid models, some groups have instead focused on more simple 2D multilineage models that involving combining different neuronal cell types as separate cell populations.[43,44] While the use of these models has so far been limited, as our understanding of the etiology of ASD using reductionist single cell models becomes clearer, these more complex 2D and 3D cell models are likely to become more salient.

## ASD-associated phenotypes observed in patient iPSC-derived models of neurodevelopment

Among the cellular phenotypes that have been associated with ASD in human subject-derived iPSC models, common alterations include changes in the metabolic and proliferative properties of these models during their specification and/or differentiation into neural restricted progenitors and into neurons or glia. Other common phenotypes include alterations to neuronal function, including changes in synaptic activity, as well as alterations of excitatory or inhibitory neuron development. All of these can more generally affect the balance of neuronal excitation versus inhibition in ASD-associated models. Finally, while these have not yet been extensively characterized in cellular models of ASD, disrupted glial development and function has been observed in a number of extant ASD models, and undoubtedly represents a still under-characterized contributor to ASD phenotypes. Examples of these phenotypes have been summarized in Table 1 and Fig. 3 and are drawn from some of the extant ASD cellular modeling literature.

**TABLE 1** Core phenotypes identified in cellular models of ASD associated mutations.[4,16,41,43–90]

| ASD-linked mutation | PSC cell type | Neuronal cell type/s | Model generation | Core phenotypes | | | | | References |
|---|---|---|---|---|---|---|---|---|---|
| | | | | Metabolism | Proliferation, differentiation | Synapses | Function | Glia | |
| TCS1/2 | iPSC | N, O | DP | | | | ↑ | X | 16, 45 |
| HRAS | iPSC | A | DP | | | | | X | 46 |
| NRXN1 | iPSC | N, A | DP | | | | ↑ | X | 47-50 |
| FMR1 | ESC | N, A | DP | | X | | ↓ | X | 51, 52 |
| FMR1 | iPSC | NS | DP | | | | | | 53 |
| MECP2 | ESC, iPSC | N, A | DP | X | X | ↓ | ↓ | X | 41, 54-59 |
| CDKL5 | iPSC | N | DP | | | ↓ | | | 60 |
| UBE3A | iPSC | N, A | DP | | | | ↓ | | 61 |
| UBE3A | ESC | N | DD | | | | ↑ | | 62 |
| CACNA1C | iPSC | N | DP | | X | | | | 63 |
| CACNA1C | iPSC | Org | DP | | X | | | | 64 |
| SHANK3 | ESC, iPSC | N | DP | | X | ↓ | | | 65-68 |
| SHANK3 | ESC | N | DD | | | ↓ | ↓ | | 87 |
| EHMT1 | iPSC | N | DP | | | | ↓ | | 69 |
| SHANK2 | iPSC | N | DP | | | ↑ | ↑ | | 44 |
| NLGN4 | iPSC | N | DD | | | ↑ | ↑ | | 70 |

*Continued*

**TABLE 1** Core phenotypes identified in cellular models of ASD associated mutations [4,16,41,43–86]—cont'd

| | | | | | | | | | |
|---|---|---|---|---|---|---|---|---|---|
| NRXN1 | iPSC | N | DP | | X | | ↓ | X | 71,72 |
| 16p11.2 deletion | iPSC | N | DP | | X | ↑ | ↑ | | 73 |
| 16p11.2 duplication | iPSC | N | DP | | X | ↓ | ↓ | | 73 |
| TRPC6 | iPSC | N | DP | | | ↓ | | | 88 |
| PTCHD1 | iPSC | N | DP | | | ↑ | ↓ | | 74 |
| SCN2A | iPSC | N | DD | | | | ↓ | | 89 |
| ATRX | iPSC | N | DD | | | | ↓ | | 89 |
| AFF2 | iPSC | N | DD | | | | ↓ | | 89 |
| KCNQ2 | iPSC | N | DD | | | | ↓ | | 89 |
| ASTN2 | iPSC | N | DD | | | | ↓ | | 89 |
| Idiopathic | iPSC | N, A | DP | X | | ↓ | ↓ | X | 43 |
| Idiopathic | iPSC | N | DP | | | | ↓ | | 75 |
| Idiopathic | iPSC | N | DP | | | | ↓ | | 76 |
| Idiopathic | iPSC | N | DP | | X | ↓ | ↓ | | 4 |
| Idiopathic | iPSC | N | DP | | X | | | | 77 |
| Idiopathic | iPSC | Org | DP | | X | ↑ | | | 78 |
| RAB39b | iPSC | Org | DP | | X | | | | 90 |
| Idiopathic | iPSC | N | DP | | | | ↑ | | 79 |
| EHMT2 | iPSC | N | DD | | | | ↑ | | 80, 81 |
| CNTN5 | iPSC | N | DD | | | | ↑ | | 80, 81 |
| CDKL5 | iPSC | N | DP | X | | | | | 82 |
| NF1 | iPSC | N, Org | DP | | X | | | X | 83 |
| Idiopathic | iPSC | N | DP | | X | | | | 84 |
| Idiopathic | iPSC | N | DP | | X | | | | 85 |
| VPS13B | iPSC | N | DP | | X | ↓ | | | 86 |

N = neurons, O = oligodendrocytes, A = astrocytes, Org = organoids, NS = neurospheres, DP = developmental patterning, DD = direct differentiation. X indicates the phenotyping categories described in each study and the arrows and color coding indicates increased (green) versus decreased (red) changes in synapse production or neuronal function.

## Altered cellular metabolism: Oxidative stress in ASD models

Alterations of oxidative stress that may contribute to ASD pathogenesis involve imbalances between the synthesis of reactive oxygen species (ROS) and the body's ability to block their deleterious effects using antioxidative systems. As central regulators of oxygen metabolism,

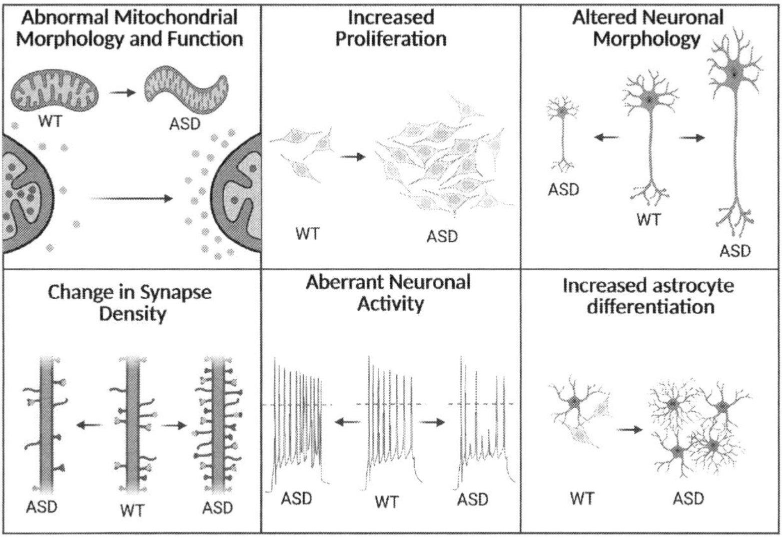


**FIG. 3** Major classes of cellular phenotypes associated with ASD. Abnormal mitochondrial morphology and function has been observed by both electron microscopy and by using fluorescent markers of mitochondrial membrane potential. Increased NPC proliferation is also commonly observed in ASD models. Altered neuronal morphology, often involving changes in soma and dendrite size, has been observed in ASD models; however, the directionality of this phenotype (e.g., reduced or increased size) is largely linked to the model being assessed. Changes in synapse density are also commonly observed by measuring dendritic spine density and examining the expression pattern of synaptic markers. However, synapse density has also been shown to both increase and decrease in ASD cellular models, depending on the particular model under investigation. Aberrant neuronal activity is likewise a common feature of ASD cellular models, with both increased and decreased neuronal and neuronal network activity observed, depending on the mutation being studied. Finally, there is limited evidence for association of increased astrocyte differentiation with ASD.

mitochondria are responsible for both production and elimination of ROS, while deficits in mitochondrial function affect this process. Commonly alterations in mitochondrial morphology and mitochondrial membrane potential are seen as hallmarks of abnormal mitochondrial function which are likely to result in abnormal ROS production or elimination.

Studying two hESC-derived models, one with a patient derived mutation in methyl-CpG binding protein 2 (*MECP2*) and other with *MECP2* knockout (both achieved using CRISPR/Cas9 mediated mutation), Bu et al.[54] established that both models showed an increase in mitochondrial fragmentation and a reduction in mitochondrial membrane potential.[54] Taken together these phenotypes suggest that mitochondrial health has been compromised in these models. Similarly, in an iPSC model carrying a heterozygous mutation in cyclin-dependent kinase-like 5 (*CDKL5*) that is associated with ASD, Jagtap et al. reported a similar decrease in mitochondrial membrane potential and abnormal mitochondrial morphology.[82] Extending this further, Jagtap et al. also reported that *CDKL5* mutant cells had increased oxygen consumption compared to controls. This result further confirms that *CDKL5* mutation caused abnormal mitochondrial function that was likely to result in increased ROS production. Therefore, while oxidative stress phenotypes have not yet been broadly characterized in ASD iPSC models, there is preliminary evidence from limited studies in cellular models to suggest that this is an important area for future exploration.

## Altered neuronal development: Abnormalities in neuronal production and morphology

Data from multiple iPSC models of neurodevelopmental disorders including ASD suggest that altered proliferative control of neural progenitor cells occurs often and is a frequent contributor to patient phenotypes, particularly in cases of brain growth disorders such as macrocephaly.[91] For example, in a study of neurofibromatosis type I, an inherited neurocutaneous disorder associated with neurodevelopmental disorders including ASD, Anastasaki et al. suggested that multiple forms of the neurofibromin 1 (*NF1*) germline mutation result in increased RAS activity and elevated NPC proliferation.[83] Likewise, Mariani et al. found that iPSC-derived brain organoids from idiopathic autism patients exhibited an accelerated cell cycle and subsequently overproduced GABAergic inhibitory neurons.[78] Increases to proliferation were also experimentally observed by Moore et al. in an iPSC-derived NPC model derived from patients with idiopathic ASD.[84] An accelerated cell cycle was also reflected by increasing rates of DNA damage in ASD iPSC-derived NPC models derived from macrocephalic ASD patients.[77,85] In particular, by comparison with normal NPCs, Wang observed that macrocephalic NPCs exhibited higher than average rates of DNA damage at replication stress-susceptible genes with higher rates of double-strand breaks.[85] This was observed in combination with acceleration of the S phase of cell division. Likewise, after differentiating iPSCS into excitatory microtubule-associated protein 2 (MAP2)-expressing neurons, Shaefer et al. observed dysregulation of specific gene networks associated with acceleration of growth, with the expression of specific genes associated with synapse organization and neuron generation affected (including BR serine/threonine kinase 1, calcium voltage-gated channel auxiliary subunit beta 1, RAS-associated protein RAB3A, and glypican 2). These gene expression changes were linked to altered chromatin accessibility of these genes at early stages of NPC development. Likewise, epigenetic analysis of four lines of iPSCs derived from males diagnosed with fragile X syndrome, a neurodevelopmental disease frequently co-diagnosed with autism, found changes to methylation patterns in genes that control neuronal cell maturation.[52] In particular, this resulted in hypermethylation of the fragile X mental retardation 1 (*FMR1*) gene, which reduced its expression. As another example, neural cells derived from individuals with idiopathic autism exhibited increased NPC proliferation, which was linked to dysregulation of a β-catenin/BRN2 transcriptional cascade; this dysregulation also contributed to later functional neuronal deficits.[4]

While the studies summarized above highlight a frequent finding of increased rates of proliferation in ASD patient-derived iPSC models, it should be noted that this is not universally observed: in some cases, ASD iPSC-derived NPCs instead displayed reduced or unaltered proliferation. For example, an iPSC line derived from a patient with Cohen syndrome, a rare autosomal disorder associated with mutations in the vacuolar protein sorting 13 homolog C (*VPS13*) gene, a novel compound heterozygous mutation in *VPS13* was linked to reduced proliferation in SRY-box transcription factor 2 (SOX2)-expressing neural progenitor cells.[86] As another example, Adhya et al. observed no difference in the proliferation and differentiation potential of ASD iPSC models from patients with macrocephaly versus control iPSCs although the ASD-derived cells exhibited neurodevelopmental impairment, failing to form the neural rosette structures into which neuroepithelial progenitors self-organize in culture.[92] Given the lack of proliferative phenotypes in these models, the authors suggested that the observed differentiation-related anomalies may occur independently of the macrocephaly associated alterations in cell proliferation that were presumed to underpin the patient phenotype.

Beyond altered NPC proliferation, multiple studies have also reported deficits in neuronal development that result in abnormal neuronal morphology. For example, mutations in SH3 and multiple ankyrin repeat domains 2 (*SHANK2*) have been associated with ASD and have been shown to promote neuronal hyperconnectivity in iPSC-derived cortical neurons carrying mutations in *SHANK2*.[44] This model developed increased dendrite complexity and length and exhibited impaired plasticity, with an impaired transcriptional response to neuronal activity.[44] A similar set of experiments examined iPSC lines with deletions in the 16p11.2 region of the human genome, which is also associated with increased risk of developing ASD, demonstrating that these cells exhibited both increased soma size and dendrite length.[73]

As SH3 and multiple ankyrin repeat domains 3 (*SHANK3*) deletion also contributes to ASD, similar experiments have also focused on iPSC lines derived from patients with SHANK3 mutations.[65] However, rather than increased dendrite complexity, neurons derived from these lines instead exhibited reduced dendrite length and complexity. Related deficits in synaptic transmission were observed, as well as impaired early and late-stage neurodevelopment. Contrasting with the increased soma size observed in models derived from patients with deletions at the 16p11.2 locus, Deshpandi et al. observed that 16p11.2 duplication (also associated with an increased risk of ASD) instead caused decreased neuron soma size and dendrite length. Similar results were observed in an iPSC model of Rett syndrome (RTT), with iPSC-derived neurons exhibiting reduced dendrite length as well as reduced soma size by comparison with controls.[55] Together, these results suggest that both deficits in proliferation and altered neuronal differentiation are hallmarks of ASD pathology. However, while there is mounting evidence for an increase in proliferation associated with ASD patient-derived models, specific alterations of neuronal morphology presently appear to be more strongly associated with the genetic risk factor under examination than with the diagnosis of ASD.

## Altered neuronal function: Changes in synapse production associated with ASD

Neuronal phenotypes involving altered synaptic development or function are also frequently observed in ASD cellular models. Among the most prominent phenotypes are changes in density of dendritic spines and changes in gene expression associated with synaptic development. Dendritic spines are small protrusions from dendrites, which are the location of over 90% of all excitatory synapses; as such, changes in their density and morphology have long been used to infer deficits in synapse production. More recent work has also focused on measuring synapse production more directly, by focusing on the expression of markers of the presynaptic and postsynaptic densities (either scaffold proteins such as post-synaptic density protein-95 (PSD-95) or synaptic transporters such as vesicular glutamate transporter 1 (VGLUT1)).

Models of multiple neurodevelopmental disorders exhibit altered dendritic spine density at glutamatergic synapses, including either increases or decreases in density. This is concordant with the observation that the genomes of individuals with ASD are overrepresented for CNVs that disrupt genes associated with postsynaptic density.[93] For example, mutations in *CDLK5*, critical for maintaining stability among excitatory and inhibitory synapses, have been associated with ASD. Patient iPSC models of *CDLK5* disruption exhibited reduction in presynaptic (VGLUT1) and postsynaptic (PSD-95) positive puncta and a corresponding increase in the size of dendritic spines in this patient iPSC-derived neuronal model, suggesting a strengthening of the remaining synapses.[60] Similar effects have been seen in models of *MECP2* mutation,[55] 16p11.2 duplication,[73] and transient receptor potential cation channel subfamily C member 6 (*TRPC6*) mutation.[94]

By contrast, studies have also shown an increase in synapse production associated with ASD risk genes. For example, a mutation in Neuroligin 4 X-Linked (*NLGN4X*) that was identified in an ASD patient and modeled in hESCs was associated with increased production of synapses, as measured by the postsynaptic marker PSD-95.[70] No other significant changes in neuronal morphology were observed in this model. In examining mutations in patched domain containing 1 (*PTCHD1*) in iPSC-derived neurons, Ross et al. similarly observed an increased synaptic density in one of the patient models, as measured with both a presynaptic (Synapsin I, SYN1) and a postsynaptic (homer scaffold protein 1, HOMER1) marker.[74] Similar results have also been observed in iPSC-derived neurons carrying mutations in *SHANK2*[44] or a deletion at the 16p11.2 locus.[73]

In examining idiopathic ASD in iPSC-derived neuronal models, Marchetto et al.[4] found decreased synapse production, as measured with the presynaptic markers (VGLUT1 and SYN1). However, in examining a similar idiopathic ASD patient population in a ventral telencephic organoid model, Mariani et al. instead showed an increase in synapse production (specifically an increase in punctae expressing SYN1 and the vesicular GABA transporter, VGAT) with no change in VGLUT1 + punctae. Alterations in the regulation of gene expression programs involved in synaptic development represent another contributor to altered synapse formation and function in ASD. For example, in examining the effects of mutations in *CDKL5, MECP2,* or forkhead box G1 (*FOXG1*), neurodevelopmental syndromes all associated with ASD, Livide et al. and Patriarchi et al. found increased expression of the ionotropic glutamate receptor glutamate delta-1 (GluD1).[95,96] GluD1 does not function as an ion transporter, but instead acts as a cell adhesion molecule that facilitates the formation of GABAergic synapses.[97] While these studies used divergent cellular models, the different results may suggest that, while disruptions in synapse development are associated with ASD, the nature of these disruptions does not necessarily correlate across ASD cases or etiologies.

## Altered neuronal function: Disruption of the balance between neuronal excitation and inhibition

The precise balance between excitatory signaling from glutamatergic neurons and inhibitory signaling from GABAergic neurons is critical for the proper functioning of the cortex. Dysfunction in either cell type can result in an imbalance between these two signals (E/I imbalance) and a hyper- or hypoactive network. This type of dysfunction can be observed in ASD patients[98] and is thought to be the result of many of the cellular phenotypes that have been described above.

Phenotypes involving altered neuronal function have frequently been detected in hPSC models of ASD. For example, using a mixed culture of iPSC-derived excitatory and inhibitory neurons from patients with RTT, Marchetto et al. detected decreased excitatory neuron activity, as measured both by calcium transients and as a decreased frequency of spontaneous excitatory postsynaptic currents (sEPSCs), findings also recapitulated by Djuric et al..[55,56] Evidence was also presented that these phenotypes are likely driven by decreased synaptogenesis in RTT neurons. In this study, while the synaptogenesis phenotype could be rescued with IGF-1 treatment, this did not correct the diminished electrophysiological activity. However, the presence of inhibitory GABAergic neurons in this model may confound this explanation, as changes in this population were not assessed in this work and may have significant effects on the excitability of neuronal cultures. In a model of 22q13 deletion syndrome, Shcheglovitov et al. similarly demonstrated decreased synaptogenesis, which they also linked to decreased neuronal activity.[68] In assessing the basis of this phenotype, Shcheglovitov et al. also showed abnormal neuronal responses to both NMDA and AMPA. Like Marchetto et al., they attempted to rescue this phenotype with IGF-1 treatment, coupled with replacement of *SHANK3*, a key gene within the 22q13 locus.[55] In this case, this rescue was effective in reversing both the synaptogenesis phenotype and corresponding electrophysiological deficits. Both of these cellular models of ASD demonstrate a link to decreased neuronal activity in excitatory neurons driven by abnormal synaptogenesis.

In further work by Marchetto et al., DeRosa et al., and Amatya et al., iPSC models from idiopathic ASD individuals exhibited decreased neuronal network activity in multielectrode array (MEA) analyses of excitatory and inhibitory neuronal co-cultures.[4,76,79] Marchetto et al. demonstrated that this phenotype was underpinned by significant reduction in all measured synaptic markers and GABAergic neuronal production, suggesting that the reduced neuronal activity is unlikely to be driven solely by deficits in a single neuronal cell population.[4] As in the work above, rescue was attempted by using IGF-1 supplementation; this resulted in a detectable but minor increase in neuronal activity. Interestingly, this rescue was attempted at the later stages of functional development, after the establishment of neuronal networks; the relatively modest rescue obtained may suggest that, once deficits in E/I imbalance are established, they are less pharmacologically tractable. Deneault et al. also modeled the effects of heterozygous loss of function of 10 ASD risk genes by CRISPR/Cas9-mediated gene disruption.[80,81] In MEA analysis, only one of these gene knockout models (sodium voltage-gated channel alpha subunit 2, *SCN2A*) showed reduced neuronal activity; this knockout alone also exhibited diminished synchronized network behavior. However, in addition to *SCN2A*, another three of these models [ATRX chromatin remodeler (*ATRX*), AF4/FMR2 family member 2 (*AFF2*), and potassium voltage-gated channel subfamily Q member 2 (*KCNQ2*) knockout] exhibited decreased neuronal network activity, as measured by bursting behavior. Despite the varied presentation of these phenotypes in MEA analyses, Deneault et al. also found that five of the ten gene knockouts had a reduced frequency of spontaneous EPSCs.[80,81] Taken together, these results suggest that there may be some common alterations of neuronal function visible even when using complex functional assessment approaches such as MEAs and when the particular ASD cellular model differs. However, it is also important to note that not all models used by Deneault et al. showed significant changes in either neuronal function or network behavior.

Despite the apparent convergence of evidence for ASD model-associated decreased neuronal activity, which is suggested from the work above, a recent study demonstrated increased neuronal network activity in two models of ASD.[80] In each case, patient-derived models carrying either gene variants that encoded truncated contactin 5 (*CNTN5*) or a mutant form of euchromatic histone-lysine *N*-methyltransferase 2 (*EHMT2*) showed a more complex phenotype than that shown in a heterozygous knockout model. In the iPSC model carrying the *CNTN5* patient variant, increased network activity appeared relatively early, as neuronal networks began to form, and persisted throughout the period of analysis. However, heterozygous knockout of the same gene instead resulted in only a transient increase in network activity at very late stages of neuronal network maturation.[80] The patient model of *EHMT2* mutation initially exhibited increased network activity, which trended toward control levels as the system aged, while the heterozygous knockout model instead exhibited an increasingly pronounced increase in neuronal network activity relative to controls as the system aged.[80] Likewise, in examining a patient mutation in the *SHANK2* gene associated with ASD, Zaslavsky et al. showed an increase in spontaneous EPSCs; a similar but much more muted effect was seen in a *SHANK2* gene knockout model by comparison.[44] These studies in particular illustrate the often-divergent phenotypes seen in patient models, by comparison with genetically engineered gene knockout models, particularly with respect to complex functional phenotypes. This divergence may involve the specific genetic background present in the patient-derived models or may be caused by differential effects of particular mutations on gene expression and function.

Recent work by Alsaqati et al.[16] examined a patient-derived neuronal model of TSC complex subunit 2 (*TSC2*) loss and demonstrated similarly increased neuronal network activity by using excitatory and inhibitory co-cultures and MEA assays. However, in this study, the authors further assessed the complexity of the phenotypes observed and concluded that, while their model showed neuronal hyperexcitability, this activity was less organized than that seen in control cells. By contrast with the findings of diminished synaptic activity for the RTT model described above ([55]), here Alsaqati et al. found increased expression of many synaptic and GABA and glutamate signaling genes. Attempting to pharmacologically correct the deficits observed in this model by targeting mammalian target of rapamycin (mTOR) signaling after they were established, these authors also demonstrated a significant phenotype reversal of the mutant models toward the control; however, like the findings of Marchetto et al., this correction was incomplete.[4] This indicates that complex phenotypes may be less tractable to pharmacologic intervention at later stages of development.

Taken together, these studies indicate that imbalanced neuronal excitation and inhibition may often contribute to aberrant neuronal network behavior associated with ASD. However, there is currently little consensus regarding the directionality of these changes, with some studies pointing toward increased and others toward decreased neuronal activity. Further work is necessary to understand the basis of these differences and their association with ASD etiology. Furthermore, the underlying cause of this aberrant neuronal network behavior and whether this involves alterations of neurodevelopmental mechanisms in a single neuronal cell type or more global alterations of neurodevelopment remain unclear.

## Altered glial production and function: An emerging role of glia in the pathogenesis of ASD

Another aspect of iPSC models of ASD that has yet to be explored extensively is the role of disrupted glial development and function. Glial cells play essential roles in maintaining brain homeostasis and providing support and protection for neurons. Mutations that alter the density and function of different glial cell types, including astrocytes, oligodendrocytes, and microglia, can contribute to autism spectrum disorder (ASD), primarily by affecting neuron–glia interactions and thus influencing synaptic activity. Although protocols exist for producing PSC-based glial cell cultures for disease modeling, most research to date that has studied the roles of ASD-associated mutations has been conducted using animal-derived glial cell cultures. Thus, until glial differentiation is more prominently performed by using iPSC models of ASD, its contribution to pathogenesis in humans remains unclear in most instances.

Relative to the other two main types of glial cells, astrocyte development has been more widely modeled in iPSC models of ASD. Astrocytes support neural networks and axons, provide trophic support to neurons, respond to inflammation, and, along with other cells, form the blood–brain barrier. In examining the effect of a mutation in HRas proto-oncogene

GTPase (*HRAS*) in iPSC-derived astrocytes, Krencik et al. found that cells carrying the *HRAS* mutation precociously differentiated into astrocytes and that these astrocytes overproduced extracellular matrix proteins including proteoglycans.[46] Using a mouse model of the same mutation, Krencik et al. suggested that these phenotypes were likely to disrupt cortical maturation.[46] Studies in hPSC models of ASD examining the effect of *NRXN1* heterozygous deletion[47] and mutation in the *FMR1* gene[51] also showed increased astrocyte production. This result was further supported by a study from Zuiki et al., which modeled the effect of immune activation, a risk factor for ASD development, in an iPSC model; this was also associated with increased astrocyte production.[99] Russo et al. used an iPSC-derived astrocyte model of idiopathic autism to assess neuron-astrocyte interactions in co-cultures and found that ASD subject-derived astrocytes interfered with neuronal development, decreasing synaptogenesis through increased interleukin-6 (IL-6) secretion.[43] This result was particularly interesting, as Zuiki et al. used IL-6 as a proxy for immune activation, suggesting a possible positive feedback loop. While a majority of studies to date associated increased astrocyte production with ASD risk, models of *MECP2* mutation[57] and of *NRXN1* knockdown mediated by shRNA[72] were both associated with decreased astrocyte production. Therefore, while there is presently a lack of consensus regarding the effects of ASD-associated genetic abnormalities on astrocyte differentiation and function, it is clear that deficits in this cell type should be further investigated in the context of ASD pathology.

Recent findings have indicated that ASD is associated with alterations in white matter and myelin production in diverse areas across the brain.[100] However, there is presently little evidence from cellular models of a link between ASD pathogenesis and altered oligodendrocyte function. Recent work from Nadadhur et al.[45] began investigating this link in iPSC models carrying *TSC* mutations that were differentiated into both neurons and oligodendrocytes. This work suggested that, while the presence of *TSC* mutant oligodendrocytes did not alter the neuronal morphological phenotypes that were observed directly, they did block pharmacological rescue of these phenotypes. Finally, in examining oligodendrocyte development in this model, Nadadhur et al. found increased production of oligodendrocyte progenitors (marked by OLIG2) but no significant increase in production of functional (MBP expressing) oligodendrocytes, suggesting an alteration of the oligodendrocyte developmental program. While further investigation of the role of oligodendrocyte dysfunction in ASD is needed, this study provides one line of evidence to suggest that these studies will be valuable.

Finally, like oligodendrocytes, microglia have yet to be investigated in hPSC models of ASD; however, there is significant evidence from both animal and human studies to suggest a role for this cell type in ASD.[101,102]

Microglia are critically important for mediating the immune response in the CNS and therefore may play roles similar to those indicated for astrocytes in the Russo et al. study.[43] As microglia also play a role in synaptic pruning, microglial deficits may also alter synaptic density, reminiscent of the neuronal studies described above. Therefore, while cellular modeling of microglia associated with ASD risk mutations has yet to be the focus of significant investigation, it is an area of increasing interest.

## Limitations of modeling neurodevelopmental disorders with iPSCs

iPSC-derived neurons, glia, and organoids provide useful and experimentally manipulable models to recapitulate aspects of human fetal brain development that are otherwise not available for study. These include genetic liabilities and neurodevelopmental processes that are human-specific and not readily modeled in animals. However, it is important to be aware of the limitations inherent in these models. Importantly, iPSC-derived neurons share developmental trajectories with and recapitulate key features of early human neuronal development, most closely recapitulating aspects of brain development that occur during mid- to late-gestation. Accordingly, these models may be most useful for understanding neurodevelopmental anomalies that may have occurred during gestation, while being more challenging to extrapolate to later contributors to liability. Despite this potential limitation, at a simplistic level iPSC-derived neurons and glia can model major functional behaviors of the target cells (e.g. neuronal activity/networks, tripartite synapses, myelination, and phagocytosis/cytokine production). Thus, while many of these behaviors may be less developed than those present in adult humans, deficits observed in cellular models may still parallel some of those present in more mature versions of the same neurological processes.

It is also very important to consider experimental design when assessing the cellular pathologies identified by studies on human cellular models of ASD. Many studies focus on a single cell type of interest, thus limiting confounding factors and allowing the elucidation of often subtle phenotypes. However, this reductionist model may miss more complex phenotypes, which are often only observable in more complex systems encompassing multiple neuronal cell types. It is also possible that under more "normal" physiological conditions, other neuronal cell types can compensate for deficits seen in a reductionist, single neuronal cell type model, and thus that the phenotypes obtained may be less relevant to the etiology of ASD. By contrast, complex cellular model systems such as organoids and complex multilineage cell cultures provide a much closer facsimile of physiological conditions. However, this complexity can render it more difficult to assess observed phenotypes, as these may involve deficits in multiple cell types or may specifically involve a confluence of deficits across multiple cell types. Thus, it is critical when examining phenotypes observed in human cellular models to consider how the neurodevelopmental model utilized for these comparisons may affect the ASD-associated phenotypes observed.

## Conclusions

Recent analyses have revealed ASD to be a complex disorder, with mutations in hundreds of genes associated with increased ASD risk. A number of ASD risk-associated variants have now been modeled in hPSCs and these studies have provided insights into cellular phenotypes that are associated with and may contribute to ASD. However, further work is still needed in most cases, to understand how the disrupted development and function of different neuronal and glial cell types contributes to patient phenotypes. In particular, since most studies to date have characterized these models in only one hPSC-derived neuronal cell type, most frequently cortical excitatory neurons, expanding these analyses to glial and to more complex multicellular models is likely to provide further insight into how these cellular phenotypes compare across models and may relate to altered physiological function.

Existing cellular models of ASD have identified key hubs of dysfunction that are commonly associated with mutations in multiple ASD risk genes. These include altered mitochondrial function, early cortical neuron production, synapse production, and glial differentiation. Ultimately, dysfunction in several of these general neurodevelopmental categories is likely to contribute to altering the balance of neuronal excitation and inhibition. However, the effect of particular ASD-associated gene variants on these phenotypic hubs appears to differ between models and to be related most frequently to the particular mutation under study. Further work is needed to better understand how divergent cellular phenotypes seen in comparisons between hPSC models nonetheless are associated with a shared diagnosis of ASD.

Finally, the nature of ASD as a spectrum that involves differential clinical presentation among individual patients presents a unique challenge to cellular modeling efforts that has yet to be addressed. Much of the extant literature presented here focuses on syndromic forms of autism, because these involve patient populations with a similar genetic risk factor and shared clinical features, often including diagnoses for other co-occurring conditions such as intellectual disability. However, these syndromic cases may be more representative of the particular syndrome under investigation, rather than representative of the broader range of genetic liabilities that contribute to ASD. More complex study designs encompassing both syndromic and nonsyndromic forms of ASD, as well as meta-comparisons of data from prior studies, could begin to define cellular and molecular phenotypes that are more closely associated with ASD, versus other co-occurring diagnoses present in syndromic forms of the disorder. Efforts to link the clinical presentation to particular cellular phenotypes across cohorts of patient-derived cellular models may also more broadly inform efforts to connect phenotypes obtained in cellular models to particular aspects of the clinical presentation.

In summary, while cellular modeling of ASD remains an emerging area of study, the increasing availability of a wealth of sequencing data from ASD patients, and the ability to relate the data obtained in cellular modeling studies to clinical ASD phenotypes, provide fertile ground for future studies. Efforts to characterize human cellular models from a broad range of ASD cases, encompassing diverse genetic contributors, and to conduct meta-analyses of the data obtained will be critical to define core aspects of neurodevelopmental dysfunction underlying ASD pathology. These resources will also provide greater scope for and will enhance the use of ASD cellular models and their accompanying phenotypes as platforms for developing therapeutic interventions.

## Acknowledgment of funding sources

This work was supported by National Institutes of Health grants R01NS114551, R01MH124808, U01HG007530 (NINDS/NIH Common Fund, subaward), U54HD087011 (administrative supplement), P50HD129966 (subaward), P50HD103525 (subaward), and by awards from the M-CM Network, Jakob Gene Fund, and Washington University Center for Regenerative Medicine, WU Children's Discovery Institute (CDI-LI-2019-819), and WU Institute for Clinical and Translational Sciences to K.L.K.

## Declaration of competing interests

None.

## Author contributions

G.C. and K.L.K. conceptualized and supervised this project, G.C., I.A., M.N., R.S., and R.E. reviewed the literature, G.C. created tables and figures, and G.C., I.A., M.N., R.S., R.E., and K.L.K wrote the manuscript.

## References

1. Molnár Z, Métin C, Stoykova A, et al. Comparative aspects of cerebral cortical development. *Eur J Neurosci*. 2006;23(4):921–934. https://doi.org/10.1111/j.1460-9568.2006.04611.x.
2. Drakulic D, Djurovic S, Syed YA, et al. Copy number variants (CNVs): a powerful tool for iPSC-based modelling of ASD. *Mol Autism*. 2020;11(1):42. https://doi.org/10.1186/s13229-020-00343-4.

3. Autism Spectrum Disorder Working Group of the Psychiatric Genomics Consortium, BUPGEN, Major Depressive Disorder Working Group of the Psychiatric Genomics Consortium, 23andMe Research Team, et al. Identification of common genetic risk variants for autism spectrum disorder. *Nat Genet.* 2019;51(3):431–444. https://doi.org/10.1038/s41588-019-0344-8.
4. Marchetto MC, Belinson H, Tian Y, et al. Altered proliferation and networks in neural cells derived from idiopathic autistic individuals. *Mol Psychiatry.* 2017;22(6):820–835. https://doi.org/10.1038/mp.2016.95.
5. Yamanaka S. Induced pluripotent stem cells: past, present, and future. *Cell Stem Cell.* 2012;10(6):678–684. https://doi.org/10.1016/j.stem.2012.05.005.
6. Ananiev G, Williams EC, Li H, Chang Q. Isogenic pairs of wild type and mutant induced pluripotent stem cell (iPSC) lines from rett syndrome patients as in vitro disease model. *PLoS One.* 2011;6(9). https://doi.org/10.1371/journal.pone.0025255, e25255.
7. Barrangou R, Doudna JA. Applications of CRISPR technologies in research and beyond. *Nat Biotechnol.* 2016;34(9):933–941. https://doi.org/10.1038/nbt.3659.
8. Cho SW, Kim S, Kim Y, et al. Analysis of off-target effects of CRISPR/Cas-derived RNA-guided endonucleases and nickases. *Genome Res.* 2014;24(1):132–141. https://doi.org/10.1101/gr.162339.113.
9. Qi LS, Larson MH, Gilbert LA, et al. Repurposing CRISPR as an RNA-guided platform for sequence-specific control of gene expression. *Cell.* 2013;152(5):1173–1183. https://doi.org/10.1016/j.cell.2013.02.022.
10. Chambers SM, Fasano CA, Papapetrou EP, Tomishima M, Sadelain M, Studer L. Highly efficient neural conversion of human ES and iPS cells by dual inhibition of SMAD signaling. *Nat Biotechnol.* 2009;27(3):275–280. https://doi.org/10.1038/nbt.1529.
11. Ho S-M, Hartley BJ, Tcw J, et al. Rapid Ngn2-induction of excitatory neurons from hiPSC-derived neural progenitor cells. *Methods.* 2016;101:113–124. https://doi.org/10.1016/j.ymeth.2015.11.019.
12. Young-Pearse TL, Morrow EM. Modeling developmental neuropsychiatric disorders with iPSC technology: challenges and opportunities. *Curr Opin Neurobiol.* 2016;36:66–73. https://doi.org/10.1016/j.conb.2015.10.006.
13. Cusco I, Medrano A, Gener B, et al. Autism-specific copy number variants further implicate the phosphatidylinositol signaling pathway and the glutamatergic synapse in the etiology of the disorder. *Hum Mol Genet.* 2009;18(10):1795–1804. https://doi.org/10.1093/hmg/ddp092.
14. Sgadò P, Dunleavy M, Genovesi S, Provenzano G, Bozzi Y. The role of GABAergic system in neurodevelopmental disorders: a focus on autism and epilepsy. *Int J Physiol Pathophysiol Pharmacol.* 2011;3(3):223–235.
15. Zhang S-C, Wernig M, Duncan ID, Brüstle O, Thomson JA. In vitro differentiation of transplantable neural precursors from human embryonic stem cells. *Nat Biotechnol.* 2001;19(12):1129–1133. https://doi.org/10.1038/nbt1201-1129.
16. Alsaqati M, Heine VM, Harwood AJ. Pharmacological intervention to restore connectivity deficits of neuronal networks derived from ASD patient iPSC with a TSC2 mutation. *Mol Autism.* 2020;11(1):80. https://doi.org/10.1186/s13229-020-00391-w.
17. Crawford TQ, Roelink H. The Notch response inhibitor DAPT enhances neuronal differentiation in embryonic stem cell-derived embryoid bodies independently of sonic hedgehog signaling. *Dev Dyn.* 2007;236(3):886–892. https://doi.org/10.1002/dvdy.21083.
18. Kemp PJ, Rushton DJ, Yarova PL, et al. Improving and accelerating the differentiation and functional maturation of human stem cell-derived neurons: role of extracellular calcium and GABA: enhancing functional neuronal differentiation of stem cells. *J Physiol.* 2016;594(22):6583–6594. https://doi.org/10.1113/JP270655.
19. Qi Y, Zhang X-J, Renier N, et al. Combined small-molecule inhibition accelerates the derivation of functional cortical neurons from human pluripotent stem cells. *Nat Biotechnol.* 2017;35(2):154–163. https://doi.org/10.1038/nbt.3777.

20. Li X-J, Zhang X, Johnson MA, Wang Z-B, LaVaute T, Zhang S-C. Coordination of sonic hedgehog and Wnt signaling determines ventral and dorsal telencephalic neuron types from human embryonic stem cells. *Development.* 2009;136(23):4055–4063. https://doi.org/10.1242/dev.036624.
21. Yang N, Chanda S, Marro S, et al. Generation of pure GABAergic neurons by transcription factor programming. *Nat Methods.* 2017;14(6):621–628. https://doi.org/10.1038/nmeth.4291.
22. Edmonson C, Ziats MN, Rennert OM. Altered glial marker expression in autistic post-mortem prefrontal cortex and cerebellum. *Mol Autism.* 2014;5(1):3. https://doi.org/10.1186/2040-2392-5-3.
23. Kim YS, Choi J, Yoon B-E. Neuron-glia interactions in neurodevelopmental disorders. *Cell.* 2020;9(10):2176. https://doi.org/10.3390/cells9102176.
24. Shaltouki A, Peng J, Liu Q, Rao MS, Zeng X. Efficient generation of astrocytes from human pluripotent stem cells in defined conditions. *Stem Cells.* 2013;31(5):941–952. https://doi.org/10.1002/stem.1334.
25. Tcw J, Wang M, Pimenova AA, et al. An efficient platform for astrocyte differentiation from human induced pluripotent stem cells. *Stem Cell Rep.* 2017;9(2):600–614. https://doi.org/10.1016/j.stemcr.2017.06.018.
26. Leferink PS, Dooves S, Hillen AEJ, et al. Astrocyte subtype vulnerability in stem cell models of vanishing white matter. *Ann Neurol.* 2019;86(5):780–792. https://doi.org/10.1002/ana.25585.
27. Canals I, Ginisty A, Quist E, et al. Rapid and efficient induction of functional astrocytes from human pluripotent stem cells. *Nat Methods.* 2018;15(9):693–696. https://doi.org/10.1038/s41592-018-0103-2.
28. Windrem MS, Osipovitch M, Liu Z, et al. Human iPSC glial mouse chimeras reveal glial contributions to schizophrenia. *Cell Stem Cell.* 2017;21(2):195–208.e6. https://doi.org/10.1016/j.stem.2017.06.012.
29. Douvaras P, Wang J, Zimmer M, et al. Efficient generation of myelinating oligodendrocytes from primary progressive multiple sclerosis patients by induced pluripotent stem cells. *Stem Cell Rep.* 2014;3(2):250–259. https://doi.org/10.1016/j.stemcr.2014.06.012.
30. Douvaras P, Fossati V. Generation and isolation of oligodendrocyte progenitor cells from human pluripotent stem cells. *Nat Protoc.* 2015;10(8):1143–1154. https://doi.org/10.1038/nprot.2015.075.
31. Matjusaitis M, Wagstaff LJ, Martella A, et al. Reprogramming of fibroblasts to oligodendrocyte progenitor-like cells using CRISPR/Cas9-based synthetic transcription factors. *Stem Cell Rep.* 2019;13(6):1053–1067. https://doi.org/10.1016/j.stemcr.2019.10.010.
32. Ehrlich M, Mozafari S, Glatza M, et al. Rapid and efficient generation of oligodendrocytes from human induced pluripotent stem cells using transcription factors. *Proc Natl Acad Sci U S A.* 2017;114(11):E2243–E2252. https://doi.org/10.1073/pnas.1614412114.
33. García-León JA, Kumar M, Boon R, et al. SOX10 single transcription factor-based fast and efficient generation ofoligodendrocytes from human pluripotent stem cells. *Stem Cell Rep.* 2018;10(2):655–672. https://doi.org/10.1016/j.stemcr.2017.12.014.
34. Wurm J, Konttinen H, Andressen C, Malm T, Spittau B. Microglia development and maturation and its implications for induction of microglia-like cells from human iPSCs. *Int J Mol Sci.* 2021;22(6):3088. https://doi.org/10.3390/ijms22063088.
35. Abud EM, Ramirez RN, Martinez ES, et al. IPSC-derived human microglia-like cells to study neurological diseases. *Neuron.* 2017;94(2):278–293.e9. https://doi.org/10.1016/j.neuron.2017.03.042.
36. Douvaras P, Sun B, Wang M, et al. Directed differentiation of human pluripotent stem cells to microglia. *Stem Cell Rep.* 2017;8(6):1516–1524. https://doi.org/10.1016/j.stemcr.2017.04.023.

37. McQuade A, Coburn M, Tu CH, Hasselmann J, Davtyan H, Blurton-Jones M. Development and validation of a simplified method to generate human microglia from pluripotent stem cells. *Mol Neurodegener.* 2018;13(1):67. https://doi.org/10.1186/s13024-018-0297-x.
38. Lancaster MA, Renner M, Martin C-A, et al. Cerebral organoids model human brain development and microcephaly. *Nature.* 2013;501(7467):373–379. https://doi.org/10.1038/nature12517.
39. Ormel PR, Vieira de Sá R, van Bodegraven EJ, et al. Microglia innately develop within cerebral organoids. *Nat Commun.* 2018;9(1):4167. https://doi.org/10.1038/s41467-018-06684-2.
40. Bagley JA, Reumann D, Bian S, Lévi-Strauss J, Knoblich JA. Fused cerebral organoids model interactions between brain regions. *Nat Methods.* 2017;14(7):743–751. https://doi.org/10.1038/nmeth.4304.
41. Kim H, Xu R, Padmashri R, et al. Pluripotent stem cell-derived cerebral organoids reveal human oligodendrogenesis with dorsal and ventral origins. *Stem Cell Rep.* 2019;12(5):890–905. https://doi.org/10.1016/j.stemcr.2019.04.011.
42. Song L, Yuan X, Jones Z, et al. Functionalization of brain region-specific spheroids with isogenic microglia-like cells. *Sci Rep.* 2019;9(1):11055. https://doi.org/10.1038/s41598-019-47444-6.
43. Russo FB, Freitas BC, Pignatari GC, et al. Modeling the interplay between neurons and astrocytes in autism using human induced pluripotent stem cells. *Biol Psychiatry.* 2018;83(7):569–578. https://doi.org/10.1016/j.biopsych.2017.09.021.
44. Zaslavsky K, Zhang W-B, McCready FP, et al. SHANK2 mutations associated with autism spectrum disorder cause hyperconnectivity of human neurons. *Nat Neurosci.* 2019;22(4):556–564. https://doi.org/10.1038/s41593-019-0365-8.
45. Nadadhur AG, Alsaqati M, Gasparotto L, et al. Neuron-glia interactions increase neuronal phenotypes in tuberous sclerosis complex patient iPSC-derived models. *Stem Cell Rep.* 2019;12(1):42–56. https://doi.org/10.1016/j.stemcr.2018.11.019.
46. Krencik R, Hokanson KC, Narayan AR, et al. Dysregulation of astrocyte extracellular signaling in Costello syndrome. *Sci Transl Med.* 2015;7(286):286ra66. https://doi.org/10.1126/scitranslmed.aaa5645.
47. Raciti M, Salma J, Spulber S, et al. NRXN1 deletion and exposure to methylmercury increase astrocyte differentiation by different notch-dependent transcriptional mechanisms. *Front Genet.* 2019;10. https://doi.org/10.3389/fgene.2019.00593.
48. Avazzadeh S, McDonagh K, Reilly J, et al. Increased Ca2+ signaling in NRXN1α+/− neurons derived from ASD induced pluripotent stem cells. *Mol Autism.* 2019;10(1):52. https://doi.org/10.1186/s13229-019-0303-3.
49. Lam M, Moslem M, Bryois J, et al. Single cell analysis of autism patient with bi-allelic NRXN1-alpha deletion reveals skewed fate choice in neural progenitors and impaired neuronal functionality. *Exp Cell Res.* 2019;383(1):111469. https://doi.org/10.1016/j.yexcr.2019.06.014.
50. Pak C, Danko T, Zhang Y, et al. Human neuropsychiatric disease modeling using conditional deletion reveals synaptic transmission defects caused by heterozygous mutations in NRXN1. *Cell Stem Cell.* 2015;17(3):316–328. https://doi.org/10.1016/j.stem.2015.07.017.
51. Telias M, Segal M, Ben-Yosef D. Neural differentiation of fragile X human embryonic stem cells reveals abnormal patterns of development despite successful neurogenesis. *Dev Biol.* 2013;374(1):32–45. https://doi.org/10.1016/j.ydbio.2012.11.031.
52. Boland MJ, Nazor KL, Tran HT, et al. Molecular analyses of neurogenic defects in a human pluripotent stem cell model of fragile X syndrome. *Brain J Neurol.* 2017;140(3):582–598. https://doi.org/10.1093/brain/aww357.
53. Achuta VS, Möykkynen T, Peteri U-K, et al. Functional changes of AMPA responses in human induced pluripotent stem cell–derived neural progenitors in fragile X syndrome. *Sci Signal.* 2018;11(513). https://doi.org/10.1126/scisignal.aan8784.

54. Bu Q, Wang A, Hamzah H, et al. CREB signaling is involved in Rett syndrome pathogenesis. *J Neurosci.* 2017;37(13):3671–3685. https://doi.org/10.1523/JNEUROSCI.3735-16.2017.
55. Marchetto MC, Carromeu C, Acab A, et al. A model for neural development and treatment of Rett syndrome using human induced pluripotent stem cells. *Cell.* 2010;143(4):527–539. https://doi.org/10.1016/j.cell.2010.10.016.
56. Djuric U, Cheung AYL, Zhang W, et al. MECP2e1 isoform mutation affects the form and function of neurons derived from Rett syndrome patient iPS cells. *Neurobiol Dis.* 2015;76:37–45. https://doi.org/10.1016/j.nbd.2015.01.001.
57. Kim JJ, Savas JN, Miller MT, et al. Proteomic analyses reveal misregulation of LIN28 expression and delayed timing of glial differentiation in human iPS cells with MECP2 loss-of-function. *PLoS One.* 2019;14(2). https://doi.org/10.1371/journal.pone.0212553, e0212553.
58. Williams EC, Zhong X, Mohamed A, et al. Mutant astrocytes differentiated from Rett syndrome patients-specific iPSCs have adverse effects on wild-type neurons. *Hum Mol Genet.* 2014;23(11):2968–2980. https://doi.org/10.1093/hmg/ddu008.
59. Mellios N, Feldman DA, Sheridan SD, et al. MeCP2-regulated miRNAs control early human neurogenesis through differential effects on ERK and AKT signaling. *Mol Psychiatry.* 2018;23(4):1051–1065. https://doi.org/10.1038/mp.2017.86.
60. Ricciardi S, Ungaro F, Hambrock M, et al. CDKL5 ensures excitatory synapse stability by reinforcing NGL-1–PSD95 interaction in the postsynaptic compartment and is impaired in patient iPSC-derived neurons. *Nat Cell Biol.* 2012;14(9):911–923. https://doi.org/10.1038/ncb2566.
61. Fink JJ, Robinson TM, Germain ND, et al. Disrupted neuronal maturation in Angelman syndrome-derived induced pluripotent stem cells. *Nat Commun.* 2017;8(1):15038. https://doi.org/10.1038/ncomms1.
62. Sun AX, Yuan Q, Fukuda M, et al. Potassium channel dysfunction in human neuronal models of Angelman syndrome. *Science.* 2019;366(6472):1486–1492. https://doi.org/10.1126/science.aav5386.
63. Paşca SP, Portmann T, Voineagu I, et al. Using iPSC-derived neurons to uncover cellular phenotypes associated with Timothy syndrome. *Nat Med.* 2011;17(12):1657–1662. https://doi.org/10.1038/nm.2576.
64. Birey F, Andersen J, Makinson CD, et al. Assembly of functionally integrated human forebrain spheroids. *Nature.* 2017;545(7652):54–59. https://doi.org/10.1038/nature22330.
65. Huang G, Chen S, Chen X, et al. Uncovering the functional link between SHANK3 deletions and deficiency in neurodevelopment using iPSC-derived human neurons. *Front Neuroanat.* 2019;13. https://doi.org/10.3389/fnana.2019.00023.
66. Gouder L, Vitrac A, Goubran-Botros H, et al. Altered spinogenesis in iPSC-derived cortical neurons from patients with autism carrying de novo SHANK3 mutations. *Sci Rep.* 2019;9(1):94. https://doi.org/10.1038/s41598-018-36993-x.
67. Kathuria A, Nowosiad P, Jagasia R, et al. Stem cell-derived neurons from autistic individuals with SHANK3 mutation show morphogenetic abnormalities during early development. *Mol Psychiatry.* 2018;23(3):735–746. https://doi.org/10.1038/mp.2017.185.
68. Shcheglovitov A, Shcheglovitova O, Yazawa M, et al. SHANK3 and IGF1 restore synaptic deficits in neurons from 22q13 deletion syndrome patients. *Nature.* 2013;503(7475):267–271. https://doi.org/10.1038/nature12618.
69. Frega M, Linda K, Keller JM, et al. Neuronal network dysfunction in a model for Kleefstra syndrome mediated by enhanced NMDAR signaling. *Nat Commun.* 2019;10(1):4928. https://doi.org/10.1038/s41467-019-12947-35038.
70. Marro SG, Chanda S, Yang N, et al. Neuroligin-4 regulates excitatory synaptic transmission in human neurons. *Neuron.* 2019;103(4):617–626.e6. https://doi.org/10.1016/j.neuron.2019.05.043.
71. Flaherty E, Zhu S, Barretto N, et al. Neuronal impact of patient-specific aberrant NRXN1α splicing. *Nat Genet.* 2019;51(12):1679–1690. https://doi.org/10.1038/s41588-019-0539-z.

72. Zeng L, Zhang P, Shi L, Yamamoto V, Lu W, Wang K. Functional impacts of NRXN1 knockdown on neurodevelopment in stem cell models. *PLoS One.* 2013;8(3). https://doi.org/10.1371/journal.pone.0059685, e59685.
73. Deshpande A, Yadav S, Dao DQ, et al. Cellular phenotypes in human iPSC-derived neurons from a genetic model of autism spectrum disorder. *Cell Rep.* 2017;21(10):2678–2687. https://doi.org/10.1016/j.celrep.2017.11.037.
74. Ross PJ, Zhang W-B, Mok RSF, et al. Synaptic dysfunction in human neurons with autism-associated deletions in PTCHD1-AS. *Biol Psychiatry.* 2020;87(2):139–149. https://doi.org/10.1016/j.biopsych.2019.07.014.
75. Liu X, Campanac E, Cheung H-H, et al. Idiopathic autism: cellular and molecular phenotypes in pluripotent stem cell-derived neurons. *Mol Neurobiol.* 2017;54(6):4507–4523. https://doi.org/10.1007/s12035-016-9961-8.
76. DeRosa BA, El Hokayem J, Artimovich E, et al. Convergent pathways in idiopathic autism revealed by time course transcriptomic analysis of patient-derived neurons. *Sci Rep.* 2018;8(1):8423. https://doi.org/10.1038/s41598-018-26495-1.
77. Schafer ST, Paquola ACM, Stern S, et al. Pathological priming causes developmental gene network heterochronicity in autistic subject-derived neurons. *Nat Neurosci.* 2019;22(2):243–255. https://doi.org/10.1038/s41593-018-0295-x.
78. Mariani J, Coppola G, Zhang P, et al. FOXG1-dependent dysregulation of GABA/glutamate neuron differentiation in autism spectrum disorders. *Cell.* 2015;162(2):375–390. https://doi.org/10.1016/j.cell.2015.06.034.
79. Amatya DN, Linker SB, Mendes APD, et al. Dynamical electrical complexity is reduced during neuronal differentiation in autism spectrum disorder. *Stem Cell Rep.* 2019;13(3):474–484. https://doi.org/10.1016/j.stemcr.2019.08.001.
80. Deneault E, Faheem M, White SH, et al. CNTN5- /+ or EHMT2- /+ human iPSC-derived neurons from individuals with autism develop hyperactive neuronal networks. *Elife.* 2019;8. https://doi.org/10.7554/eLife.40092.
81. Deneault E, White SH, Rodrigues DC, et al. Complete disruption of autism-susceptibility genes by gene editing predominantly reduces functional connectivity of isogenic human neurons. *Stem Cell Rep.* 2019;12(2):427–429. https://doi.org/10.1016/j.stemcr.2019.01.008.
82. Jagtap S, Thanos JM, Fu T, et al. Aberrant mitochondrial function in patient-derived neural cells from CDKL5 deficiency disorder and Rett syndrome. *Hum Mol Genet.* 2019;28(21):3625–3636. https://doi.org/10.1093/hmg/ddz208.
83. Anastasaki C, Wegscheid ML, Hartigan K, et al. Human iPSC-derived neurons and cerebral organoids establish differential effects of germline NF1 gene mutations. *Stem Cell Rep.* 2020;14(4):541–550. https://doi.org/10.1016/j.stemcr.2020.03.007.
84. Moore D, Meays BM, Madduri LSV, et al. Downregulation of an evolutionary young miR-1290 in an iPSC-derived neural stem cell model of autism spectrum disorder. *Stem Cells Int.* 2019;2019:8710180. https://doi.org/10.1155/2019/8710180.
85. Wang M, Wei P-C, Lim CK, et al. Increased neural progenitor proliferation in a hiPSC model of autism induces replication stress-associated genome instability. *Cell Stem Cell.* 2020;26(2):221–233.e6. https://doi.org/10.1016/j.stem.2019.12.013.
86. Lee Y-K, Hwang S-K, Lee S-K, et al. Cohen syndrome patient iPSC-derived neurospheres and forebrain-like glutamatergic neurons reveal reduced proliferation of neural progenitor cells and altered expression of synapse genes. *J Clin Med.* 2020;9(6). https://doi.org/10.3390/jcm9061886.
87. Yi F, Danko T, Botelho SC, et al. Autism-associated SHANK3 haploinsufficiency causes Ih channelopathy in human neurons. *Science.* 2016;352(6286):aaf2669. https://doi.org/10.1126/science.aaf2669.
88. Griesi-Oliveira K, Acab A, Gupta AR, et al. Modeling non-syndromic autism and the impact of TRPC6 disruption in human neurons. *Mol Psychiatry.* 2015;20(11):1350–1365. https://doi.org/10.1038/mp.2014.141.

89. Deneault E, White SH, Rodrigues DC, et al. Complete disruption of autism-susceptibility genes by gene editing predominantly reduces functional connectivity of isogenic human neurons. *Stem Cell Rep.* 2018;11(5):1211–1225. https://doi.org/10.1016/j.stemcr.2018.10.003.
90. Zhang W, Ma L, Yang M, et al. Cerebral organoid and mouse models reveal a RAB39b-PI3K-mTOR pathway-dependent dysregulation of cortical development leading to macrocephaly/autism phenotypes. *Genes Dev.* 2020;34(7–8):580–597. https://doi.org/10.1101/gad.332494.119.
91. Ernst C. Proliferation and differentiation deficits are a major convergence point for neurodevelopmental disorders. *Trends Neurosci.* 2016;39(5):290–299. https://doi.org/10.1016/j.tins.2016.03.001.
92. Adhya D, Swarup V, Nagy R, et al. Atypical neurogenesis in induced pluripotent stem cells from autistic individuals. *Biol Psychiatry.* 2021;89(5):486–496. https://doi.org/10.1016/j.biopsych.2020.06.014.
93. Gai X, Xie HM, Perin JC, et al. Rare structural variation of synapse and neurotransmission genes in autism. *Mol Psychiatry.* 2012;17(4):402–411. https://doi.org/10.1038/mp.2011.10.
94. Griesi-Oliveira K, Suzuki AM, Alves AY, et al. Actin cytoskeleton dynamics in stem cells from autistic individuals. *Sci Rep.* 2018;8(1):11138. https://doi.org/10.1038/s41598-018-29309-6.
95. Livide G, Patriarchi T, Amenduni M, et al. GluD1 is a common altered player in neuronal differentiation from both MECP2-mutated and CDKL5-mutated iPS cells. *Eur J Hum Genet.* 2015;23(2):195–201. https://doi.org/10.1038/ejhg.2014.81.
96. Patriarchi T, Amabile S, Frullanti E, et al. Imbalance of excitatory/inhibitory synaptic protein expression in iPSC-derived neurons from FOXG1(+/-) patients and in foxg1(+/-) mice. *Eur J Hum Genet.* 2016;24(6):871–880. https://doi.org/10.1038/ejhg.2015.216.
97. Yasumura M, Yoshida T, Lee S-J, Uemura T, Joo J-Y, Mishina M. Glutamate receptor δ1 induces preferentially inhibitory presynaptic differentiation of cortical neurons by interacting with neurexins through cerebellin precursor protein subtypes. *J Neurochem.* 2012;121(5):705–716. https://doi.org/10.1111/j.1471-4159.2011.07631.x.
98. Dickinson A, Jones M, Milne E. Measuring neural excitation and inhibition in autism: different approaches, different findings and different interpretations. *Brain Res.* 2016;1648:277–289. https://doi.org/10.1016/j.brainres.2016.07.011.
99. Zuiki M, Chiyonobu T, Yoshida M, et al. Luteolin attenuates interleukin-6-mediated astrogliosis in human iPSC-derived neural aggregates: a candidate preventive substance for maternal immune activation-induced abnormalities. *Neurosci Lett.* 2017;653:296–301. https://doi.org/10.1016/j.neulet.2017.06.004.
100. Galvez-Contreras AY, Zarate-Lopez D, Torres-Chavez AL, Gonzalez-Perez O. Role of oligodendrocytes and myelin in the pathophysiology of autism spectrum disorder. *Brain Sci.* 2020;10(12). https://doi.org/10.3390/brainsci10120951.
101. Kim JW, Hong JY, Bae SM. Microglia and autism spectrum disorder: overview of current evidence and novel immunomodulatory treatment options. *Clin Psychopharmacol Neurosci.* 2018;16(3):246–252. https://doi.org/10.9758/cpn.2018.16.3.246.
102. Liao X, Yang J, Wang H, Li Y. Microglia mediated neuroinflammation in autism spectrum disorder. *J Psychiatr Res.* 2020;130:167–176. https://doi.org/10.1016/j.jpsychires.2020.07.013.

CHAPTER

# 11

# Overview of autism interventions

*Erin Kang*[a], *Rachel G. McDonald*[a], *and Susan W. White*[b]

**[a]Psychology Department, Montclair State University, Montclair, NJ, United States, [b]Department of Psychology, The University of Alabama, Tuscaloosa, AL, United States**

## Overview of autism interventions

Given the rising prevalence of autism spectrum disorder (ASD), it is crucial to develop effective treatments for individuals with ASD. Just as ASD is a markedly heterogeneous condition with a diverse range of presenting problems, there are various treatment options with varying degrees of empirical support. A growing body of literature on treatments for ASD demonstrates that efficacious and effective interventions produce reductions in ASD symptoms, as well as improved health, well-being, and quality of life for individuals with ASD. While early intervention for young children with ASD may focus on core ASD symptoms to improve social function, language ability, and functional communication, focus of treatment may shift as the individual gets older to other problems that are impairing the individual's life rather than core ASD symptoms. Therefore, effectively addressing secondary, co-occurring symptoms (e.g., anxiety) can also lead to meaningful changes and reduce impairment.

Due to a variety of intervention methods available for individuals with ASD with varying treatment targets, determination of empirically supported treatments for ASD may be different than other disorders. The criteria for "empirically validated" treatments were initially established by the 1995 report from the Society of Clinical Psychology (Division 12 of the American Psychological Association) Task Force on Promotion and Dissemination of Psychological Treatment Procedures.[1] Evidence-based

*The Neuroscience of Autism*
https://doi.org/10.1016/B978-0-12-816393-1.00004-X

treatments (EBT) are treatments that have been proven effective (to some degree) through outcome evaluations with following criteria according to Chambless and Hollon: (a) Has the treatment been shown to be beneficial in controlled research? (efficacy); (b) Is the treatment useful in applied clinical settings and, if so, with what patients and under what circumstances? (effectiveness); and (c) Is the treatment efficient in the sense of being cost-effective relative to other alternative interventions?[2]

Although it is beyond the scope of this chapter to fully review them, there are several resources on EBT practices for ASD. For example, the National Clearinghouse on Autism Evidence and Practice (NCAEP) also released a report identifying 28 evidence-based practices in ASD and 10 manualized interventions that also met criteria from the literature published from 1990 to 2017 (See Resources at the end of the chapter for additional resources). Given the focus of the present chapter, we provide an overview of interventions for ASD, and describe treatment approaches that are evidence-based and/or promising in terms of efficacy for the common challenges for children and adolescents with ASD, including intervention approaches for core (i.e., diagnostic of ASD) and secondary (i.e., co-occurring) symptoms.

## Behavioral/cognitive interventions

### Applied behavioral analysis (ABA)

One of the most frequently used behavioral interventions for ASD are early interventions based in applied behavioral analysis (ABA) techniques.[3,4]According to the US Surgeon General and the American Psychological Association, ABA is considered an evidence-based best practice treatment and the most empirically-supported treatment for core communication deficits in ASD. ABA refers to a set of principles that form the basis for many behavioral treatments.[5] Specifically, ABA is a highly structured data-driven approach that uses operant and classical conditioning to modify behavior through the reinforcement of positive behavioral response.[6] Early Intensive Behavioral Interventions (EIBI) is an example of a well-established ABA intervention.[7] Discrete Trial Training (DTT) is one of the most common techniques within a behavior analytic framework, using a structured one-to-one approach to reinforce correct response to a cue from a therapist.[8] Pivotal Response Training (PRT) and Naturalistic Developmental Behavioral Interventions (NDBIs) are also variations of an ABA-based model.[4,9,10] PRT and NDBIs approach reinforcing positive behaviors in less structured play-based or natural environments.[11] Further, rather than targeting specific behaviors, PRT targets developmental areas such as motivation, responding to multiple cues, self-management, and self-initiations.[4,9,10] Similarly, NDBIs are centered in the reinforcement of behaviors that are produced spontaneously in naturalistic environments.[11] NDBIs combine ABA and developmental principles, whereby the child and therapist share control and natural spontaneous responses are heavily reinforced.[10] While this technique is often more flexible than traditional ABA approaches (cf. DTT), it still has specific targeted behaviors, contingent feedback, and a clear data-oriented goal-tracking.[6,9,10] The Early Start Denver Model (ESDM) is an example of a NDBI that combines naturalistic teaching methods into a comprehensive intervention package to target a range of developmental domains.[12]

### *Symptoms targeted*

EIBIs are often used to target core skills deficits and behavioral challenges.[13] Language deficits, developmental delays, and adaptive behaviors are often targeted by both traditional ABA and NDBIs.[6] For example, ESDM targets a range of developmental domains, such as communication, cognitive, social, language, motor, and adaptive behaviors.[12]

### *State of the evidence*

Both efficacy and effectiveness of ABA approaches and DTT, PRT, and NDBI are supported by a number of empirical studies and in systematic reviews and metaanalyses.[6,9,14,15] Studies have demonstrated effects of ABA approaches in reducing problem behaviors and improving academics, adaptive skills, communication, and social behaviors.[16,17] Most evidence base for ABA comes from children younger than 8 years old receiving high doses of intensive therapy (up to 40 hours per week).[18] Specifically, NDBIs have shown small-to-moderate effect sizes for treating autism symptoms, social engagement, cognitive functioning, expressive, and receptive language.[6,12,19]

## Cognitive-behavioral therapy (CBT)

CBT is a widely used treatment in psychotherapy that works to create improvements in psychological functioning by targeting cognitions, behaviors, and environment.[20,21] CBT focuses on replacing negative or ineffective patterns of thought and behaviors (e.g., maladaptive or distorted automatic thoughts) with more adaptive and effective ones (efficient problem-solving and coping strategies, and accurately identifying other's thoughts, feelings, and behaviors).[20–22] The therapist often works with the client to be able to accurately identify and utilize these skills in their day-to-day life. Behavioral strategies, such as exposures, where the client works on facing and noticing natural reduction in distress rather than avoiding fearful or uncomfortable experiences, and behavioral experiments (e.g., what-if exercises) are often utilized. Sometimes this behavioral work is paired with the use of relaxation techniques and training in adaptive coping skills.[20] These experiences are tailored to the person's current situation and to help the individual successfully experience previously feared or avoided environments, improving quality of life.

### *Symptoms targeted*

In ASD interventions, CBT approaches have been adapted to target problems such as anxiety, anger, depression, and social deficits by helping individuals with ASD learn to accurately monitor their own behaviors and regulate their behaviors appropriately.[23–25] CBT for anxiety disorders often has adaptations in the following categories to allow for better understanding and ease of delivery of the treatment: (1) concrete language; (2) incorporation of tools and supports (i.e., visuals); (3) incorporation of special interests; (4) use of hierarchies addressing both anxiety and ASD symptoms; (5) increased psychoeducation; and (6) parental involvement.[20,22–24,26] Additionally, reliance on primarily behavioral strategies (rather than cognitive) may be useful when treating individuals with reduced verbal abilities or cognitive inflexibility. These approaches reduce the cognitive burden on the client and instead target skills such as adaptive behaviors, social communication, and daily living skills, allowing the client to address anxiety and ASD symptoms through targeted behavioral changes.[20,22] While these adaptations are focused on anxiety, considering these adaptations in CBT for other internalizing disorders may optimize outcomes. A recent systematic review of CBT found that the most common CBT interventions used to treat anxiety are *Facing Your Fears*,[25] *Multimodal Anxiety and Social Skills Intervention*,[23] and *Behavioral Interventions for Anxiety in Children with Autism*.[22,24] Each of these manualized treatments has been adapted or designed for children and adolescents with ASD.

### *State of the evidence*

CBT has recently begun to garner attention of researchers and clinicians for the treatment of co-occurring disorders in ASD. The majority of studies conducted on CBT in ASD focus on the treatment of anxiety disorders, with moderate-to-large effects.[23–25,27] There is limited evidence on the effects of CBT in targeting depression, obsessive-compulsive disorder, emotion regulation, and anger problems in ASD.[28–31] Of note, most CBT literature has focused on children and adolescents with IQs above 70. That said, some research suggests that CBT may be effective for treating anxiety and emotion regulation in children under 8 years old.[32]

## Mindfulness-based approaches

Mindfulness-based Interventions (MBIs) promote nonjudgmental awareness, decreased emotional avoidance and use of helpful coping strategies.[33,34] MBIs often utilize meditations, relaxation techniques, and mindful awareness to promote resilience and discourage avoidance of emotional plan and distress.[35–37] Studies examining MBIs have mainly been conducted in adolescents and adults with average cognitive functioning.[33,36–42] MBIs may be an effective intervention strategy to address underlying deficits with cognitive and emotional control leading to generalized improvements and can be an alternative for CBT-based treatments.

## Symptoms targeted

Many MBIs focus on general quality of life improvements combined with specific symptom targets, such as anxiety, depression, emotion regulation, social communication, and aggressive behaviors.[31,33,35,37,40,41] MBIs may improve internalizing and externalizing symptoms through targeting the underlying emotional dysregulation and promoting emotional control.[36]

## Modifications for ASD

While MBIs provide strategies that are not as cognitively demanding as CBT, some modifications may be helpful when treating individuals with ASD. Metaphors and the incorporation of abstract thoughts are often eliminated or simplified when MBIs are being used with individuals with ASD.[20,22,35] It is also suggested to start with meditations that focus on physical awareness or external stimuli (e.g., sounds in the room) and then move to internal awareness (e.g., of one's breath) once the skill has been significantly practiced.[35] Further, activities and meditations are often reduced in length to account for limited attention, and language is simplified. Due to heightened sensory and emotional experiences in some individuals with ASD, mindfulness-based practices may be an overwhelming experience. Clinicians should be vigilant of this possibility, and model nonjudgmental awareness of the individual's experience and sensations, focusing on practicing the present-centered awareness, skills growth, and providing encouragement.[35,43]

## State of the evidence

Preliminary evidence suggests that MBIs may improve prosocial behaviors, co-occurring internalizing symptoms (anxiety and depression) and emotion regulation in adolescents and adults with ASD,[33,36,39–41] as well as reduce externalizing behaviors such as aggression.[37,40] Even though MBIs are in the preliminary stages of research, one study compared MBI to CBT and found similar reductions in anxiety and depression symptoms.[44] Further, some recent evidence has shown positive results with the addition of yoga techniques.[37] Overall, MBIs are a promising approach in this population and warrant further research.

## Social skills interventions

Social skills interventions (SSI) are widely used approaches to improve social functioning in ASD. Specifically, group-based SSIs are frequently used, as they provide in vivo opportunity for practicing learned skills in a naturalistic setting.[45,46] SSIs can take several different approaches to interventions involving different content and methodologies. Two of the most common are structured-learning and social-performance-based approaches.[45,47–49] Structured-learning SSIs often take a didactic approach where skills are explicitly taught by a provider, then practiced in vivo where direct feedback can be provided (e.g., UCLA Program for the Educational and Enrichment of Relational Skills; PEERS).[49] Social performance SSIs do not actively teach social skills with didactic learning. Rather, these skills are implicitly learned through naturalistic social experiences provided in an enriched, supported group setting with peers (e.g., Socio-Dramatic Affective-Relational Intervention,[45,50] SENSE Theater[51]).

### Symptoms targeted

SSIs often focus on improving social competence, social skills, peer, and/or romantic relationships in children and adults with ASD. Some specific targets of treatment are skills relating to Theory of Mind, emotion recognition, self-awareness, acquisition of skills to understand nonliteral language, among other skills relating to social engagement and peer relationship,[45,51] whereas others focus on appropriate nonverbal communication strategies (e.g., eye contact), appropriate conversation topics and starters.[49,52] In some approaches, both caregivers and children are often provided with psychoeducation about social skills, and caregivers are involved in implementing learned skills outside of the intervention setting to facilitate generalization and skill maintenance posttreatment.[52,53]

### State of the evidence

Individual and group-based SSIs have both been shown to be effective and efficacious for treating social skills deficits in ASD, as reported in several reviews and metaanalytic studies.[45–47,54] Further, these treatments often show improvements in the frequency of peer interaction and number of friendships an individual has.[53,54] Other secondary improvements have also been observed from SSI treatments, such as improvements in anxiety, and depression.[23] However, findings from some SSIs are often limited to parent-report and by differences across interventions models. A recent metaanalysis of group-based SSIs suggests an overall medium effect size in improvement in social competence for youth with ASD.[47] However, the effects seem to differ by informants. For example, while effects are the largest for self-report, they are attributable entirely to improved social knowledge, not self-reported changes in social behavior.[47] Moreover, some studies report rather small effects, especially for observer-reported outcomes.[55] It is also worth noting that the evidence around long-term transfer or generalization of intervention effects is limited and should be further examined in future research.[55,56]

## Biological/pharmaceutical interventions

### Pharmaceutical approaches

While there is no medication that has demonstrated efficacy for directly treating core ASD symptoms in social communicative challenges, many individuals with ASD receive pharmacological treatment, that fall into many different subcategories of medications to address co-occurring symptoms: antipsychotics, stimulants, glutamatergic and gamma-aminobutyric acid (GABA) agents, and selective serotonin reuptake inhibitors (SSRI).[57] The most commonly used and most studied medication type in ASD is antipsychotics. Two antipsychotics have been approved by US Food and Drug Administration (FDA) for treatment of irritability (e.g., aggression) in children with ASD—risperidone and aripiprazole; however, most other medications are prescribed "off-label" (without FDA approval) to treat ASD and other co-occurring symptoms.[58–60] Many individuals with ASD who are placed on a medication in childhood continue to be medicated into adulthood.[61]

#### *Symptoms targeted*

Antipsychotics, such as risperidone, aripiprazole, and haloperidol, are often used for treating behavioral problems and irritability in adolescents with ASD.[60,62,63] Psychostimulants can help treat symptoms of attention deficit/hyperactivity disorder (ADHD) such as hyperactivity and impulsivity.[58,64,65] SSRIs are often utilized to address repetitive and restrictive behaviors with careful monitoring of possible adverse side effects.[66–68]

#### *State of the evidence*

Although pharmaceutical approaches in ASD are very common (with over one-half of individuals with ASD receiving treatment), these approaches are extremely understudied and are often not approved for use by the FDA.[58] Risperidone, aripiprazole, and haloperidol have shown some effectiveness for treating behavioral symptoms and irritability in adolescents with ASD, but come with significant side effects (e.g., breast enlargement and lactation, weight gain).[58,62,63] Clonidine, guanfacine, methylphenidate, and atomoxetine have demonstrated efficacy in improving ADHD symptoms with minimal side effects.[58,64,65] There is no clear evidence reflecting effectiveness of SSRIs in treating repetitive and stereotyped behaviors in ASD.[58,67,68] While glutamatergic agents have shown little-to-no effects, GABA agents (e.g., Bumetanide) have shown tentative improvement.[67,69,70] However, these are early-stage trials and further research is needed on possible side effects, as individuals with ASD are generally more likely to experience side effects.[57]

## Alternative medical approaches

Alternative medical approaches have gained attention in the past few years. These approaches include use of oxytocin, melatonin, sulforaphane, as well as treatments targeting the gut microbiota.[38,59,71,72] These approaches are used as either complementary (i.e., in addition to other approaches) or alternative to other medical interventions. Oxytocin is a neuropeptide hormone that plays a major role in many physiological and neurological processes. It has gained recent attention related to the treatment of ASD due its role in social affiliation and influence on social behavior.[59] Although results are mixed, recent studies have shown improvements in repetitive behaviors, social communication, and social recognition with minimal side effects for most participants.[73,74] Melatonin is a naturally produced hormone in the human body that relates to sleep behaviors. Sleep disturbances are common in individuals with ASD; evidence suggests that melatonin increases sleep duration and latency with few side effects.[71] Further, melatonin has been shown to improve anxiety, communication, and rigidity.[75,76] Sulforaphane is a naturally produced phytochemical found in some foods and seeds.[72] A recent study suggests that high doses of sulforaphane taken orally may improve cognition and behavioral symptoms in youth with ASD.[77] While sulforaphane seems to be well-tolerated by most participants, it is important to note that some participants experienced significant side effects.[72,77] Several treatments regarding the gut have emerged in recent literature in response to theories relating to inflammation in the gut and anomalies in the gut-brain axis in individuals with ASD.[38,78] For example, microbiota transfer therapy targets the gut through implantation of healthy bacteria. While studies investigating this approach have shown significant improvement behavioral problems and symptoms of ASD after treatment, there is still very limited research on this topic in ASD.[38,78,79]

### *State of the evidence*

Evidence for alternative medical treatments in ASD is still quite new and understudied. For each approach discussed, most studies have small sample sizes and findings are not universally supported.[58,78] While many of these approaches appear to be effective for treating ASD symptoms they should be further studied in order to establish effectiveness.

# Other approaches

## Parent-mediated approaches

Parent training approaches or parent-mediated interventions (PMI) are skills-based approaches that use psychoeducation and parenting skills training to manage child's behavior.[66,80] PMIs can be effective as parents often play an integral role in helping children generalize newly learned skills. Moreover, PMIs may help increase parental self-efficacy and reduce parenting stress. PMIs are used to target various behaviors in children with ASD, including aggressive behaviors, restrictive eating, improving communication skills, parent-child interactions, and decreased parental stress.[81,82] These approaches often involve theories of behavior and social learning in order to train parents on implementing behavioral changes through the identification of antecedents and consequences of their child's behavior. Some studies have suggested PMIs to be effective for treating behavioral problems, ASD symptoms, poor self-regulation, and for training adaptive behaviors in children and adolescents. Specifically, Parent Management Training (PMT) and the RUBI Autism Network Parent Training programs have been shown to be effective in treating disruptive and hyperactive behaviors in children with ASD.[83,84] Both PMT and RUBI focus on addressing disruptive behaviors through parent training to improve behavioral management and psychoeducation about ASD and the interpretation of expressed behaviors.[83,85] However, PMT also has components focused on the management of anxiety and rigidity, while RUBI's training focuses mainly on behavioral management strategies and maintenance. These treatments are unique in the regard that they are designed specifically for children with ASD who are experiencing behavioral problems.[83,85] Other PMIs, such as Floortime techniques, have shown to exert improvements in self-regulation, language development, and improved parent-child engagement.[86,87] Floortime is named as such because the parent gets down on the floor with the child to meet them at their level, and focuses on building parent-child relationships using play-based activities to improve parent engagement, child and parent communication, and skills deficits in the child.[86,87] While these treatments have all demonstrated effectiveness, most research focuses on parents of young children and limited research investigates parental outcomes.[88]

## Technology-based approaches

Technology-based approaches have been gaining in popularity in recent years, and are diverse in format (e.g., use of virtual reality, multiplayer gaming) and technology employed (e.g., iPad, robots).[89] There has been mixed evidence presented about the efficacy of these treatment approaches, although there is a fair amount of usability research suggesting feasibility and acceptability of these approaches.[89–91] Those that have shown positive effects have target social communication deficits, language, social skills, and facilitating learning.[91,92] However, it is important to note that most trials of these approaches were conducted in very small groups of children and adolescence, and the maintenance of effects of these treatments has only been established in some studies.[89] To gain more perspective on the utility of these treatments, further research should be conducted on a larger scale.

### Special education and related services

Many children with ASD receive special education services and have their Individualized Education Program (IEP) at school. There are also additional comprehensive special education programs for students with ASD. TEACCH Autism Program is a method that provides structured tools and strategies to teachers in the classroom setting, such as external/physical organizational supports, individualized schedules, visual or written information, and structured support for social communication.[93] TEACCH has a substantial research base.[94] Other disciplines such as speech-language, occupational, and physical therapy also provide specific interventions for individuals with ASD, often in home or school settings.[95–98] Speech-language therapy addresses challenges in language and communication, including verbal, nonverbal, and pragmatic communication.[99] Interventions targeting communication deficits have the most literature supporting effectiveness.[95] Occupational therapy targets skills that help individuals participate in a range of day-to-day activities, such as independent dressing, eating, and fine motor skills.[100] Physical therapy and sensory integration activities target deficits in behavior or movements.[101] These interventions have been shown to be effective in treating these symptoms; however, there is a disparity of evidence.[95,96,100] In conclusion, these approaches provide an effective tool for the treatment of some ASD and other impairing symptoms, although they require further research.[101]

## Interventions for adults with ASD

ASD is a lifelong, chronic condition that typically persists through adulthood.[102] However, there is great paucity of evidence-based interventions for adults with ASD. Of all therapeutic intervention studies conducted in ASD, only 8% of participants were older than 18 years old, and only 16% of studies included adults with ASD.[103] Of those studies, most were for pharmaceutical or behavioral interventions targeting core ASD symptoms.[103] A limited number of studies have begun to focus on job or employment training, mental health interventions, or quality of life outcomes.[103] More studies are now ongoing to examine effects of services and supports (e.g., job or employment training, health management) for transition-age youth and adults with ASD in improving the functioning and community integration of adults on the spectrum.

## Implications for researchers and clinicians

The literature on evidence-based interventions for ASD has grown tremendously, reflecting promising evidence for individuals with ASD and their families. While treatments for ASD have traditionally focused on young children and school-aged children, there has also been an increase in efforts to provide appropriate and effective interventions for adolescents and adults on the spectrum. Overall, it is important to acknowledge that there is no "one-size-fits-all" intervention method for individuals with ASD. Also, most individuals with ASD and their families receive a combination of interventions that often impact multiple domains of life, underscoring the importance of multidisciplinary collaboration (e.g., psychologists, therapists, social workers, primary care providers, psychiatrists, teachers, school administrators, as well as family) in coordinating intervention planning and care. The field of autism research is increasingly recognizing the importance of meaningfully including autistic people, their families, and those who work directly with persons on the spectrum as stakeholders in research (participatory action research).[104,105] Particularly for intervention research, academic researchers and clinicians can collaborate and participate in community-engaged research to develop and implement effective interventions in community settings (e.g., Fortuna et al.[106]). In autism research, guidelines for participatory research might include leadership by or partnership with autistic people and promoting inclusiveness to improve engagement with the diverse community of stakeholders.[107–109]

In addition, it is particularly important for researchers and clinicians to be well-informed of evidence-based treatments, and as there are potentially harmful treatments that are still frequently administered in clinical and educational settings that warrant caution.[110,111] Clinical psychology, as a field, has historically focused on demonstration of clinical impact, or therapeutic benefit, arguably at the exclusion of adequately considering potential harmful impacts.[112] Some interventions that have been implemented for ASD do indeed pose "obvious" physical risks (e.g., chelation therapy; hyperbaric oxygen therapy).[113] Many more treatment approaches, however, pose risks that are less obvious in nature (e.g., excessive cost or time involvement, which could preclude other treatments). Critical consumption of the literature, in order to make evidence-based decisions about treatment, requires clinicians (and families) to evaluate the quality of the scientific evidence for benefit, as well as the risk for burden and harm.[114]

Despite advancements, there are still challenges for improving interventions for individuals with ASD. Substantial heterogeneity in core and secondary symptom presentation in ASD can complicate accurate assessment of treatment response. Recent advancement in identifying meaningful subtypes within ASD and their implications for personalized treatment underscores flexible intervention strategies that adapt to the diverse needs of individuals with ASD.[115–117] Also, many intervention studies failed to assess generalization of skills posttreatment, or report that it is difficult to achieve when individuals no longer receive clinical support and in vivo reinforcement. Thus, future studies should address the issue of sustainability of effects.[56] Furthermore, examining the trajectory of social development and mechanistic processes (as opposed to focusing on outcomes at posttreatment) via prospective, longitudinal studies would provide insights into optimal windows of time (or critical periods) for specific intervention, as well how interventions may reorganize neural pathways across development, which in turn may be useful in the formulation of more effective intervention.

Moreover, there is an increasing need to move beyond the questions of "Does the intervention work?" to understanding mechanisms of change by examining mediators (factors that can be responsible for the effects of a given intervention) and moderators (i.e., "for whom" and "under what conditions") of treatment response, which will help advance the field toward a precision medicine approach.[118] For example, as the field has recognized the impact of frequently co-occurring conditions in individuals with ASD, it is important to examine how the efficacy of treatment may be hampered by comorbid conditions like ADHD and anxiety.[119]

To better assess effects of intervention for ASD, issues around assessment tools should also be addressed. A recent systematic review of 406 clinical trials identified a lack of standardization and harmonization of assessment tools and specific target domains across outcome studies, making it difficult to draw comparisons across studies or to effectively synthesize the findings.[120] Treatments should be evaluated using a multiinformant, multimethod approach, integrating across biological, behavioral, and psychophysiological measures. Recent developments have focused on use of more objective neuroscience methods that are less reliant on subjective perceptions of change.[121] Such an approach can offer specific insights into the mechanisms that are impacted by a given intervention and provides a way to identify potential processes supporting maintenance of effects over time, particularly during childhood and adolescence when dynamic neurophysiological changes occur. Putative biomarkers associated with symptoms of ASD (e.g., latency of the N170 event-related potential) may serve as predictors of treatment response, thereby providing insights to clinicians for identifying who will most likely benefit from the intervention.[122,123] Indeed, research suggests that such biomarkers may be used to indicate change in the neural processes related to symptoms in ASD, thereby bridging the gap between basic research and clinical assessment and pointing toward personalized treatments.[124–128] In addition, collaboration potential to translate preclinical models, such as animal models of ASD, to the clinical setting can also provide insight into etiology and mechanisms underlying ASD to identify targets for novel therapeutic approaches.[129] Such practices will be vital for improving evidence-based practices for individuals with ASD and their families.

## Resources on evidence-based treatments for ASD

- **American Psychological Association (APA)** https://www.apa.org/
- **Association for Behavioral and Cognitive Therapies (ABCT)** https://www.abct.org/
- **Autistica** https://www.autistica.org.uk/
- **British Association for Behavioral and Cognitive Psychotherapies (BABCP)** https://babcp.com/
- **British Psychological Society (BPS)** https://www.bps.org.uk/
- **Center for Disease Control and Prevention (CDC)** https://www.cdc.gov/
- **Cochrane Library** https://www.cochranelibrary.com/
- **Effective Child Therapy** (by the Society of Clinical Child & Adolescent Psychology) https://effectivechildtherapy.org/concerns-symptoms-disorders/disorders/autism/
- **National Autism Center/National Standards Project** https://www.nationalautismcenter.org/national-standards-project/
- **National Autistic Society (NAS)** https://www.autism.org.uk/
- **National Professional Development Center on Autism Spectrum Disorder** https://autismpdc.fpg.unc.edu/evidence-based-practices

## References


1. Steinbrenner JR, Hume K, Odom SL, et al. *Evidence-Based Practices for Children, Youth, and Young Adults with Autism.* The University of North Carolina at Chapel Hill, Frank Porter Graham Child Development Institute, National Clearinghouse on Autism Evidence and Practice Review Team; 2020. Published online.
2. Chambless DL, Hollon SD. Defining empirically supported therapies. *J Consult Clin Psychol.* 1998;66(1). https://doi.org/10.1037/0022-006X.66.1.7.
3. Lovass O. *Teaching Individuals with Developmental Delays: Basic Intervention Techniques.* PRO-ED; 2003.

4. Chahin SS, Apple RW, Kuo KH, Dickson CA. Autism spectrum disorder: psychological and functional assessment, and behavioral treatment approaches. *Transl Pediatr.* 2020;9(S1):S66–S75. https://doi.org/10.21037/tp.2019.11.06.
5. U.S. Departmemt of Health and Human Services. *Mental Health: Culture, Race, and Ethnicity: A Supplement to Mental Health: A Report of the Surgeon General.* US public health service: Substance abuse and mental health services administration; 2001. Published online.
6. Tiede G, Walton KM. Meta-analysis of naturalistic developmental behavioral interventions for young children with autism spectrum disorder. *Autism.* 2019;23(8):2080–2095. https://doi.org/10.1177/1362361319836371.
7. Lovaas OI. Behavioral treatment and normal educational and intellectual functioning in young autistic children. *J Consult Clin Psychol.* 1987;55(1):3–9. https://doi.org/10.1037/0022-006X.55.1.3.
8. Lei J, Ventola P. Pivotal response treatment for autism spectrum disorder: current perspectives. *Neuropsychiatr Dis Treat.* 2017;13. https://doi.org/10.2147/NDT.S120710.
9. Fuller EA, Kaiser AP. The effects of early intervention on social communication outcomes for children with autism spectrum disorder: a meta-analysis. *J Autism Dev Disord.* 2020;50(5):1683–1700. https://doi.org/10.1007/s10803-019-03927-z.
10. Nahmias AS, Pellecchia M, Stahmer AC, Mandell DS. Effectiveness of community-based early intervention for children with autism spectrum disorder: a meta-analysis. *J Child Psychol Psychiatry Allied Discip.* 2019;60(11):1200–1209. https://doi.org/10.1111/jcpp.13073.
11. Schreibman L, Dawson G, Stahmer AC, et al. Naturalistic developmental behavioral interventions: empirically validated treatments for autism spectrum disorder. *J Autism Dev Disord.* 2015;45(8). https://doi.org/10.1007/s10803-015-2407-8.
12. Rogers SJ, Estes A, Lord C, et al. A multisite randomized controlled two-phase trial of the early start Denver model compared to treatment as usual. *J Am Acad Child Adolesc Psychiatry.* 2019;58(9). https://doi.org/10.1016/j.jaac.2019.01.004.
13. Myers SM, Johnson CP, Lipkin PH, et al. Management of children with autism spectrum disorders. *Pediatrics.* 2007;120(5). https://doi.org/10.1542/peds.2007-2362.
14. Reichow B, Barton EE, Boyd BA, Hume K. Early intensive behavioral intervention (EIBI) for young children with autism spectrum disorders (ASD). *Cochrane Database Syst Rev.* 2012. https://doi.org/10.1002/14651858.cd009260.pub2.
15. Smith T, Iadarola S. Evidence base update for autism spectrum disorder. *J Clin Child Adolesc Psychol.* 2015;44(6). https://doi.org/10.1080/15374416.2015.1077448.
16. Koegel LK, Carter CM, Koegel RL. Teaching children with autism self-initiations as a pivotal response. *Top Lang Disord.* 2003;23(2). https://doi.org/10.1097/00011363-200304000-00006.
17. Pierce K, Schreibman L. Increasing complex social behaviors in children with autism: effects of peer-implemented pivotal response training. *J Appl Behav Anal.* 1995;28(3). https://doi.org/10.1901/jaba.1995.28-285.
18. Eikeseth S, Smith T, Jahr E, Eldevik S. Outcome for children with autism who began intensive behavioral treatment between ages 4 and 7: a comparison controlled study. *Behav Modif.* 2007;31(3). https://doi.org/10.1177/0145445506291396.
19. Lake JK, Tablon Modica P, Chan V, Weiss JA. Considering efficacy and effectiveness trials of cognitive behavioral therapy among youth with autism: a systematic review. *Autism.* 2020;24(7):1590–1606. https://doi.org/10.1177/1362361320918754.
20. White SW, Simmons GL, Gotham KO, et al. Psychosocial treatments targeting anxiety and depression in adolescents and adults on the autism spectrum: review of the latest research and recommended future directions. *Curr Psychiatry Rep.* 2018;20(10). https://doi.org/10.1007/s11920-018-0949-0.
21. Farmer RF, Chapman AL, Farmer RF, Chapman AL. Changing behavior by building skills. In: *Behavioral Interventions in Cognitive Behavior Therapy: Practical Guidance for Putting Theory into Action.* 2nd ed; 2015. https://doi.org/10.1037/14691-006.

22. Keefer A, White SW, Vasa RA, Reaven J. Psychosocial interventions for internalizing disorders in youth and adults with ASD. *Int Rev Psychiatry.* 2018;30(1):62–77. https://doi.org/10.1080/09540261.2018.1432575.
23. White SW, Ollendick T, Albano AM, et al. Randomized controlled trial: multimodal anxiety and social skill intervention for adolescents with autism spectrum disorder. *J Autism Dev Disord.* 2013;43(2). https://doi.org/10.1007/s10803-012-1577-x.
24. Wood JJ, Drahota A, Sze K, Har K, Chiu A, Langer DA. Cognitive behavioral therapy for anxiety in children with autism spectrum disorders: a randomized, controlled trial. *J Child Psychol Psychiatry Allied Discip.* 2009;50(3). https://doi.org/10.1111/j.1469-7610.2008.01948.x.
25. Reaven J, Blakeley-Smith A, Culhane-Shelburne K, Hepburn S. Group cognitive behavior therapy for children with high-functioning autism spectrum disorders and anxiety: a randomized trial. *J Child Psychol Psychiatry Allied Discip.* 2012;53(4). https://doi.org/10.1111/j.1469-7610.2011.02486.x.
26. Moree BN, Davis TE. Cognitive-behavioral therapy for anxiety in children diagnosed with autism spectrum disorders: modification trends. *Res Autism Spectr Disord.* 2010;4(3). https://doi.org/10.1016/j.rasd.2009.10.015.
27. Vasa RA, Carroll LM, Nozzolillo AA, et al. A systematic review of treatments for anxiety in youth with autism spectrum disorders. *J Autism Dev Disord.* 2014;44(12):3215–3229. https://doi.org/10.1007/s10803-014-2184-9.
28. McGillivray JA, Evert HT. Group cognitive behavioural therapy program shows potential in reducing symptoms of depression and stress among young people with ASD. *J Autism Dev Disord.* 2014;44(8). https://doi.org/10.1007/s10803-014-2087-9.
29. Santomauro D, Sheffield J, Sofronoff K. Depression in adolescents with ASD: a pilot RCT of a group intervention. *J Autism Dev Disord.* 2016;46(2). https://doi.org/10.1007/s10803-015-2605-4.
30. Storch EA, Arnold EB, Lewin AB, et al. The effect of cognitive-behavioral therapy versus treatment as usual for anxiety in children with autism spectrum disorders: a randomized, controlled trial. *J Am Acad Child Adolesc Psychiatry.* 2013;52(2). https://doi.org/10.1016/j.jaac.2012.11.007.
31. Conner CM, White SW, Beck KB, Golt J, Smith IC, Mazefsky CA. Improving emotion regulation ability in autism: the emotional awareness and skills enhancement (EASE) program. *Autism.* 2019;23(5):1273–1287. https://doi.org/10.1177/1362361318810709.
32. Scarpa A, Reyes NM. Improving emotion regulation with CBT in young children with high functioning autism spectrum disorders: a pilot study. *Behav Cogn Psychother.* 2011;39(4):495–500. https://doi.org/10.1017/S1352465811000063.
33. Hartley M, Dorstyn D, Due C. Mindfulness for children and adults with autism spectrum disorder and their caregivers: a meta-analysis. *J Autism Dev Disord.* 2019;49(10):4306–4319. https://doi.org/10.1007/s10803-019-04145-3.
34. Kabat-Zinn J, Lipworth L, Burney R. The clinical use of mindfulness meditation for the self-regulation of chronic pain. *J Behav Med.* 1985;8(2). https://doi.org/10.1007/BF00845519.
35. Beck KB, Conner CM, White SW, Mazefsky CA. Mindfulness "here and now": strategies for helping adolescents with autism. *J Am Acad Child Adolesc Psychiatry.* 2020;59(10):1125–1127. https://doi.org/10.1016/j.jaac.2020.07.004.
36. Gu J, Strauss C, Bond R, Cavanagh K. How do mindfulness-based cognitive therapy and mindfulness-based stress reduction improve mental health and wellbeing? A systematic review and meta-analysis of mediation studies. *Clin Psychol Rev.* 2015;37. https://doi.org/10.1016/j.cpr.2015.01.006.
37. de Bruin EI, Blom R, Smit FMA, van Steensel FJA, Bögels SM. MYmind: mindfulness training for youngsters with autism spectrum disorders and their parents. *Autism.* 2015;19(8). https://doi.org/10.1177/1362361314553279.

38. Fattorusso A, di Genova L, Dell'isola GB, Mencaroni E, Esposito S. Autism spectrum disorders and the gut microbiota. *Nutrients.* 2019;11(3). https://doi.org/10.3390/nu11030521.
39. Beck KB, Greco CM, Terhorst LA, Skidmore ER, Kulzer JL, McCue MP. Mindfulness-based stress reduction for adults with autism spectrum disorder: feasibility and estimated effects. *Mind.* 2020;11(5):1286–1297. https://doi.org/10.1007/s12671-020-01345-2.
40. Ridderinkhof A, de Bruin EI, Blom R, Bögels SM. Mindfulness-based program for children with autism spectrum disorder and their parents: direct and long-term improvements. *Mind.* 2018;9(3). https://doi.org/10.1007/s12671-017-0815-x.
41. Semple RJ. Review: yoga and mindfulness for youth with autism spectrum disorder: review of the current evidence. *Child Adolesc Mental Health.* 2019;24(1):12–18. https://doi.org/10.1111/camh.12295.
42. Juliano AC, Alexander AO, DeLuca J, Genova H. Feasibility of a school-based mindfulness program for improving inhibitory skills in children with autism spectrum disorder. *Res Dev Disabil.* 2020;101. https://doi.org/10.1016/j.ridd.2020.103641.
43. White SW, Conner CM, Beck KB, Mazefsky CA. Clinical update: the implementation of evidence-based emotion regulation treatment for clients with Autism. *Evid-Based Pract Child Adolesc Ment Health.* 2020. https://doi.org/10.1080/23794925.2020.1796551.
44. Sizoo BB, Kuiper E. Cognitive behavioural therapy and mindfulness based stress reduction may be equally effective in reducing anxiety and depression in adults with autism spectrum disorders. *Res Dev Disabil.* 2017;64. https://doi.org/10.1016/j.ridd.2017.03.004.
45. Lerner M, McMahon C, Britton N. Group-based social skills interventions for adolescents with higher-functioning autism spectrum disorder: a review and looking to the future. *Adolesc Health Med Ther.* 2013. https://doi.org/10.2147/ahmt.s25402.
46. Williams White S, Keonig K, Scahill L. Social skills development in children with autism spectrum disorders: a review of the intervention research. *J Autism Dev Disord.* 2007;37(10). https://doi.org/10.1007/s10803-006-0320-x.
47. Gates JA, Kang E, Lerner MD. Efficacy of group social skills interventions for youth with autism spectrum disorder: a systematic review and meta-analysis. *Clin Psychol Rev.* 2017;52:164–181. https://doi.org/10.1016/j.cpr.2017.01.006.
48. Lerner MD, Mikami AY. A preliminary randomized controlled trial of two social skills interventions for youth with high-functioning autism spectrum disorders. *Focus Autism Other Dev Disabl.* 2012;27(3). https://doi.org/10.1177/1088357612450613.
49. Laugeson EA, Frankel F, Gantman A, Dillon AR, Mogil C. Evidence-based social skills training for adolescents with autism spectrum disorders: the UCLA PEERS program. *J Autism Dev Disord.* 2012;42(6). https://doi.org/10.1007/s10803-011-1339-1.
50. Marro BM, Kang E, Hauschild KM, Normansell KM, Abu-Ramadan TM, Lerner MD. Social performance-based interventions promote gains in social knowledge in the absence of explicit training for youth with autism spectrum disorder. *Bull Menninger Clin.* 2019;83(3):301–325. https://doi.org/10.1521/bumc.2019.83.3.301.
51. Corbett BA, Swain DM, Coke C, et al. Improvement in social deficits in autism spectrum disorders using a theatre-based, peer-mediated intervention. *Autism Res.* 2014;7(1). https://doi.org/10.1002/aur.1341.
52. Leaf JB, ed. *Handbook of Social Skills and Autism Spectrum Disorder: Assessment, Curricula, and Intervention.* New York: Springer; 2017.
53. Laugeson EA, Frankel F, Mogil C, Dillon AR. Parent-assisted social skills training to improve friendships in teens with autism spectrum disorders. *J Autism Dev Disord.* 2009;39(4). https://doi.org/10.1007/s10803-008-0664-5.
54. Reichow B, Steiner AM, Volkmar F. Social skills groups for people aged 6 to 21 with autism spectrum disorders (ASD). *Cochrane Database Syst Rev.* 2012;2012(7). https://doi.org/10.1002/14651858.CD008511.pub2.

55. Kamps D, Thiemann-Bourque K, Heitzman-Powell L, et al. A comprehensive peer network intervention to improve social communication of children with autism Spectrum disorders: a randomized trial in kindergarten and first grade. *J Autism Dev Disord.* 2015;45(6). https://doi.org/10.1007/s10803-014-2340-2.
56. Rao PA, Beidel DC, Murray MJ. Social skills interventions for children with Asperger's syndrome or high-functioning autism: a review and recommendations. *J Autism Dev Disord.* 2008;38(2). https://doi.org/10.1007/s10803-007-0402-4.
57. Cassidy S, Cassidy S. Medications to treat co-occurring psychiatric conditions in autism spectrum disorder. In: *The Oxford Handbook of Autism and Co-Occurring Psychiatric Conditions*; 2020. https://doi.org/10.1093/oxfordhb/9780190910761.013.19.
58. Goel R, Hong JS, Findling RL, Ji NY. An update on pharmacotherapy of autism spectrum disorder in children and adolescents. *Int Rev Psychiatry.* 2018;30(1). https://doi.org/10.1080/09540261.2018.1458706.
59. Cai Q, Feng L, Yap KZ. Systematic review and meta-analysis of reported adverse events of long-term intranasal oxytocin treatment for autism spectrum disorder. *Psychiatry Clin Neurosci.* 2018;72(3):140–151. https://doi.org/10.1111/pcn.12627.
60. Fung LK, Mahajan R, Nozzolillo A, et al. *Pharmacologic Treatment of Severe Irritability and Problem Behaviors in Autism: A Systematic Review and Meta-Analysis.* vol 137; 2016. www.aappublications.org/news.
61. Mandell DS, Morales KH, Marcus SC, Stahmer AC, Doshi J, Polsky DE. Psychotropic medication use among medicaid-enrolled children with autism spectrum disorders. *Pediatrics.* 2008;121(3). https://doi.org/10.1542/peds.2007-0984.
62. McCracken JT, McGough J, Shah B, et al. Risperidone in children with autism and serious behavioral problems. *N Engl J Med.* 2002;347(5). https://doi.org/10.1056/nejmoa013171.
63. Bartram LA, Lozano J, Coury DL. Aripiprazole for treating irritability associated with autism spectrum disorders. *Expert Opin Pharmacother.* 2019;20(12):1421–1427. https://doi.org/10.1080/14656566.2019.1626825.
64. Arnold LE, Aman MG, Cook AM, et al. Atomoxetine for hyperactivity in autism spectrum disorders: placebo-controlled crossover pilot trial. *J Am Acad Child Adolesc Psychiatry.* 2006;45(10).
65. Sturman N, Deckx L, van Driel ML. Methylphenidate for children and adolescents with autism spectrum disorder. *Cochrane Database Syst Rev.* 2017;2017(11). https://doi.org/10.1002/14651858.CD011144.pub2.
66. Liu Q, Hsieh WY, Chen G. A systematic review and meta-analysis of parent-mediated intervention for children and adolescents with autism spectrum disorder in mainland China, Hong Kong, and Taiwan. *Autism.* 2020;24(8):1960–1979. https://doi.org/10.1177/1362361320943380.
67. Chugani DC, Chugani HT, Wiznitzer M, et al. Efficacy of low-dose buspirone for restricted and repetitive behavior in young children with autism spectrum disorder: a randomized trial. *J Pediatr.* 2016;170. https://doi.org/10.1016/j.jpeds.2015.11.033.
68. Hollander E, Chaplin W, Soorya L, et al. Divalproex sodium vs placebo for the treatment of irritability in children and adolescents with autism spectrum disorders. *Neuropsychopharmacology.* 2010;35(4). https://doi.org/10.1038/npp.2009.202.
69. Lemonnier E, Villeneuve N, Sonie S, et al. Effects of bumetanide on neurobehavioral function in children and adolescents with autism spectrum disorders. *Transl Psychiatry.* 2017;7(3). https://doi.org/10.1038/tp.2017.10.
70. Veenstra-Vanderweele J, Cook EH, King BH, et al. Arbaclofen in children and adolescents with autism spectrum disorder: a randomized, controlled, phase 2 trial. *Neuropsychopharmacology.* 2017;42(7). https://doi.org/10.1038/npp.2016.237.
71. Rzepka-Migut B, Paprocka J. Efficacy and safety of melatonin treatment in children with autism spectrum disorder and attention-deficit/hyperactivity disorder-a review of the literature. *Brain Sci.* 2020;10(4). https://doi.org/10.3390/brainsci10040219.

72. McGuinness G, Kim Y. Sulforaphane treatment for autism spectrum disorder: a systematic review. *EXCLI J.* 2020;19:892–903. https://doi.org/10.17179/excli2020-2487.
73. Parker KJ, Oztan O, Libove RA, et al. Intranasal oxytocin treatment for social deficits and biomarkers of response in children with autism. *Proc Natl Acad Sci U S A.* 2017;114(30). https://doi.org/10.1073/pnas.1705521114.
74. Phaik Ooi Y, Weng SJ, Kossowsky J, Gerger H, Sung M. Oxytocin and autism spectrum disorders: a systematic review and meta-analysis of randomized controlled trials. *Pharmacopsychiatry.* 2017;50(1). https://doi.org/10.1055/s-0042-109400.
75. Wasdell MB, Jan JE, Bomben MM, et al. A randomized, placebo-controlled trial of controlled release melatonin treatment of delayed sleep phase syndrome and impaired sleep maintenance in children with neurodevelopmental disabilities. *J Pineal Res.* 2008;44(1). https://doi.org/10.1111/j.1600-079X.2007.00528.x.
76. Wright B, Sims D, Smart S, et al. Melatonin versus placebo in children with autism spectrum conditions and severe sleep problems not amenable to behaviour management strategies: a randomised controlled crossover trial. *J Autism Dev Disord.* 2011;41(2). https://doi.org/10.1007/s10803-010-1036-5.
77. Singh K, Connors SL, Macklin EA, et al. Sulforaphane treatment of autism spectrum disorder (ASD). *Proc Natl Acad Sci U S A.* 2014;111(43). https://doi.org/10.1073/pnas.1416940111.
78. Nitschke A, Deonandan R, Konkle ATM. The link between autism spectrum disorder and gut microbiota: a scoping review. *Autism.* 2020;24(6):1328–1344. https://doi.org/10.1177/1362361320913364.
79. Kang DW, Adams JB, Coleman DM, et al. Long-term benefit of microbiota transfer therapy on autism symptoms and gut microbiota. *Sci Rep.* 2019;9(1). https://doi.org/10.1038/s41598-019-42183-0.
80. Althoff CE, Dammann CP, Hope SJ, Ausderau KK. Parent-Mediated interventions for children with autism spectrum disorder: a systematic review. *Am J Occup Ther.* 2019;73(3). https://doi.org/10.5014/ajot.2019.030015. 7303205010p1-7303205010p13.
81. Sharp WG, Burrell TL, Jaquess DL. The autism MEAL plan: a parent-training curriculum to manage eating aversions and low intake among children with autism. *Autism.* 2014;18(6). https://doi.org/10.1177/1362361313489190.
82. Wetherby AM, Guthrie W, Woods J, et al. Parent-implemented social intervention for toddlers with autism: an RCT. *Pediatrics.* 2014;134(6). https://doi.org/10.1542/peds.2014-0757.
83. Sofronoff K, Leslie A, Brown W. Parent management training and Asperger syndrome. A randomized controlled trial to evaluate a parent based intervention. *Autism.* 2004;8(3). https://doi.org/10.1177/1362361304045215.
84. Tarver J, Palmer M, Webb S, et al. Child and parent outcomes following parent interventions for child emotional and behavioral problems in autism spectrum disorders: a systematic review and meta-analysis. *Autism.* 2019;23(7). https://doi.org/10.1177/1362361319830042.
85. Bearss K, Johnson C, Smith T, et al. Effect of parent training vs parent education on behavioral problems in children with autism spectrum disorder: a randomized clinical trial. *JAMA.* 2015;313(15). https://doi.org/10.1001/jama.2015.3150.
86. Solomon R, van Egeren LA, Mahoney G, Huber MSQ, Zimmerman P. PLAY project home consultation intervention program for young children with autism spectrum disorders: a randomized controlled trial. *J Dev Behav Pediatr.* 2014;35(8). https://doi.org/10.1097/DBP.0000000000000096.
87. Praphatthanakunwong N, Kiatrungrit K, Hongsanguansri S, Nopmaneejumruslers K. Factors associated with parent engagement in DIR/Floortime for treatment of children with autism spectrum disorder. *Gen Psychiatry.* 2018;31(2). https://doi.org/10.1136/gpsych-2018-000009.

88. Bearss K, Burrell TL, Stewart L, Scahill L. Parent training in autism spectrum disorder: what's in a name? *Clin Child Fam Psychol Rev.* 2015;18(2). https://doi.org/10.1007/s10567-015-0179-5.
89. Robinson NL, Cottier TV, Kavanagh DJ. Psychosocial health interventions by social robots: systematic review of randomized controlled trials. *J Med Internet Res.* 2019;21(5). https://doi.org/10.2196/13203.
90. Alves FJ, de Carvalho EA, Aguilar J, de Brito LL, Bastos GS. Applied behavior analysis for the treatment of autism: a systematic review of assistive technologies. *IEEE Access.* 2020;8:118664–118672. https://doi.org/10.1109/ACCESS.2020.3005296.
91. Beaumont R, Walker H, Weiss J, Sofronoff K. Randomized controlled trial of a video gaming-based social skills program for children on the autism spectrum. *J Autism Dev Disord.* 2021. https://doi.org/10.1007/s10803-020-04801-z.
92. Hopkins IM, Gower MW, Perez TA, et al. Avatar assistant: improving social skills in students with an asd through a computer-based intervention. *J Autism Dev Disord.* 2011;41(11). https://doi.org/10.1007/s10803-011-1179-z.
93. Mesibov GB, Shea V, Schopler E, et al. *The Teacch Approach to Autism Spectrum Disorders;* 2004. https://doi.org/10.1007/978-0-306-48647-0.
94. Mesibov GB, Shea V. The TEACCH program in the era of evidence-based practice. *J Autism Dev Disord.* 2010;40(5). https://doi.org/10.1007/s10803-009-0901-6.
95. Sandbank M, Bottema-Beutel K, Crowley S, et al. Intervention effects on language in children with autism: a project AIM meta-analysis. *J Speech Lang Hear Res.* 2020;63(5):1537–1560. https://doi.org/10.1044/2020_JSLHR-19-00167.
96. Busti Ceccarelli S, Ferrante C, Gazzola E, et al. Fundamental motor skills intervention for children with autism spectrum disorder: a 10-year narrative review. *Children.* 2020;7(11):250. https://doi.org/10.3390/children7110250.
97. Schoen SA, Lane SJ, Mailloux Z, et al. A systematic review of ayres sensory integration intervention for children with autism. *Autism Res.* 2019;12(1):6–19. https://doi.org/10.1002/aur.2046.
98. Tse ACY. Brief report: impact of a physical exercise intervention on emotion regulation and behavioral functioning in children with autism Spectrum disorder. *J Autism Dev Disord.* 2020;50(11):4191–4198. https://doi.org/10.1007/s10803-020-04418-2.
99. O'Hare A, Bremner L. Management of developmental speech and language disorders: part 1. *Arch Dis Child.* 2016;101(3). https://doi.org/10.1136/archdischild-2014-307394.
100. Novak I, Honan I. Effectiveness of paediatric occupational therapy for children with disabilities: a systematic review. *Aust Occup Ther J.* 2019;66(3). https://doi.org/10.1111/1440-1630.12573.
101. American Physical Therapy Association. Guide to Physical Therapist Practice. Second Edition. American Physical Therapy Association. *Physical Therapy.* 2001;81(1).
102. Lewis AS, van Schalkwyk GI. Systematic review: distribution of age and intervention modalities in therapeutic clinical trials for autism Spectrum disorder. *J Autism Dev Disord.* 2020;50(6):2208–2216. https://doi.org/10.1007/s10803-019-03942-0.
103. Benevides TW, Shore SM, Andresen ML, et al. Interventions to address health outcomes among autistic adults: a systematic review. *Autism.* 2020;24(6):1345–1359. https://doi.org/10.1177/1362361320913664.
104. Cornwall A, Jewkes R. What is participatory research? *Soc Sci Med.* 1995;41(12). https://doi.org/10.1016/0277-9536(95)00127-S.
105. Baum F, MacDougall C, Smith D. Participatory action research. *J Epidemiol Community Health.* 2006;60(10):854–857. https://doi.org/10.1136/jech.2004.028662.
106. Fortuna K, Barr P, Goldstein C, et al. Application of community-engaged research to inform the development and implementation of a peer-delivered mobile health intervention for adults with serious mental illness. *J Particip Med.* 2019;11(1). https://doi.org/10.2196/12380.

107. Frazier TW, Dawson G, Murray D, Shih A, Sachs JS, Geiger A. Brief report: a survey of autism research priorities across a diverse community of stakeholders. *J Autism Dev Disord.* 2018;48(11):3965–3971. https://doi.org/10.1007/s10803-018-3642-6.
108. Fletcher-Watson S, Adams J, Brook K, et al. Making the future together: shaping autism research through meaningful participation. *Autism.* 2019;23(4):943–953. https://doi.org/10.1177/1362361318786721.
109. Nicolaidis C, Raymaker D, Kapp SK, et al. The AASPIRE practice-based guidelines for the inclusion of autistic adults in research as co-researchers and study participants. *Autism.* 2019;23(8):2007–2019. https://doi.org/10.1177/1362361319830523.
110. Lilienfeld SO, Marshall J, Todd JT, Shane HC. The persistence of fad interventions in the face of negative scientific evidence: facilitated communication for autism as a case example. *Evid-Based Commun Assess Interv.* 2014;8(2). https://doi.org/10.1080/17489539.2014.976332.
111. FDA. Be Aware of Potentially Dangerous Products and Therapies that Claim to Treat Autism. Consumer Updates, (n.d.).
112. McKay D, Jensen-Doss A. Harmful treatments in psychotherapy. *Clin Psychol Sci Pract.* 2021;28(1):2–4. https://doi.org/10.1037/cps0000023.
113. Lilienfeld SO. Psychological treatments that cause harm. *Perspect Psychol Sci.* 2007;2(1):53–70. https://doi.org/10.1111/j.1745-6916.2007.00029.x.
114. Teachman BA, White BA, Lilienfeld SO. Identifying harmful therapies: setting the research agenda. *Clin Psychol Sci Pract.* 2021;28(1):101–106. https://doi.org/10.1037/cps0000002.
115. Kang E, Lerner MD, Gadow KD. Atypical communication characteristics among clinic-referred youth with and without autism spectrum disorder: stability and associations with clinical correlates. *Dev Psychopathol.* 2020;32(4). https://doi.org/10.1017/S095457942000070X.
116. Lerner MD, de Los RA, Drabick DAG, Gerber AH, Gadow KD. Informant discrepancy defines discrete, clinically useful autism spectrum disorder subgroups. *J Child Psychol Psychiatry Allied Discip.* 2017;58(7). https://doi.org/10.1111/jcpp.12730.
117. Lord C, Luyster R, Guthrie W, Pickles A. Patterns of developmental trajectories in toddlers with autism spectrum disorder. *J Consult Clin Psychol.* 2012;80(3). https://doi.org/10.1037/a0027214.
118. Lerner MD, White SW, McPartland JC. Mechanisms of change in psychosocial interventions for autism spectrum disorders. *Dialogues Clin Neurosci.* 2012;14(3). https://doi.org/10.31887/dcns.2012.14.3/mlerner.
119. Antshel KM, Polacek C, McMahon M, et al. Comorbid ADHD and anxiety affect social skills group intervention treatment efficacy in children with autism spectrum disorders. *J Dev Behav Pediatr.* 2011;32(6). https://doi.org/10.1097/DBP.0b013e318222355d.
120. Provenzani U, Fusar-Poli L, Brondino N, et al. What are we targeting when we treat autism spectrum disorder? A systematic review of 406 clinical trials. *Autism.* 2020;24(2):274–284. https://doi.org/10.1177/1362361319854641.
121. Aldao A, de Los RA. Commentary: a practical guide for translating basic research on affective science to implementing physiology in clinical child and adolescent assessments. *J Clin Child Adolesc Psychol.* 2015;44(2). https://doi.org/10.1080/15374416.2014.895942.
122. Kang E, Keifer CM, Levy EJ, Foss-Feig JH, McPartland JC, Lerner MD. Atypicality of the N170 event-related potential in autism spectrum disorder: a meta-analysis. *Biol Psychiatry: Cogn Neurosci.* 2018;3(8). https://doi.org/10.1016/j.bpsc.2017.11.003.
123. McPartland JC. Developing clinically practicable biomarkers for autism spectrum disorder. *J Autism Dev Disord.* 2017;47(9). https://doi.org/10.1007/s10803-017-3237-7.
124. van Hecke AV, Stevens S, Carson AM, et al. Measuring the plasticity of social approach: a randomized controlled trial of the effects of the PEERS intervention on EEG asym-

metry in adolescents with autism spectrum disorders. *J Autism Dev Disord.* 2015;45(2). https://doi.org/10.1007/s10803-013-1883-y.

125. Faja S, Webb SJ, Jones E, et al. The effects of face expertise training on the behavioral performance and brain activity of adults with high functioning autism spectrum disorders. *J Autism Dev Disord.* 2012;42(2). https://doi.org/10.1007/s10803-011-1243-8.
126. Dawson G, Jones EJH, Merkle K, et al. Early behavioral intervention is associated with normalized brain activity in young children with autism. *J Am Acad Child Adolesc Psychiatry.* 2012;51(11). https://doi.org/10.1016/j.jaac.2012.08.018.
127. Stavropoulos KKM. Using neuroscience as an outcome measure for behavioral interventions in autism spectrum disorders (ASD): a review. *Res Autism Spectr Disord.* 2017;35. https://doi.org/10.1016/j.rasd.2017.01.001.
128. Baker E, Veytsman E, Martin AM, Blacher J, Stavropoulos KKM. Increased neural reward responsivity in adolescents with ASD after social skills intervention. *Brain Sci.* 2020;10(6):1–11. https://doi.org/10.3390/brainsci10060402.
129. Chahrour M, Kleiman RJ, Manzini MC. Translating genetic and preclinical findings into autism therapies. *Dialogues Clin Neurosci.* 2017;19(4). https://doi.org/10.31887/dcns.2017.19.4/cmanzini.

# Index

Note: Page numbers followed by *f* indicate figures, *t* indicate tables, and *b* indicate boxes.

## D



## E



## F



## G

## O



## P



## Q



## R



## S

Made in the USA
Monee, IL
13 September 2026

63138378R00164